Functional somatic syndromes are defined as physical syndromes without an organic disease explanation, demonstrable structural changes or established biochemical abnormalities. The reality of these disorders has been accepted by clinicians and intensive scientific inquiry continues to reveal their multiple biological aspects. This book reviews the state of scientific and clinical understanding of the nine most common functional somatic syndromes, conditions which disable patients and often frustrate clinicians through the absence of consistently effective therapeutic interventions.

For each syndrome, expert authors provide a brief historical perspective, a current definition, a case presentation, confirmatory and contradictory research findings, a discussion of the leading pathogenetic hypotheses, and guidelines for diagnosis and treatment. Advice is given for the determination of disability of patients with these medically unexplained disorders, and both medical and psychiatric interventions are described.

Stressing the importance of a sound therapeutic relationship as a basis for treatment, this is a sympathetic, innovative and scientifically sophisticated account of a range of conditions that are as perplexing to clinicians as they are distressing to affected patients. For professionals in primary care and many other disciplines, this book will enlighten, inform and encourage good practice.

PETER MANU is Associate Professor of Medicine and Psychiatry, Albert Einstein College of Medicine, Yeshiva University, and Director of Medical Services, Hillside Hospital, Long Island Jewish Medical Center, New York.

Functional Somatic Syndromes: Etiology, Diagnosis and Treatment

EDITED BY

PETER MANU

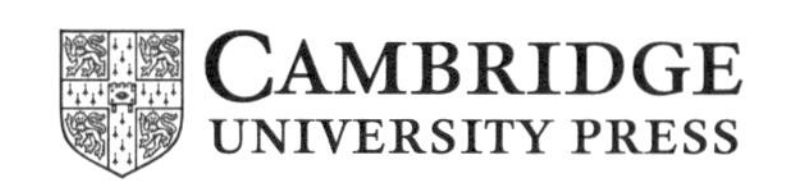

PUBLISHED BY THE PRESS SYNDICATE OF THE UNIVERSITY OF CAMBRIDGE
The Pitt Building, Trumpington Street, Cambridge CB2 1RP, United Kingdom

CAMBRIDGE UNIVERSITY PRESS
The Edinburgh Building, Cambridge CB2 2RU, UK http://www.cup.cam.ac.uk
40 West 20th Street, New York, NY 10011-4211, USA http://www.cup.org
10 Stamford Road, Oakleigh, Melbourne 3166, Australia

First published 1998

Printed in the United Kingdom at the University Press, Cambridge

Typeset in Palatino 10/12 pt [VN]

A catalogue record for this book is available from the British Library

Library of Congress Cataloguing in Publication data

Functional somatic syndromes / edited by Peter Manu.
p. cm.
Includes indes.
ISBN 0 521 59130 9. – ISBN 0 521 63491 1 (pbk.)
1. Syndromes. I. Manu, Peter, 1967– .
RC69 F86 1998
616–dc21 98–24733 CIP

ISBN 0 521 59130 9 hardback
ISBN 0 521 63491 1 paperback

Every effort has been made in preparing this book to provide accurate and up-to-date information which is in accord with accepted standards and practice at the time of publication. Nevertheless, the authors, editors and publisher can make no warranties that the information contained herein is totally free from error, not least because clinical standards are constantly changing through research and regulation. The authors, editors and publisher therefore disclaim all liability for direct or consequential damages resulting from the use of material contained in this book. Readers are strongly advised to pay careful attention to information provided by the manufacturer of any drugs or equipment that they plan to use.

Contents

Contributors

MICHA ABELES
Division of Rheumatology
University of Connecticut Health Center
Farmington, CT 06030-1310
USA

CAROL M. GRECO
Pain Evaluation and Treatment Institute
University of Pittsburgh
4601 Baum Boulevard
Pittsburgh, PA 15213-1217
USA

ANDREW HERLICH
University of Pittsburgh School of Medicine
4601 Baum Boulevard
Pittsburgh, PA 15213-1217
USA

NGOC HO
Department of Epidemiology
University of Washington
1959 Pacific Street
Seattle, WA 98195-3820
USA

JAMES A. KOZIOL
Department of Molecular and Experimental Medicine
311N The Scripps Research Institute
10550 North Torrey Pines Road
La Jolla, CA 92037-1000
USA

GEORGE F. LONGSTRETH
Kaiser Permanente
4647 Zion Avenue
San Diego, CA 92120-2507
USA

PETER MANU
Hillside Hospital
Long Island Jewish Medical Center
Glen Oaks, NY 11004
USA

DALE A. MATTHEWS
Department of Medicine
Georgetown University Medical Center
3800 Reservoir Road NW
Washington, DC 20007-2196
USA

C. LOWELL PARSONS
Department of Urology
University of California at San Diego
University Hospital
225 West Dickinson Street
San Diego, CA 92103-8897
USA

TERI PEARLSTEIN
Brown University School of Medicine
Women's Treatment Program
Butler Hospital
345 Blackstone Boulevard
Providence, RI 02906-4861
USA

ARTHUR RIFKIN
Hillside Hospital
Long Island Jewish Medical Center
Glen Oaks, NY 11004
USA

THOMAS E. RUDY
University of Pittsburgh School of Medicine
4601 Baum Boulevard
Pittsburgh, PA 15213
USA

GARY TAERK
Toronto Hospital
300 St Clair Avenue West
Suite 102, Toronto
Ontario
Canada M4V 1S4

ABBA I. TERR
Department of Medicine
Division of Immunology
Room S-021
Stanford University Medical Center
Stanford, CA 94305
USA

STEPHEN P. TYRER
Pain Management Unit
Royal Victoria Infirmary
Queen Victoria Road
Newcastle upon Tyne
NE1 4LP
UK

LAWSON R. WULSIN
231 Bethesda Avenue
ML559
Cincinnati, OH 45267-0559
USA

Preface

This book describes the clinical characteristics and the available treatments for a group of nine conditions often seen in primary care practice. The entities are chronic fatigue syndrome, fibromyalgia, irritable bowel syndrome, premenstrual syndrome, temporomandibular joint pain and dysfunction syndrome, interstitial cystitis, nonischemic chest pain syndrome, repetitive strain injuries and multiple chemical sensitivities. Their common denominators are the presence of multiple somatic symptoms, the lack of defining structural defects or laboratory abnormalities, the frequent association with psychiatric disorders, the absence of proven pathophysiological mechanisms and the paucity of effective therapeutic interventions.

The book is addressed to primary care physicians, because they are seeing patients with these vexing, puzzling and disabling conditions every day in the office and clinic; to physicians practicing psychiatry, neurology and physical rehabilitation, to whom these patients are often referred for consultation and treatment; to the postgraduate trainees in the above-mentioned fields; and to the relatively large number of patients with one or more of these syndromes who perceive the need to educate themselves and their families.

In selecting the format for the presentation of the state of the science we have been guided by the principles of evidence-based medicine and combined in-depth review of the best available publications with the rich clinical experience of our group of expert collaborators. We start with the definition of functional symptoms, syndromes and illnesses and the evaluation of the way in which paradigmatic shifts of the past decade have influenced perception and practice. Data regarding the individual syndromes are then presented according to a common descriptive sequence which includes a brief history, the standard definition, a clinical case presentation, prevalence, economic costs, research confirmations (i.e., similar findings obtained by at least two independent groups of investigators), research contradictions (i.e., unequivocally opposite findings in independent studies with comparable methodologies), a discussion of the leading pathogenetic hypotheses, diagnostic and treatment approaches, and a summary of the clinically relevant facts. As much of the available treatment modalities focus on the associated psychiatric symptomatology, we offer separate chapters on the psychopharmacology and psychotherapy of functional somatic syndromes. A distinct contribution analyzes the difficult process of assessing the occupational disability claimed by patients with these diagnoses. Finally, we examine the extent to which research data have identified common denominators of these syndromes.

This project brought together a group of academic physicians who selflessly gave their time despite the unceasing demands of their heavy clinical workload. I acknowledge with gratitude the efforts of my collaborators for their lucid appraisals and their help in obtaining a degree of homogeneity for data of such diversity. I am also indebted to Richard Barling of Cambridge University Press for his tenacity, patience and kindness in assisting my attempts to clarify the objectives and to shape the content of this book. Thanks are also extended to Glenn Affleck, Javier Escobar, Victor Hesselbrock, Hank Kranzler, Howard Tennen and Simon Wessely, mentors, colleagues and friends during my struggle to begin to understand some of the complexities of the interfaces between psychology, psychiatry and medicine.

Peter Manu

1

Definition and Etiological Theories

PETER MANU

Definitions

Functional somatic syndromes are physical illnesses without an organic disease explanation and devoid of demonstrable structural lesion or established biochemical change (Lipkin, 1969; Smith, 1991; Sharpe et al., 1995). Alternative modern descriptors are somatoform disorders and medically unexplained symptoms; other terms which implied occult disease (hysteria), imagined illness ((hypochondriasis), or psychogenesis (psychosomatic syndrome, somatization and abnormal illness behavior) are only rarely used (Sharpe et al., 1995).

The term functional is often misinterpreted to mean that the illness is not very significant, that the suffering is not real, that the treatment will be difficult, time-consuming and likely to fail, and that the patients are unhappy and dull (Lipkin, 1969). In contrast to these misperceptions stands a vast body of recent research that has accepted the reality of functional disorders and has accorded them equal status as targets for serious scientific inquiry into their multiple biological dimensions. A search of the literature published from 1990 to 1996 identified nine syndromes which were intensely studied by numerous and prolific researchers; there were 1051 publications on chronic fatigue syndrome, 728 on fibromyalgia, 656 on irritable bowel syndrome, 609 on premenstrual syndrome, 598 on temporomandibular pain and dysfunction syndrome, 263 on interstitial cystitis, 133 on atypical (noncardiac) chest pain, 112 on multiple chemical sensitivities and 48 on repetitive strain injury. The analysis of the yearly scientific output indicated a steady rate of publications, undoubtedly reflecting continuous interest and the availability of funding.

The degree to which these syndromes have been characterized as unique entities is variable. On one end of the spectrum one can find fibromyalgia, a condition defined exclusively in objective terms. The diagnosis is made only if the subject has muscle pain at 11 of 18 specified anatomical locations; the amount of digital or instrumental pressure to be applied is defined and the technique of measuring pain responses carefully described to ensure reproducibility. As described by Abeles (Chapter 3), this definition has been the result of a prospective clinical study conducted by a group of experts with documented nationwide recognition and has been endorsed by the American College of Rheumatology (Wolfe et al., 1990). At the other end of the spectrum is the syndrome of multiple chemical sensitivities, a condition said to consists of multiple symptoms produced by exposure to multiple chemicals at levels below those known to cause morbid effects in the general population. This completely subjective construct is popular with patients and some health care practitioners but, as Abba Terr indicates in his contribution to this volume (Chapter 10), major professional associations and the World Health Organization have not endorsed the definition and have not legitimized the syndrome (UNEP-ILO-WHO, 1996). Somewhere in the middle of the spectrum is the definition of premenstrual syndrome, which requires an assessment of severity of a specified type of affective disturbance that is restricted to the luteal phase of the menstrual cycle. Although the clinical description is based on subjective data, the aggregation during the luteal phase offers a degree of objectivity. As indicated by Pearlstein's contribution (Chapter 5), the definition has been extensively used in research studies and has been included among the diagnostic standards of the American Psychiatric Association (American Psychiatric Association, 1994). An unusual case is the repetitive strain injury syndrome which includes conditions with demonstrable pathology (and therefore not functional) such as carpal tunnel syndrome, but also ill-defined muscle weakness, cramping and tenderness. In his contribution, Tyrer (Chapter 9) points out that this heterogeneity might be due to workmen's compensation and social security disability systems that have focused on the relationship between complaints and job-related activities rather than on the association between complaints and objective clinical findings (Bammer & Bignault, 1988).

Etiological theories

A number of paradigmatic theoretical approaches have been formulated during the past decade and anchored by three major postulates: that functional somatic syndromes represent atypical forms of established psychiatric disorders, that they represent expressions of psychoemotional distress in a somatic language influenced by sociological trends, or that they are distinct disorders with specific dysfunctions and individualized genetic and biological abnormalities.

Functional somatic syndromes as forms of affective spectrum disorder with a common biological causation

In 1989 two Harvard Medical School researchers published an analysis of the association between fibromyalgia and psychopathology (Hudson & Pope, 1989). This association was documented, according to the authors, by work belonging to six distinct lines of evidence:

(1) symptoms of depression, anxiety, irritability, poor concentration, loss of interest and difficulty with concentration;
(2) results of psychological testing or rating scales consistently similar to those usually observed in patients with affective, anxiety and somatoform disorders;
(3) elevated rates of specific psychiatric disorders, significantly higher than those found among patients with the disabling painful condition of rheumatoid arthritis;
(4) high lifetime rates of major depressive disorder in the relatives of patients with fibromyalgia;
(5) encouraging response of fibromyalgia symptoms to treatment with antidepressant drugs;
(6) high rates of psychiatric disorders, predominantly from the mood disorder category, among patients with chronic fatigue syndrome, a disorder displaying features similar to those of fibromyalgia.

Hudson and Pope then formulated the three explanatory hypotheses for the association between fibromyalgia and psychopathology: fibromyalgia is the cause of psychopathology; fibromyalgia is the effect of psychopathology; fibromyalgia and psychopathology are the result of a common underlying morbid process. The first hypothesis was rejected by the authors' findings that the onset of the psychiatric disorder had preceded the onset of fibromyalgia syndrome in a majority of patients and that many of these patients' relatives had a history of major depressive disorder. The second hypothesis was ruled out by the fact that a substantial number of patients with fibromyalgia did not satisfy criteria for any psychiatric diagnosis at any time during their illness; the possibility that fibromyalgia is a factitious or hysterical disorder was dismissed, given fibromyalgia's display of stable, stereotyped symptom pattern. The outcome of this analysis was to strengthen the third hypothesis, which postulated that fibromyalgia is a member of a cluster of associated and overlapping disorders that included chronic fatigue syndrome and irritable bowel syndrome and that the entities of this cluster are all caused by a common pathophysiological process.

In addition to the three functional somatic syndromes mentioned, the cluster identified by Hudson and Pope comprised migraine headache and the psychiatric disorders major depression, bulimia, cataplexy, panic disorder, obsessive compulsive disorder and attention deficit disorder with hyperactivity. The cluster was named 'affective spectrum disorder'. The common features of its component syndromes were high comorbidity with each other; high rates of major depression or another component syndrome in first-degree relatives; and therapeutic response to antidepressant agents belonging to three or more pharmacological classes (Hudson & Pope, 1989). The antidepressant classes considered were tricyclic agents, monoamine oxidase inhibitors, serotonin uptake inhibitors and atypical agents and the treatment–response model implied that these patients had a disordered neurotransmission (Hudson & Pope, 1990). Sleep abnormalities and hypercortisolism were mentioned as possible common biological markers, but the precise nature of the underlying pathophysiological process was not defined (Hudson & Pope, 1989).

Functional somatic syndromes as expressions of somatization with a common psychosocial causation

In 1990, a University of Toronto clinical scientist reported her observations on 50 patients who carried the diagnosis of 'environmental sensitivity', one of the names of the functional somatic syndrome described in this book as multiple chemical sensitivities (Stewart, 1990). The hypothesis tested in the study postulated that the patients with multiple chemical sensitivities are 'chronic somatizers' who tend to have many nonspecific and vague symptoms such as fatigue, headache, muscle and joint pains, digestive complaints, dizziness, irritability and difficulty with concentration. It was also hypothesized that these patients adopt newly described diseases (or 'diseases of fashion') as the explanation for their long-standing ailments.

The median age of the group was 39 years and 74% of the patients had a college education. Forty-two (88%) of the study patients were women. All patients had stopped working and most were receiving long-term disability payments through their previous employers. The patients provided their past medical histories and had their medical records reviewed. The results indicated that 64% of patients had also been diagnosed with chronic fatigue syndrome (often named postinfectious neuromyasthenia or chronic Epstein–Barr virus infection), 50% with severe premenstrual syndrome, 18% with fibromyalgia and 12% with temporomandibular joint syndrome. Besides, many patients carried the diagnoses of food allergy causing psychological symptoms (76%), candidiasis hypersensitivity syndrome (58%), idiopathic hypoglycemia (46%) and vitamin or mineral deficiency (24%). Only 10% of the patients had had none of these other conditions diagnosed at some time during the ten years prior to the diagnosis of multiple chemical sensitivities. Over the three years of the study, the patients' own diagnostic attribution showed common trends; in 1985 a majority thought that their symptoms were allergic responses to food or environmental agents, in 1986 the cause was considered by many to be *Candida albicans* and in 1987 many patients believed that their suffering was the result of reactivated Epstein–Barr virus infection. Only 20% of the patients had been diagnosed by a physician. The majority (62%) of patients first considered the diagnosis of multiple chemical sensitivities themselves based on information obtained from popular books for the layperson or through the broadcast or print media. The remaining patients (18%) had been 'diagnosed' by a relative, friend or nonphysician health care provider.

These findings were interpreted to confirm the fact that patients with one functional somatic syndrome, multiple chemical sensitivities, have a tendency to endorse other disorders with uncertain etiology and multiple symptoms. They seek explanations in the lay literature and actively incorporate poorly substantiated theories such as immune dysfunction, environmental allergies, overgrowth of *Candida albicans* and reactivation of dormant Epstein–Barr virus as the cause of their illness. Other characteristics of this population include the over-representation of 'well-educated women at the end of their child-bearing years who have unhappy personal and marital relationships', the high prevalence of psychiatric disorders pre-dating their functional somatic syndrome by many years, and the increased utilization of health care services for symptoms of somatization. A biological explanation for these features appeared unlikely; instead, these patients were considered to be suggestible and 'at high risk for acquiring diagnoses that are popularized by the media'.

Functional somatic syndromes as distinct entities with variable biological and psychosocial causations

This construct was published in 1994 by the late Robert Kellner, a University of New Mexico psychiatrist who had devoted decades of clinical research to the understanding of psychosomatic processes (Kellner, 1994). His approach consisted in a careful analysis of the published data and an attempt to define the major contributing factors to the causation of these syndromes. For fibromyalgia, he suggested that physical disease, psychopathology and low serotonin concentration cause abnormalities in nonrapid eye movement sleep. The sleep abnormality decreases the pain threshold and thus produces the main clinical features of the syndrome. He understood chronic fatigue syndrome as having multiple causations. For some patients, he postulated an immunological complication of a viral infection; others seemed to have acquired their illness because they had experienced postviral fatigue, avoided physical activity and ended up with impaired fitness and exercise intolerance; for yet another group of chronic fatigue patients, the main cause was a depressive disorder. For irritable bowel syndrome, he believed that the biological factor consisted in an increased sensitivity to gas and feces, with consequent pain and enhanced bowel motility. The psychiatric symptoms, like the majority of all the noncolonic complaints, were considered to be related to patterns of seeking medical help rather than as necessary factors for the development or maintenance of the irritable bowel. On the other hand he suggested that the causation of the noncardiac chest pain was closely related to one or more psychiatric disorders, those frequently represented being panic disorder, major depression and hyperventilation.

Kellner also addressed the tendency for clustering of functional somatic syndromes, a prominent feature of the work of Hudson & Pope (1989) and Stewart (1990). The operational concept was the relationship between the number and severity of symptoms and the severity of both emotional disturbance and psychopathology. Clustering was, understood to reflect the process of somatization (i.e. an individual tendency to express emotional distress as physical symptoms and to seek medical attention for them), as well as the clinical expression of stress-induced physiological changes in multiple organs and systems.

Kellner's work has been continued and expanded in the latest contribution to the evolution of ideas regarding the etiology of these syndromes (Mayou et al., 1995). This group of clinician–investigators from the Warneford Hospital and John Radcliffe Hospital, Oxford avoided a unifying causal construct; instead, they attempted to structure the problem by highlighting the predisposing, precipitating and perpetuating factors that are believed to contribute to the clinical presentation and outcome of these syndromes. Prominent predisposing factors include abnormal personality traits (such as excessive health consciousness), illness beliefs, personal or family history of major physical illness and genetic predispositions. Among the precipitating factors the authors included physiological variability in arousal, muscle tension, quality of sleep, physical performance, respiratory rate, and the effect of diet, alcohol and drugs; anatomical changes, such as benign tissue lumps and inconsistencies; minor physical illnesses; psychiatric disorders; stressful events and chronic difficulties; and the lack of social support and problems in coping. Important perpetuating factors are primary or secondary psychiatric disorders; perceived functional disability and its relationship with litigation and long-term disability benefits; the side-effects of inappropriate therapeutic interventions, such as avoidance of physical activities or restricted diets; and the realization that suffering is not taken seriously by relatives, friends and health care providers.

In the following chapters we allow the scientific evidence to demonstrate biological and psychological abnormalities in patients with functional somatic syndromes. This approach is dictated by clinical realities, as we need to provide the knowledge base for the understanding of these disorders and their logical treatment rather than solutions to the unknown of their causes.

References

American Psychiatric Association (1994). *Diagnostic and Statistical Manual for Mental Disorders*, 4th edn (DSM-IV). Washington, DC: American Psychiatric Press.

Bammer G & Bignault L (1988). More than a pain in the arms: a review of the consequences of developing overuse syndromes. *Journal of Occupational Health of Australia and New Zealand*, **4**, 389–97.

Hudson JI & Pope HG Jr (1989). Fibromyalgia and psychopathology: is fibromyalgia a form of 'affective spectrum disorder'? *Journal of Rheumatology*, **16**, (supp. 19) 15–22.

Hudson JI & Pope HG Jr (1990). Affective spectrum disorder: does antidepressant response identify a family of disorders with common pathophysiology? *American Journal of Psychiatry*, **147**, 552–64.

Kellner R (1994). Psychosomatic syndromes, somatization and somatoform disorders. *Psychotherapy and Psychosomatics*, **61**, 4–24.

Lipkin M (1969). Functional or organic? A pointless question. *Annals of Internal Medicine*, **5**, 1013–17.

Mayou R, Bass C & Sharpe M (1995). Overview of epidemiology, classification and aetiology. In *Treatment of Functional Somatic Symptoms*, ed. R. Mayou, C. Bass & M. Sharpe, pp. 42–65. Oxford: Oxford University Press.

Sharpe M, Mayou R & Bass C (1995). Concepts, theories and terminology. In *Treatment of Functional Somatic Symptoms*, ed. R. Mayou, C. Bass & M. Sharpe, pp. 3–16. Oxford: Oxford University Press.

Smith RC (1991). Somatization disorder: defining its role in clinical medicine. *Journal of General Internal Medicine*, **6**, 168–75.

Stewart D (1990). The changing faces of somatization. *Psychosomatics*, **31**, 153–8.

Wolfe F, Smythe HA, Yunus B, Bennett R, Bombardier C, Goldenberg DL, Tugwell P, Campbell S, Abeles M, Clark P, Fam AG, Farber SJ, Fiechtner JJ, Franklin C, Gatter RA, Hamaty D, Lessard J, Lichtbroun AA, Masi AT, McCain GA, Reynolds TJ, Russell IJ & Sheon RP (1990). The American College of Rheumatology 1990 criteria for the classification of fibromyalgia. *Arthritis and Rheumatism*, **33**, 160–72.

UNEP-ILO-WHO (1996). Conclusions and recommendations of a workshop on 'multiple chemical sensitivities' (MCS). *Regulatory Toxicology and Pharmacology*, **24**, S188–S189.

2

Chronic Fatigue Syndrome

PETER MANU AND DALE A. MATTHEWS

A syndrome of persistent or relapsing fatigue has been the focus of intense public attention and scientific research during the past two decades. From 1982 to 1987 the syndrome was considered by some investigators to be the manifestation of a reactivated Epstein–Barr virus (EBV) infection (Tobi et al., 1982; Dubois et al., 1984; Jones et al., 1985; Straus et al., 1985). As this etiological relationship could not be confirmed (Buchwald et al., 1987; Homes et al., 1987; Hellinger et al., 1988), the US Centers for Disease Control sponsored a proposal to redefine this syndrome on clinical grounds and renamed it the chronic fatigue syndrome (CFS) (Holmes, 1988*a*).

History

In 1869 the New York neurologist George M. Beard introduced the term 'neurasthenia' to describe a condition characterized by a chronic fatigue which was 'developed, fostered and perpetuated with the advance of culture and refinement, and the corresponding preponderance of labor of the brain over that of the muscles' (Beard, 1869). He observed that women were more frequently affected than men, especially 'the sensitive white woman, . . . torn and cursed by happy and unhappy love; waylaid at all hours by the cruelest of robbers, worry and ambition' (Beard, 1881).

George Beard's description of neurasthenia proved influential among psychiatrists, a fact most notably reflected in Sigmund Freud's use of the neurasthenic construct to define anxiety neurosis (Freud, 1894). A decade later, some of the phobic and obsessive features of neurasthenia were considered to indicate a specific mental disorder, psychasthenia (Janet, 1903). The firm grounding of neurasthenia as a psychiatric illness continued for most of this century with the American

Psychiatric Association (APA, 1968) defining the condition as one of 'easy fatigability and sometimes exhaustion, different from anxiety neurosis and psychophysiological disorder in the nature of the predominant complaint, and from depressive disorder in the moderateness of the depression and the chronicity of its course'. Later editions of the Association's Manual (APA, 1980, 1987) eliminated neurasthenia from the American psychiatric nomenclature and referred to it only as a variant of dysthymia, a chronic affective disorder.

Definition

The modern definition of CFS was developed in 1988 to facilitate future epidemiological, clinical and laboratory studies (Holmes et al., 1988*a*, *b*). In 1994 the Centers for Disease Control and Prevention (CDC) directed a second effort to define CFS.

The definition requires the presence of persistent or relapsing chronic fatigue that:

(1) is of new or definite onset,
(2) has remained unexplained after clinical evaluation,
(3) is not the result of ongoing exertion,
(4) is not substantially alleviated by rest,
(5) produces significant reduction in previous levels of occupational and social activities.

In addition, the definition requires the concurrent presence of at least four of the following symptoms:

(1) substantial impairment in short-term memory and concentration,
(2) sore throat,
(3) tender cervical or axillary lymph nodes,
(4) muscle pain,
(5) multijoint pain without other signs of acute arthritis,
(6) headaches of a new type, pattern and severity,
(7) unrefreshing sleep,
(8) postexertional malaise lasting more than 24 hours.

The four or more concurrent symptoms must have persisted or recurred during six or more consecutive months of the fatiguing illness and must not have pre-dated the onset of the fatigue symptom (Fukuda et al., 1994). There are no laboratory tests or imaging procedures useful for the positive identification of CFS. Such tests should be used only to exclude other diagnostic possibilities.

The 1994 definition identifies the following as conditions that *exclude* the diagnosis of CFS:

(1) any active medical condition that may explain the presence of chronic fatigue, including side-effects of prescribed medications;
(2) any previously diagnosed medical condition whose resolution has not been proven beyond reasonable clinical doubt;
(3) any past or current diagnosis of major depression with psychotic or melancholic features, bipolar affective disorder, schizophrenia, delusional disorder, dementia, and anorexia or bulimia nervosa;
(4) substance abuse within two years before the onset of fatigue and at any time afterward;
(5) morbid obesity, as defined by a body mass index (weight in kg/height in m^2) of at least 45.

The diagnosis of CFS is *allowed* in patients with a variety of disorders:

(1) conditions defined primarily by subjective complaints or for which there are no confirmatory laboratory tests, such as fibromyalgia, anxiety disorders, somatoform disorders, nonpsychotic or nonmelancholic major depression and multiple chemical sensitivities;
(2) conditions known to include fatigue among their symptoms, but for which the patient has received adequate treatment, such as hypothyroidism adequately treated with replacement therapy as documented by normal thyroid-stimulating hormone levels;
(3) conditions known to present with fatigue and other chronic symptoms, such as Lyme disease, if the patient had received adequate pharmacological therapy before developing the chronic symptoms.

Case presentation

A 31-year-old teacher's aide presented to the office for evaluation with a chief complaint of persistent 'mental and physical fatigue'. She came to the clinic well groomed and was dressed neatly in leisure clothes. She appeared healthy and animated. She readily discussed her complaints over a 45-minute period, giving a thorough chronology of what she believed were important symptoms and laboratory findings. She reported that she had 'lived a hectic life'. The last time she felt well was 2.5

years prior to the visit. Since that time she has been lethargic and has experienced chronic sore throat, enlarged cervical lymph nodes, joint and muscle pains, predominantly in the lower back area and knees. Additionally, she reported cognitive impairment. She described herself as 'not clicking' and 'living in a television box'. She claimed to have difficulty with concentration and a worsening of a previously excellent memory. Her symptoms worsened during certain periods where she couldn't move, but eased during other periods allowing her to work part-time.

Her condition had been evaluated by four physicians: a family practitioner, an orthopedic surgeon, an infectious disease specialist and a neurologist. Repeated comprehensive laboratory investigations had been within normal limits. She had received intravenous vitamins, oral preparations of zinc, and intramuscular injections of gammaglobulin and porcine liver extract. Her condition improved slightly at the onset of each therapeutic trial, but worsened again soon thereafter.

Her past medical history and family history were unremarkable. She was married and had two children. She stated that 'since this started, I have no support from my family and I disconnected myself from everyone'. She admitted to being depressed and feeling guilty regarding her illness. She also reported suicidal ideation in the recent past because she felt her 'family might be better off'.

A complete physical examination was performed and revealed the presence of ten tender fibromyalgic points with no other abnormalities. The muscle strength and the range of motion of all joints were normal.

A neuropsychological consultation was obtained to assess the nature and extent of her cognitive and affective symptoms. She performed well on many concentration tests, notably those with repeated trials. There was no indication of recent decline in her intellectual functioning. Her motor skills were quick and coordinated. She had evidence of mild memory impairment on measures of rote learning. Testing also revealed that as sentences increased in length, she appeared to miss significant details of the sentence; yet, she was able to grasp correctly the overall sense of the statement. She appeared moderately depressed and her mild cognitive deficits were considered to be related, at least in part, to her depression. The consultant recommended aggressive pharmacological treatment of depression and goal-directed, supportive psychotherapy.

The diagnoses of chronic fatigue syndrome, fibromyalgia

and dysthymia were discussed with the patient and presented to her family physician. A graded exercise program was initiated and the patient was given tricyclic antidepressant agents. Significant symptomatic improvement occurred within three months. She did not return to work in the school system, but set up her own catering business.

Prevalence

General population

A thorough investigation of the prevalence and incidence of CFS was conducted by the CDC in four geographically distinct metropolitan areas in the USA (Gunn et al., 1993). In these areas, all primary care providers for potential CFS patients were contacted and asked to participate as referral sources. A total of 408 physicians agreed to participate by identifying patients with at least six months of debilitating fatigue. Eighty-seven patients (26% of the group studied) met the published working-case definition of CFS (Holmes et al., 1988*a*). The remaining patients had a diagnosable psychiatric condition before the onset of their fatigue illness (45%), a medical condition that could explain the reported symptoms (15%), or too few signs and symptoms to meet the case-definition criteria (24%). The observed two-year period prevalence of CFS ranged from 0.007% to 0.015% across the four sites.

In contrast with the CDC investigation, a much higher prevalence of CFS was identified in a single urban community (Buchwald et al., 1995). A screening survey was mailed to 4000 randomly selected members of a managed care system to investigate whether the recipients had felt unusual fatigue or loss of energy for the six preceding months. Nineteen percent of the sample reported having fatigue that interfered significantly with their activities; however, only three individuals were given a final diagnosis of CFS after a complete clinical and psychometric evaluation. Using variable assumptions about the proportion of nonparticipants and nonrespondents, the estimated prevalence ranged from 0.08% to 0.27%.

Primary care practice setting

The prevalence of CFS among 1000 individuals receiving care in a primary care practice setting was studied at the Brigham and Women's Hospital in Boston (Bates et al., 1993). Of 270 patients who had had at least six months of fatigue that interfered with their daily activities, three were found to fulfill all necessary criteria for CFS. Therefore the observed point prevalence of CFS was 0.3%.

Specialized practice setting

The frequency of CFS among adult patients requesting evaluation for a chief complaint of persistent fatigue was studied at the Fatigue Clinic of the University of Connecticut Health Center (Manu et al., 1988). The patients underwent a complete review of their medical history and had a physical examination and comprehensive laboratory studies. Psychiatric evaluations were performed by administering the Diagnostic Interview Schedule (Robins & Helzer, 1985). Of the 141 patients enrolled in the study, 135 complained of fatigue described as new, persistent and debilitating, and that had its onset at least six months prior to being evaluated in the specialized setting. Of these individuals, 91 (67%) had clinically active psychiatric disorders, 4 (3%) had a physical disorder known to produce fatigue and 34 (25%) had an insufficient number of minor diagnostic criteria. Six patients were given the diagnosis of CFS. The prevalence of CFS in a specialized setting of an academic clinic was 5%, with a calculated 95% confidence interval ranging from a low of 0 to a high of 10%.

Economic costs

The economic impact of CFS has been completely evaluated only by an Australian team in a population-based survey conducted in the Richmond Valley, New South Wales, in 1989 (Lloyd & Pender, 1992). The prevalence of CFS among the 111 400 inhabitants was assessed at 0.037%. The sources of economic data were information provided by patients (duration and severity of symptoms, education, past and present employment, family income and use of traditional and alternative health care services) and the Medicare data regarding number and type of services and fees charged. Intensive efforts were made to separate expenditures unrelated to CFS. The main outcome variables were the direct costs, i.e. the increase in use of health care resources because of CFS and indirect costs, i.e. income foregone by patients resulting from cessation or reduction in employment, sickness benefits and invalid pensions paid by the government and income tax revenue lost to the government.

The total yearly economic cost of CFS was the Australian equivalent of US$8321 (in 1989) for each patient. Indirect costs accounted for US$7000 per patient per year, with the three largest components of the aggregated expenditure being income foregone (US$5100), income tax foregone (US$1150) and sickness benefits and invalid pensions (US$750). Office visits and laboratory tests added US$680. The cost of hospitalizations and medications was minimal. Extrapolations to the

US economy must take into account the differences in the health care practice, particularly the high cost of specialized care and use of 'high-ticket' items such as comprehensive immunological testing and MRI; it is reasonable to assume that the Australian costs would represent a very conservative estimate for the US economy. With this caveat, using the lowest limit of the estimated prevalence rate of 0.007% (Gunn et al., 1993) and adjusting individual expenditures for inflation to US$12 000, the cost of CFS in the USA today could be estimated to be at least US$200 million each year.

Confirmations

Preponderance of middle-aged and well-educated white women

Women outnumber men in every clinical report describing a series of patients with CFS, with the proportion of women ranging from 59% to 77% (Kruesi et al., 1989; Klimas et al., 1990; Peterson et al., 1990; Demitrack et al., 1991; Lane et al., 1991; Buchwald et al., 1994). Epidemiological research has confirmed these observations; the observed two-year period prevalence of CFS across four urban sites in the USA was 12.1 per 100 000 white women and 2.4 per 100 000 white men, or a white female : white male ratio of 4.3 : 1 (Gunn et al., 1993).

All clinical reports concur also in demonstrating that, with only occasional exceptions, CFS patients are predominantly white. For example, all 60 patients diagnosed to have the syndrome during an 18-month period at the Chronic Fatigue Clinic of the University of Connecticut were white (Lane et al., 1991). The proportions of whites were 94% among the 270 female patients and 92% among the 55 male patients seen at the Chronic Fatigue Clinic of the University of Washington (Buchwald et al., 1994). In the CDC-sponsored study, the two-year period prevalence prorated to all 590 patients identified by 408 physicians was 7.6 per 100 000 white individuals and 0.9 per 100 000 non-white individuals (Gunn et al., 1993).

High frequency of major depression

The first study specifically designed to characterize the psychiatric morbidity of patients with CFS was performed at the University of Toronto, Ontario, Canada (Taerk et al., 1987). The 24 patients evaluated had CFS whose onset occurred after an apparent infectious illness. A control group included healthy volunteers matched for age, sex and educational level. The instruments were a structured psychiatric interview and a self-report measure of depressive symptoms. The lifetime prevalence of major depression was 67% among CFS patients and 29% in the control group, a statistically significant difference. Half of the CFS patients had at least one major depressive episode before the onset of their fatigue illness. Self-report data indicated that 46% of patients, but none of the control subjects were in the midst of a moderate or severe depressive episode.

The next study addressing the frequency of major depression among CFS patients was conducted at the National Institutes of Health (Kruesi et al., 1989). The eligible patients were seen by a psychiatrist who administered a detailed structured psychiatric instrument. The 28 patients entered in this study were all white and had a mean age of 35 years; 71% were women. Psychiatric diagnoses were identified in 21 patients (75%). Major depression was the most common diagnosis, being given to 13 patients (46%).

The third study employing the Diagnostic Interview Schedule to identify major depression among patients with CFS was performed at the University of Connecticut (Lane et al., 1991). The 60 CFS patients were age and sex matched to control subjects with a chief complaint of chronic fatigue, but no CFS. Major depression that was symptomatic within the six months prior to the evaluation was identified in 71% of patients with the CFS and 70% of the fatigued control subjects. The onset of the depressive disorder in these patients preceded the chronic fatigue by more than one year in 81% of cases with CFS and in 59% of the cases identified among control subjects.

The fourth study using similar methodology for the detection of psychiatric disorders was conducted at The University of Washington Chronic Fatigue Clinic (Buchwald et al., 1994). The subjects were 348 consecutive patients diagnosed as having CFS. All patients received a standardized physical examination focused on detecting potential medical causes of fatigue, a comprehensive battery of laboratory tests and a highly structured psychiatric interview. A lifetime diagnosis of major depression was made in 74% of women and 64% of men.

Finally, similar findings were obtained in a well-controlled clinical and psychometric evaluation of patients with chronic fatigue conducted at the National Hospital for Nervous Diseases, London, England (Wessely & Powell, 1989). The participants included 41 adults with CFS, 33 patients with peripheral neuromuscular fatiguing illnesses and 26 inpatients with major depression. Overall, 34 (72%) of CFS patients, but only 12 (36%) of neuromuscular fatigue patients were diagnosed to have an active psychiatric disorder. The most common psychiatric disorder among the CFS patients was major depression, diagnosed in 47% of cases. Mental effort precipitated fatigue in 89% of CFS patients and 80% of inpatients with major depression, while feeling fatigued at rest was reported by 46% of CFS patients and 48% of cases with major depression.

High frequency of somatization disorder

The prospective studies that have identified a high frequency of major depression have also been instrumental in demonstrating a high frequency of somatization disorder. The frequencies reported were 10% in the National Institutes of Health report (Kruesi et al., 1989), 15% among patients studied in England (Wessely & Powell, 1989), 28% in the group studied at the University of Connecticut (Lane et al., 1991) and 25% in the patient sample investigated at the University of Seattle (Buchwald et al., 1994). In sharp contrast with these figures, the prevalence of somatization disorder as detected by the Diagnostic Interview Schedule in a large epidemiological study of a series of communities in the USA ranged from 0.1% to 0.4% (Escobar et al., 1987).

Abnormal personality traits

The first report of systematic evaluation of personality characteristics of patients with CFS originated from the University of Miami (Millon et al., 1989). The 24 patients with CFS were studied with a self-report instrument containing ten basic personality pattern scales and three pathological personality disorder scales. A substantial proportion of CFS patients had abnormally high scores for the following personality scales: histrionic (33% of patients), schizoid (29%), avoidant (25%), narcissistic (25%) and aggressive-sadistic (25%). The elevations on the histrionic, schizoid and avoidant personality scales appeared to be specific for this clinical population and were suggestive of severe personality pathology.

The Minnesota Multiphasic Personality Inventory (MMPI) and a well-validated coping scale were used in a study of 58 patients with CFS evaluated at the Otago Medical School, Dunedin, New Zealand (Blakely et al., 1991). A chronic pain control group comprised 81 individuals. A second control group included 104 healthy subjects. CFS patients indicated significantly greater escape/avoidance and distancing. They also had a marked inward direction of hostility and a pronounced degree of self-criticism and guilt. The CFS patients also scored significantly higher on scales measuring hypochondriasis, hysteria, paranoia, social introversion and anxiety. The differences between chronic fatigue and chronic pain did not appear to be illness specific, but seemed to reflect the high level of anxiety that characterized the CFS group.

The personality characteristics of 75 patients with chronic unexplained fatigue were also studied at the University of Washington (Russo et al., 1994). Two control groups were assembled; one comprised 61 subjects referred for evaluation of persistent dizziness and one that included 88 patients with disabling tinnitus. Psychiatric diagnoses and the assessments of personality traits were based on standard structured interviews. Of the personality dimensions studied, the subscales for worry/pessimism and impulsiveness were significantly related to the number of unexplained physical symptoms that constitute the clinical presentation of CFS.

Characteristics of patients with severe chronic fatigue syndrome

Data recently collected in Australia (Hickie et al., 1995) show that among the patients currently diagnosed with CFS there is a statistically homogeneous 'poor prognosis' subgroup comprising 27% of the sample. This subgroup is characterized by a greater proportion of women, more disability, higher current psychiatric morbidity, more symptoms and more hypochondriacal concerns. Similar findings were reported in a study of symptom persistence at 2.5 years after the initial evaluation in a group of CFS patients from Seattle (Clark et al., 1995). The CFS patients showing no recovery (59% of the original cohort) had a significantly higher lifetime prevalence of depression, dysthymia, generalized anxiety disorder and somatization disorder. Of interest is the fact that self-report measures obtained at the initial evaluation were predictive of recovery at follow-up; the 'poor prognosis' subgroup had higher scores on scales measuring depression, awareness of bodily function, somatization, and somatic and psychological distress. In contrast, virological, serological and immunological laboratory tests did not differ between the recovered and 'poor-prognosis' subgroups.

Contradictions

Identification of infectious processes

Herpesviruses

Epstein–Barr virus

A greater detection rate of Epstein–Barr (EBV) in a group of CFS patients was demonstrated in a controlled study performed at the Medical College of Georgia (Wray et al., 1993). Half of the patient sample had had a sudden onset. A control group included healthy and asymptomatic volunteers matched for age, sex and ethnic group. Serological studies tested the antibodies to well-defined EBV antigens. Pharyngeal scrapings were obtained from all participants and in-situ hybridization was performed to detect the EBV DNA. Usable data were available from 40 patients and 29 control subjects.

EBV DNA was detected in nine (22%) patients and in one (3%)

control subject; a significant difference. A direct comparison of the CFS patients with or without EBV DNA in their pharyngeal scrapings indicated similar proportions of cases with elevated antibody titers to the EBV capsid antigen (78% versus 100%), nuclear antigen (78% versus 100%) and early antigen (44% versus 47%).

Contrasting results were produced by an investigation conducted at the University of Washington (Gold et al., 1990). The study group included 26 patients who were known to have elevated titers of the IgG antibody to the EBV viral capsid and early antigens. Eighteen volunteers with no medical complaints comprised the control group. The EBV isolation was attempted from pharyngeal washings and blood, and in-situ hybridization on peripheral blood lymphocytes was performed.

The cultures of pharyngeal washings were negative for EBV in all participants. The virus was cultured from the peripheral blood cells of two patients and two control subjects. In-situ hybridization detected the EBV DNA in blood or pharyngeal washings in one chronic fatigue patient and three control subjects.

The evolution in understanding the limitations of EBV testing in CFS patients resembles the history of the introduction of other diagnostic tests (Matthews et al., 1991*a*). Early enthusiasm for the test in discriminating highly selected patients from healthy control subjects was later tempered by the lack of specificity in a broader population. In contrast to reliable diagnostic tests, positive EBV testing in CFS does not discover disease that is clinically silent, does not exclude other disorders, does not estimate prognosis or therapeutic progress and does not provide reassurance.

Human herpesvirus type 6

Assays for active infection with human herpesvirus type 6 (HHV-6) were conducted as part of a comprehensive evaluation of a large number of CFS patients from Nevada and California in the USA (Buchwald et al., 1992). HHV-6 serological testing was performed on 134 CFS patients and 27 healthy control subjects from the same community. Their coded sera were tested for IgG antibody reactivity against HHV-6 associated antigens by enzyme-linked immunosorbent assay. HHV-6 active replication in peripheral mononuclear cells were conducted in 113 patients and 40 healthy blood donors and laboratory personnel.

Median values for the HHV-6 IgG antibodies were similar in patients and control subjects. Positive bioassays indicating active HHV-6 replication were observed in 70% of the patients tested and 20% of the healthy control group. Polymerase chain reaction studies with HHV-6 specificity were performed in six patients who had a positive bioassay and were found to be positive in all.

The confirmation of these findings was recently attempted in a study using a highly sensitive and specific polymerase chain reaction (Secchiero et al., 1995). The method was developed because the authors considered that virus isolation from activated blood cells was unable to discriminate between active and latent HHV-6 infection. The assays were conducted on sera from 37 patients with CFS referred by one of the authors of the previous study and 37 healthy adults. The test was positive in only one patient (2.6%) of the CFS group.

Retroviruses

The presence of two human retroviruses, human T-lymphotropic virus (HTLV) types I and II in patients with CFS was the focus of two reports.

In the first report, the testing for HTLV consisted of Western immunoblotting, polymerase chain reaction and in-situ hybridization of blood sample (DeFreitas et al., 1991). The patient cohort comprised 30 adult and pediatric cases; exposed control subjects were age and sex-matched healthy individuals who had either sexual or casual contact with the patients. Blood samples were also obtained from 20 healthy nonexposure control subjects (ten from adults and ten from umbilical cords of newborns).

Western immunoblotting testing for HTLV was positive in 50% of adult and 61% of pediatric CFS patients. In contrast, only 23% of exposure control sera and none of the 20 nonexposure control sera were reactive. To clarify these findings, HTLV-I and HTLV-II specific proviral sequences were examined by polymerase chain reaction and HTLV-II gag sequences were identified in 83% of the HTLV positive patients, 38% of HTLV positive exposure control sera and none of the nonexposure control samples.

The confirmation of these findings was attempted at the CDC (Khan et al., 1993). Included were 21 adult patients identified in the Atlanta, Georgia, metropolitan area through a surveillance system in which individual physicians referred cases with at least six months of unexplained fatigue. Each patient was matched for age, sex and ethnic group with a healthy control subject and with two randomly selected individuals whose telephone number had the same prefix (neighborhood control subjects).

The 18 serum samples (nine from patients and nine from control subjects) tested for HTLV-I and HTLV-II antibodies by Western immunoblot and peptide enzyme-linked immunosorbent assay gave negative results. Polymerase chain reaction assays conducted on all CFS patients and healthy control subjects failed to amplify with the HTLV-II gag-gene-specific primers. Thus, the previously described retroviral marker was completely absent.

Enteroviruses

The presence of enteroviral infection was the object of a study involving 60 subjects selected from a large CFS patient population followed in Glasgow, Scotland (Gow & Behan, 1991). All patients had in common an acute febrile onset with respiratory or gastrointestinal symptoms followed by severe, unremitting fatigue and myalgia for at least one year. The control group comprised 41 patients from the same catchment area admitted for elective surgical procedures. None of the control subjects complained of fatigue or had evidence of muscle pathology. Serological studies were directed at the detection of antibodies to Coxsackie viruses. Polymerase chain reaction was employed to detect enteroviral sequences in leukocytes and skeletal muscle biopsies. Fifteen (25%) patients and 10 (24%) control subjects had positive serologies as evidenced by increased antibody titers. The polymerase chain reaction of leukocytes gave positive results in 16% of the patients and control subjects; the test was positive in the muscle biopsies of 32 (53%) of the patients, but only in 6 (15%) control subjects.

The presence of enteroviral persistence was also addressed in a study conducted in the Netherlands on 76 patients with CFS (Swanink et al., 1994). Control subjects were sex and age-matched healthy neighbors. Serological studies were carried out using broadly reactive antibody capture enzyme-linked immunosorbent assays. The isolation of virus from stool specimens was attempted using tissue culture of human lung fibroblasts and monkey kidney cells. Finally, the polymerase chain reaction was employed to detect fecal enteroviral RNA sequences.

Serological results were similar for patients and control subjects. No correlation was found between positive serology and acuteness of onset or severity of the fatigue illness. All cultures were negative for enteroviruses. The polymerase chain reaction visualized amplification products in one (1.3%) CFS patient.

Immunological dysfunction

Humoral immunity

The humoral immunity of patients with CFS was comprehensively studied in a CDC investigation of an alleged community outbreak (Holmes et al., 1987). Fifteen patients had persistent fatigue sufficient to cause absence from work for at least four weeks or a reduction of daily activity by 50% and no apparent explanation for the symptoms. Two control subjects were matched for sex, age and race with each patient; these subjects had no history of chronic illness, history of chronic fatigue or history of long-term therapy. Serological tests for antibodies to EBV, cytomegalovirus, herpes simplex virus

(HSV) types 1 and 2, and measles were performed in three different laboratories. The serological results were quantified as mean titers of antibodies for each group and each of the antibodies tested.

Compared with control subjects, the patients had significantly higher mean titers antibodies to EBV, cytomegalovirus, HSV type 2 and measles. Although the mean total IgG, IgA and IgM concentrations were similar in the two groups, the findings were considered to suggest a nonspecific polyclonal B lymphocytic response, viewed as an exaggerated immune response to unidentified stimuli.

The confirmatory search for a nonspecific polyclonal immune response in patients with CFS was the aim of a study of 20 patients diagnosed in an infectious diseases practice setting (Manian, 1994). Age and sex-matched healthy control subjects were selected from among hospital personnel and their acquaintances. All control subjects had a normal physical examination and denied chronic fatigue. Serological evaluations were performed to detect and quantify antibodies to multiple common viruses, including EBV, HHV-6, HSV-1 and HSV-2.

The geometric mean titers of antibodies to EBV early antigen, HHV-6 IgG antibodies, and HSV-1 and HSV-2 IgG antibodies were similar in patients and control subjects. There was no correlation between EBV antibodies titers and other herpesviruses. This lack of positive correlation was interpreted as a rejection of the research hypothesis that a nonspecific polyclonal immune response is present in CFS.

Cellular immunity

The lymphocyte phenotype and function were studied at the National Institutes of Health in a group of 18 patients who met strictly defined criteria (Holmes et al., 1988*a*) for CFS (Straus et al., 1993). Their illness had had an acute, infectious-type onset in 17 of the 18 cases. A control group comprised 17 healthy individuals who worked or studied full-time. Extensive phenotypic analyses of B and T cell subsets, natural killer cells and macrophages were performed using flow cytometry.

Compared with control subjects, the main positive findings indicated that the median percentages of CD4 T cells (41% versus 50%) and CD4, CD45RA or 'naive' T cells (17% versus 28%) were reduced. A second positive finding was the reduced proliferative response to phytohemaglutinin, concanavalin A and staphylococcal enterotoxin of the lymphocytes obtained from CFS patients. On the other hand, median percentages of the B cell subsets, natural killer cell markers and the activation markers CD11b (8% versus 6%), CD38 (5% versus 6%) and HLA-DR (4% versus 3%) were similar among CFS patients and control subjects.

Cellular immunity was also evaluated in a controlled study performed at the University of California, San Francisco (Barker et al.,

1994) on 56 patients and 46 healthy control subjects. In stark contrast to the previous study, flow cytometric analyses showed no abnormalities with regard to total T and B cells, monocytes and natural killer cell markers. There were no abnormalities noted on T cell proliferation studies. On the other hand, the percentage of lymphocytes with activation markers CD38 (54% versus 28%) and HLA-DR (28% versus 12%) were significantly increased in the CFS group.

Abnormal brain magnetic resonance images

Magnetic resonance imaging (MRI) of the brain was performed on 144 of the 259 individuals enrolled in a study of CFS in a population from Nevada and California (Buchwald et al., 1992). A majority of the patients had chronic headaches (91%) and paresthesias (75%). An MRI control group comprised 47 subjects without fatigue. As the MRI center evaluating the control group was at a different location, blind interpretation of images was not possible.

Abnormal MRI brain images described as punctate or patchy foci of high signal intensity, usually in the subcortical white matter, were noted in 78% of patients and 21% of control subjects. A relation between the clinical presentation and the abnormal anatomical MRI area, however, was established in only nine patients (6% of total cohort): seven patients with visual symptoms had high intensity areas in the occipital cortex, one patient with ataxia had abnormal cerebellar images, and a patient with paresis had a high signal intensity focus in the contralateral internal capsule.

The efficacy of MRI brain imaging was addressed a second time by the same authors in an investigation of 16 patients with neurological signs and symptoms who met the clinical criteria for CFS (Schwartz et al., 1994). A group of 15 healthy age and sex-matched volunteers comprised the control group. MRI abnormalities were identified in eight CFS subjects, compared with three of the control subjects, a difference statistically insignificant. The abnormalities consisted of small foci of increased signal intensity in the white matter; the cortex was of normal signal intensity in all cases. Averages of two abnormal foci per patient and 0.8 abnormal foci per control subject were recorded, but again the difference was insignificant. The authors concluded that these findings are nonspecific for CFS and that MRI does not have a substantial clinical utility as a screening test in the differential diagnosis of CFS.

Muscle fatigue and reduced oxidative metabolism

Muscle fatigue and a substantial decrease in exercise tolerance are ubiquitous among patients with CFS. The issue is of paramount importance for the determination of functional disability often alleged by these patients and is discussed in detail in Chapter 13. Direct measurements of muscle strength have produced contradictory results: one research group has found muscle strength, endurance and recovery to be normal (Lloyd et al., 1988), while another has demonstrated significant and persistent reductions in maximal isometric contractions (Maffulli et al., 1993). New technologies have allowed an interdisciplinary team from the USA and Italy to demonstrate subtle abnormalities in oxidative muscle metabolism (McCully et al., 1996). In an exercise study of CFS patients and sedentary control subjects, the muscle oxidative capacity, measured as the maximal rate of postexercise resynthesis of phosphocreatine in the calf muscle using magnetic resonance spectroscopy, was shown to be significantly decreased in the patient group. Two days later, metabolic studies were normal and the CFS subjects showed no evidence of a symptomatic relapse with strenuous exercise. The authors suggest that these abnormalities could be due to deconditioning as a result of the reduced activity levels by CFS patients and point out that similar bioenergetic changes are produced by inactivity in patients with multiple sclerosis and spinal cord section.

Pathogenetic hypotheses

The accumulated knowledge about CFS does not include a clear cause–effect relationship; however, our analyses of the literature indicate three pathogenetic hypotheses worthy of consideration in an effort to explain the somatic and psychological features of the condition. The first regards CFS as an expression of psychopathology occurring in individuals with a treatment-resistant depression (Gruber et al., 1996) who attribute their illnesses to an external cause (Lane et al., 1991). The second considers the disorder to have an organic cause (e.g. a viral infection or an immunological dysfunction) with the depressive features explained as a reaction to the chronic, disabling illness (Buchwald et al., 1992). Finally, a third hypothesis sees CFS to be a brain-centered pathological entity, with the depressive feature being the result of neurotransmitter deficiencies and the somatic features expressing dysregulation of the hypothalamic-pituitary-adrenal axis (Demitrack et al., 1991).

Diagnostic and treatment approaches

Clinical evaluation

Sufficient time should be devoted to obtain a complete history, with particular attention to the description of fatigue, including duration, severity, timing and provocative and palliative factors. A close examination of the patient's habits related to factors such as hours of work, exercise and sleep, and intake of medications, caffeine and alcohol should be performed. The patients' perception of disability with regard to home and marital life, professional functioning and social activities must be explored in detail.

A careful exploration of patients' experience with the medical care system is also important, including the diagnoses and treatments offered by other physicians, the use of alternative care practitioners (chiropractors, homeopaths, acupuncturists, nutritionists and clinical ecologists), and previous visits to mental health providers. Patients should be encouraged to describe their diagnostic belief regarding the etiology of their fatigue illness. Psychiatric interviews must be conducted with all patients having a chief complaint of chronic fatigue.

The aim of clinical and laboratory investigations is to evaluate the extensive differential diagnosis of chronic fatigue states. The main categories are:

(1) physiological states such as pregnancy, sleep deprivation and excessive muscular activity performed by persons in poor physical condition;
(2) physical disorders, including primary sleep disorders (obstructive sleep apnea, narcolepsy, periodic leg movements with frequent awakenings), neuromuscular disorders (multiple sclerosis, muscular dystrophy, myasthenia gravis), cardiovascular diseases producing low-output states, pulmonary or hematological conditions producing peripheral hypoxia, chronic inflammatory conditions, poorly controlled endocrinological disorders (diabetes mellitus and insipidus, hyperthyroidism, hypothyroidism, adrenal insufficiency and hyperparathyroidism), collagen vascular diseases (polymyalgia rheumatic, systemic lupus erythematosus), chronic infections (AIDS, tuberculosis, Lyme disease), and neurally mediated hypotension;
(3) psychiatric conditions characterized by persistent tiredness or easy fatigability including mood, anxiety, somatoform, substance use and eating disorders;
(4) side-effects of medications, most notably benzodiazepines, cancer chemotherapeutic agents, drugs commonly used to treat arterial hypertension (diuretics, calcium-channel blockers, beta-adrenergic blockers) and histamine-receptor (1H and 2H) blockers used to treat allergic conditions and peptic ulcer disease;
(5) unhealthy lifestyles especially those that neglect exercise and allow frequent disruptions of the normal wake–sleep cycle;

(6) chronic psychosocial stressors such as aggressive pursuit of professional advancement or material wealth, unemployment or fear of unemployment, marital miscommunication, family violence, prolonged bereavement and the delayed effects of traumatic events.

Laboratory investigations should be ordered according to the clinical findings. If the history and physical examination fail to indicate the presence of a definite pathological entity, the recommended battery of screening tests comprises a complete blood count, erythrocyte sedimentation rate, thyroid, renal and hepatic function tests, calcium, phosphorus, electrolytes, glucose, total protein and albumin levels, stool guaiac, urinalysis and Lyme antibody titers (Matthews et al., 1991*b*; Fukuda et al., 1994).

Treatment

Ineffective treatment modalities for CFS studied in a double-blind, full-dose placebo-controlled trials in the USA include the antiviral agent acyclovir (Straus et al., 1988), a naturopathic regimen of liver extract, folic acid and cyancobalamin (Kaslow et al., 1989), intravenous gammaglobulin (Peterson et al., 1990) and the antihistamine terfenadine (Steinberg et al., 1996). Placebo-controlled trials designed to test the effectiveness of antidepressant agents in CFS patients have had mixed results, possibly because only low dosages were offered. Phenelzine, a monoamine oxidase inhibitor (15 mg daily), produced a significant pattern of improvement (Natelson et al., 1996). In contrast, fluoxetine, a selective serotonin reuptake inhibitor (20 mg daily) produced no change in the subjective assessment of fatigue (Vercoulen et al., 1996).

Cognitive-behavioral therapy has been followed by encouraging results in two recent well-controlled trials. Among patients with CFS and substantial depression, significant improvement was noted not only for measures of depression but also for fatigue severity and the cognitive and emotional reaction to fatigue (Friedberg & Krupp, 1994). These results were confirmed in a larger study of the effect of 16 individual weekly sessions given in addition to their standard medical care (Sharpe et al., 1996). The assessment at 12 months found that 73% of recipients of cognitive-behavioral therapy had achieved normal daily functioning and a sustained reduction in the perceived and measured disability compared with 27% in a CFS control group. The favorable response was correctly attributed to changes in illness beliefs and maladaptive coping styles.

The etiological and symptomatic treatment of comorbid conditions must be considered a priority. The National Institutes of Health have recently published guidelines for primary care practice (NIAID, 1996).

Among the commonly suggested drugs are low-dose tricyclic agents (e.g. amitryptiline) for fibromyalgic symptoms (myalgias and insomnia) and long-acting benzodiazepines (e.g. clonazepam) for anxiety disorders. Fludrocortisone and adrenergic beta-blocking agents have been recommended for the 'vaso-vagal' symptoms of neurally mediated hypotension identified in some CFS patients (Bou-Holaigh et al., 1995). At the end of 1996, some of these modalities were being studied in controlled trials.

Finally, it is important to educate patients with regard to graded aerobic reconditioning. The research literature does not support rest as a therapeutic measure for CFS patients.

Conclusion

The term CFS describes a set of nonspecific symptoms (cognitive dysfunction, sore throat, tender lymph nodes, myalgias, arthralgias, headache, unrefreshing sleep and postexertional malaise) associated with persistent or relapsing fatigue. The diagnostic evaluation must exclude numerous medical and psychiatric conditions producing fatigue in association with some of these symptoms. Research studies have confirmed that the majority of patients with CFS are white middle-aged women with a high prevalence of current major depression and somatization disorder and abnormal personality traits. The cause of the condition is not known and effective pharmacological approaches have not been identified.

References

American Psychiatric Association (1968). *Diagnostic and Statistical Manual of Mental Disorders*, 2nd edn (DSM-II). Washington, DC: American Psychiatric Association.

American Psychiatric Association, Committee on Nomenclature and Statistics (1980). *Diagnostic and Statistical Manual of Mental Disorders*, 3rd edn (DSM-II). Washington, DC: American Psychiatric Association.

American Psychiatric Association, Committee on Nomenclature and Statistics (1987). *Diagnostic and Statistical Manual of Mental Disorders*, 3rd edn, revised (DSM III-R). Washington, DC: American Psychiatric Association.

Barker E, Fujimura SF, Fadem MB, Landay AL & Levy JA (1994). Immunologic abnormalities associated with chronic fatigue syndrome. *Clinical and Infectious Diseases*, **18** (Suppl.), S136–S141.

Bates DW, Schmitt W, Buchwald D, Ware NC, Lee J, Thoyer E, Kornish RJ & Komaroff AL (1993). Prevalence of fatigue and chronic fatigue syndrome in a primary care practice. *Archives of Internal Medicine*, **153**, 2759–65.

Beard GM (1869). Neurasthenia or nervous exhaustion. *Boston Medical and Surgical Journal*, **3**, 217–20.

Beard GM (1881). *American Nervousness, Its Causes and Consequences*. New York: GP Putnam.

Blakely AA, Howard RC, Sosich RM, Murdoch JC, Menkes DB & Spears GFS (1991). Psychiatric symptoms, personality and ways of coping in chronic fatigue syndrome. *Psychological Medicine*, **21**, 347–62.

Bou-Holaigh I, Rowe PC, Kan J & Calkins H (1995). The relationship between neurally-mediated hypotension and the chronic fatigue syndrome. *Journal of the American Medical Association*, **274**, 961–7.

Buchwald, D, Sullivan JL & Komaroff AL (1987). Frequency of 'chronic active Epstein–Barr virus infection' in a general medical practice. *Journal of the American Medical Association*, **257**, 2303–7.

Buchwald D, Cheney PR, Peterson DL, Henry B, Wormsley SB, Geiger A, Ablashi DV, Salahuddin Z, Saxinger C, Biddle R, Kikinis R, Jolesz FA, Folks T, Balachandran N, Peter JB, Gallo RC & Komaroff AL (1992). Chronic illness characterized by fatigue, neurologic and immunologic disorders, and active human herpesvirus type 6 infection. *Annals of Internal Medicine*, **116**, 103–13.

Buchwald, D, Pearlman T, Kith P & Schmaling K (1994). Gender differences in patients with chronic fatigue syndrome. *Journal of General Internal Medicine*, **9**, 397–940.

Buchwald D, Umali P, Umali J, Kith P, Pearlman T & Komaroff AL (1995). Chronic fatigue and the chronic fatigue syndrome: prevalence in a Pacific Northwest health care system. *Annals of Internal Medicine*, **123**, 81–8.

Clark MR, Katon W, Russo J, Kith P, Sintay M & Buchwald D (1995). Chronic fatigue: risk factors for symptom persistence in a $2\frac{1}{2}$-year follow-up study. *American Journal of Medicine*, **98**, 187–95.

DeFreitas E, Hilliard B, Cheney PR, Bell DS, Kiggundu E, Sankey D, Wroblewska Z, Palladino M, Woodward JP & Koprowski H (1991). Retroviral sequences related to human T-lymphotropic virus type II in patients with chronic fatigue immune dysfunction syndrome. *Proceedings of the National Academy of Sciences, USA*, **88**, 2922–6.

Demitrack MA, Dale JK, Straus SE, Laue L, Listwak SJ, Kruesi MJP, Chrousos GP & Gold PW (1991). Evidence for impaired activation of the hypothalamic-pituitary-adrenal axis in patients with chronic fatigue syndrome. *Journal of Clinical Endocrinology and Metabolism*, **73**, 1224–34.

Dubois RE, Seeley JK, Brus I, Sakamoto K, Ballow M; Harada S, Bechtold TA, Pearson G & Purtillo DT (1984). Chronic mononucleosis syndrome. *Southern Medical Journal*, **77**, 1376–82.

Escobar JI, Burnam MA & Karno M (1987). Somatization in the community. *Archives of General Psychiatry*, **14**, 713–18.

Freud S (1894). The justification for detaching from neurasthenia a particular syndrome: the anxiety syndrome. In Freud S, *Collected Papers*, vol. 1. New York: Basic Books, 1959.

Friedberg F & Krupp LB (1994). A comparison of cognitive behavioral treatment for chronic fatigue syndrome and primary depression. *Clinical and Infectious Diseases*, **18** (Suppl. 1), S105–S110.

Fukuda K, Straus SE, Hickie I, Sharpe MC, Dobbins JG & Komaroff A (1994). The chronic fatigue syndrome: a comprehensive approach to its definition and study. International Chronic Fatigue Syndrome Study Group. *Annals of Internal Medicine*, **121**, 953–9.

Gold D, Bowden R, Sixbey J, Riggs R, Katon WJ, Ashley R, Obrigewitch R & Corey L (1990). Chronic fatigue: a prospective clinical and virologic study. *Journal of the American Medical Association*, **264**, 48–53.

Gow JW & Behan WMH (1991). Amplification and identification of enteroviral sequences in the postviral fatigue syndrome. *British Medical Bulletin*, **47**, 872–85.

Gruber AJ, Hudson JI & Pope HG Jr (1996). The management of treatment-resistant depression in disorders on the interface of psychiatry and medicine. *Psychiatric Clinics of North America*, **19**, 351–69.

Gunn WJ, Connell DB & Randall B (1993). Epidemiology of chronic fatigue syndrome: the Centers for Disease Control study. In *Chronic Fatigue Syndrome*. Ciba Foundation Symposium **173**, pp. 83–101. Chichester: John Wiley.

Hellinger WC, Smith TF, Van Scoy RE, Spitzer PG, Forgacs P & Edson RS (1988). Chronic fatigue syndrome and the diagnostic utility of antibody to Epstein–Barr virus antigen. *Journal of the American Medical Association*, **260**, 971–3.

Hickie I, Lloyd A, Hadzi-Pavlovic D, Parker G, Bird K & Wakefield D (1995). Can the chronic fatigue syndrome be defined by distinct clinical features? *Psychological Medicine*, **25**, 925–35.

Holmes GP, Kaplan JE, Stewart JA, Hunt B, Pinsky PF & Schonberger LB (1987). A cluster of patients with mononucleosis-like syndrome; is Epstein–Barr virus the cause? *Journal of the American Medical Association*, **257**, 2297–302.

Holmes GP, Kaplan, JE, Gantz NM, Komaroff AL, Schonberger LB, Straus SE, Jones JF, Dubois RE, Cunningham-Rundles C, Pahwa S, Tosato G, Zegans LS, Purtillo DT, Brown N, Schooley RT & Brus I (1988*a*). Chronic fatigue syndrome: a working-case definition. *Annals of Internal Medicine*, **108**, 387–9.

Holmes GP, Kaplan JE, Schonberger LB, Straus SE, Zegans LS, Gantz NM, Brus I, Komaroff A, Jones JF, Dubois RE, Cunningham-Rundles C, Tosato G, Brown NA, Pahwa S & Schooley RT (1988*b*). Definition of the chronic fatigue syndrome. *Annals of Internal Medicine*, **109**, 512.

Janet P (1903). *Les Obsessions et la Psychasthenie*. Paris: Felix Alcan.

Jones JF, Ray CG, Minnich LL, Hicks MJ, Kibler R & Lucas DO (1985). Evidence for active Epstein–Barr virus infection in patients with persistent, unexplained illnesses: elevated early antigen antibodies. *Annals of Internal Medicine*, **102**, 1–7.

Kaslow JE, Rucker L & Onishi R (1989). Liver extract-folic acid-cyanocobalamin vs placebo for chronic fatigue syndrome. *Archives of Internal Medicine*, **149**, 2501–3.

Khan AS, Heneine WM, Chapman LE, Gary HE, Woods TC, Folks TM & Schonberger LBV (1993). Assessment of a retrovirus sequence and other possible risk factors for the chronic fatigue syndrome in adults. *Annals of Internal Medicine*, **118**, 241–5.

Klimas NA, Salvato FR, Morgan R & Fletcher MA (1990). Immunologic abnormalities in chronic fatigue syndrome. *Journal of Clinical Microbiology*, **28**, 1403–10.

Kruesi MJP, Dale J & Straus SE (1989). Psychiatric diagnoses in patients who have chronic fatigue syndrome. *Journal of Clinical Psychiatry*, **50**, 53–6.

Lane TJ, Manu P & Matthews DA (1991). Depression and somatization in the chronic fatigue syndrome. *American Journal of Medicine*, **91**, 335–44.

Lloyd AR & Pender H (1992). The economic impact of chronic fatigue syndrome. *Medical Journal of Australia*, **157**, 599–601.

Lloyd A, Hales J & Gandevia S (1988). Muscle strength, endurance, and recovery in the post-infection fatigue syndrome. *Journal of Neurology, Neurosurgery and Psychiatry*, **51**, 1316–22.

Lloyd A, Hickie I, Wakefield D, Boughton C & Dwyer J (1990). A double-blind, placebo-controlled trial of intravenous immunoglobulin therapy in patients with chronic fatigue syndrome. *American Journal of Medicine*, **89**, 561–8.

Lloyd AR, Hickie I, Brockman A, Hickie C, Wilson A, Dwyer J & Wakefield D (1993). Immunologic and psychologic therapy for patients with chronic fatigue syndrome: a double-blind, placebo-controlled trial. *American Journal of Medicine*, **94**, 197–203.

Maffuli N & Testa V, Capasso (1993). Post-viral syndrome: a longitudinal assessment in varsity athletes. *Journal of Sports Medicine and Physical Fitness*, **33**, 392–9.

Manian FA (1994). Simultaneous measurement of antibodies to Epstein–Barr virus, human herpesvirus 6, herpes simplex virus type 1 and 2, and 14 enteroviruses in chronic fatigue syndrome: is there evidence of activation of a nonspecific polyclonal immune response? *Clinical and Infectious Diseases*, **19**, 448–53.

Manu P, Lane TJ & Matthews DA (1988). The frequency of the chronic fatigue syndrome in patients with symptoms of persistent fatigue. *Annals of Internal Medicine*, **109**, 554–6.

Matthews DA, Lane TJ & Manu P (1991*a*). Antibodies to Epstein–Barr virus in patients with chronic fatigue. *Southern Medical Journal*, **84**, 832–40.

Matthews DA, Manu P & Lane TJ (1991*b*). Evaluation and management of patients with chronic fatigue. *American Journal of the Medical Sciences*, **302**, 269–77.

McCully KK, Natelson BJ, Iotti S, Sisto S & Leigh JS (1996). Reduced oxidative metabolism in chronic fatigue syndrome. *Muscle and Nerve*, **19**, 621–5.

Millon C, Salvato F, Blaney N, Morgan R, Mantero-Atienza E, Klimas N & Fletcher MA (1989). A psychological assessment of chronic fatigue syndrome/chronic Epstein–Barr virus patients. *Psychology Health*, **3**, 131–41.

Natelson BH, Cheu J, Pareja J, Ellis S, Policastro T & Findley TW (1996). Randomized, double blind, controlled placebo-phase in trial of low dose phenelzine in the chronic fatigue syndrome. *Psychopharmacology*, **124**, 226–30.

National Institute of Allergy and Infectious Diseases (1996). *Chronic Fatigue Syndrome: Information for Physicians*. Bethesda MD: National Institutes of Health, Public Health Service.

Peterson PK, Shepard J, Macres M, Schenck C, Crosson J, Rechtman D & Lurie N (1990). A controlled trial of intravenous immunoglobulin G in chronic fatigue syndrome. *American Journal of Medicine*, **89**, 554–60.

Robins LN & Helzer JE (1985). *Diagnostic Interview Schedule (DIS): version II-A*. St Louis: Department of Psychiatry, Washington University School of Medicine.

Russo J, Katon W, Sullivan M, Clark M & Buchwald D (1994). Severity of somatization and its relationship to psychiatric disorders and personality. *Psychosomatics*, **35**, 546–56.

Schwartz RB, Garada BM, Komaroff AL, Tice HM, Gleit M, Jolesz FA & Holman BL (1994). Detection of intracranial abnormalities in patients with chronic fatigue syndrome: comparison of MR imaging and SPECT. *American Journal of Radiology*, **162**, 935–41.

Secchiero P, Carrigan DB, Asano Y, Benedetti L, Crowley RW, Komaroff AL, Gallo RC & Lusso P (1995). Detection of human herpesvirus 6 in plasma of children with primary infection and immunosuppressed patients by polymerase chain reaction. *Journal of Infectious Diseases*, **171**, 273–80.

Sharpe M, Hawton K, Simkin S, Surawy C, Hacjman A, Klimes I, Peto T, Warrell D & Seagroatt V (1996). Cognitive behavior therapy for the chronic fatigue syndrome: a randomized controlled trial. *British Medical Journal*, **312**, 22–6.

Steinberg P, McNutt BE, Marshall P, Schenck C, Lurie N, Pheley A & Peterson PK (1996). Double-blind placebo-controlled study of the efficacy of oral terfenadine in the treatment of the chronic fatigue syndrome. *Journal of Allergy and Clinical Immunology*, **97**, 119–26.

Straus SE, Tosato G, Armstrong G, Lawley T, Prefle OT, Henle W, Davey R, Pearson G, Epstein J, Brus I & Blease RM (1985). Persistent illness and fatigue in adults with evidence of Epstein–Barr virus infection. *Annals of Internal Medicine*, **102**, 7–12.

Straus SE, Dale JK, Tobi M, Lawley T, Preble O, Blaese M, Hallahan C & Henle W (1988). Acyclovir treatment in the chronic fatigue syndrome: lack of efficacy in a placebo-controlled trial. *New England Journal of Medicine*, **319**, 1692–8.

Straus SE, Fritz S, Dale JK, Gould B & Strober W (1993). Lymphocyte phenotype and function in the chronic fatigue syndrome. *Journal of Clinical Immunology*, **13**, 30–40.

Swanink CMA, Melchers WJG, van der Meer JWM, Vercoulen JHMM, Bleijenberg G, Fennis JFM & Galama JMD (1994). Enteroviruses and the chronic fatigue syndrome. *Clinical and Infectious Diseases*, **19**, 860–4.

Taerk GS, Toner BB, Salit IE, Garfinkel PE & Ozersky S (1987). Depression in patients with neuromyasthenia (benign myalgic encephalomyelitis). *International Journal of Psychiatry and Medicine*, **17**, 49–56.

Tobi M, Morag A, Ravid I, Chowere I, Feldman-Weiss V, Michaeli Y, Ben-Chetrit E, Shalit M & Knobler H (1982). Prolonged atypical illness associated with serological evidence of persistent Epstein–Barr virus infection. *Lancet*, **1**, 61–4.

Vercoulen JH, Swanink CM, Zitman FG, Vreden SG, Hoofs MP, Fennis JF, Galama JM, van der Meer JW & Bleijenberg G (1996). Randomised, double-blind, placebo-controlled study of fluoxetine in chronic fatigue syndrome. *Lancet*, **347**, 858–61.

Wessely S & Powell B (1989). Fatigue syndromes: a comparison of chronic 'postviral' fatigue with neuromuscular and affective disorders. *Journal of Neurology, Neurosurgery and Psychiatry*, **52**, 940–8.

Wray BB, Gaugh C, Chandler FW, Berry SS, Latham JE & Durant RH (1993). Detection of Epstein–Barr virus and cytomegalovirus in patients with chronic fatigue. *Annals of Allergy*, **71**, 223–6.

3

Fibromyalgia Syndrome

MICHA ABELES

Fibromyalgia syndrome (FMS) is characterized by complaints of generalized musculoskeletal pain and the finding on physical examination of tenderness in characteristic regions. Although accepted now as a standard rheumatological entity, the condition still raises basic questions. Do tender points truly define FMS syndrome? Are the number of tender points critical to the diagnosis? Does generalized tenderness indicate a state of increased somatic awareness, hypervigilance or just a lack of discriminatory validity? Do the overlap of FMS symptoms with those of other syndromes indicate a relationship and, if so, what is the relationship? Is the diagnosis of fibromyalgia useful or does it condemn the patient to a sickness? Is FMS the final outcome of one etiological process or of numerous etiological possibilities?

For the most part, the available literature does little justice to the enormity of the questions. Bias is often evidenced by selective reference, inability or refusal to address contradictory findings and the obstinate maintenance of pet theories. Methodological problems leading to questionable results include a small number of patients, lack of appropriate controls and unique, often poorly categorized, patient populations in a tertiary setting. The study of fibromyalgia thus poses a formidable task not only for the investigator but for the physician trying to make sense of the available literature. Nevertheless, the establishment of standard diagnostic criteria has allowed investigations of a defined group of chronic pain patients. This, in turn, has shown that FMS is fairly common (Wolfe et al., 1995), can obfuscate symptoms of other diseases, and is costly in terms of medical care (Wolfe et al., 1996) and long-term disability payment. Fibromyalgia has also been a model for the investigation of chronic musculoskeletal pain as well as a model for which the biopsychosocial model of illness, in contrast to the medical model of disease, is important.

History

The present-day concept of fibromyalgia evolves from the early twentieth century work of Gowers and Stockman (Gowers, 1904; Stockman, 1904*a*). Some authors suggest that the initial framework of fibromyalgia can be found in George Beard's writings on neurasthenia (Goldenberg, 1996). Beard did describe chronic fatigue, heaviness and aching of the extremities and body as part of neurasthenia, but also attributed such a formidable number and variety of symptoms to neurasthenia that over 40 different diseases had to be ruled out before neurasthenia could be invoked (Beard, 1869, 1900). In 1904 Sir William Gowers hypothesized that fibrous or connective tissue was highly 'susceptible' to 'rheumatism', resulting in inflammation of the fibrous tissue. He suggested that by following the analogy of 'cellulitis' the designation of inflamed fibrous tissue should be 'fibrositis' (Gowers, 1904). Given its ubiquity, fibrous tissue when inflamed in the form of fibrositis, could produce local or widespread pain. 'Lumbago', sciatica (by involvement of the sciatic fibrous sheath), shoulder pain, brachial neuritis, stiff neck, pharyngeal pain, and even pleurodynia were cited as examples of fibrositis. Stockman's studies on rheumatism published that same year lent credence to Gower's hypothesis (Stockman, 1904*a*,*b*). Stockman attempted to bring some sense to the 'chaotic' understanding of 'chronic rheumatism'. He argued that the central pathological feature of chronic rheumatism was 'confined to white fibrous tissue'. As a result, 'aponeuroses, tendons, sheaths of muscles and nerves, periosteum, fascia, and fibrous ligamentous structures of the joints' were affected. The lesion was 'inflammatory' with resultant proliferation of fibrous tissue which could be both palpable and tender. If there was enough proliferation and if this proliferation was circumscribed in the form of a nodule, neuralgia or sciatica occurred as a result of pressure on a nerve. The degree, severity and extent of symptoms depended on which fibrous tissue was involved. The major symptoms produced included 'pain, aching, stiffness, muscular fatigue, and very often a want of energy and vigor' (Stockman, 1904*a*). Stockman also noted 'difficulty in locating the exact spot of the pain or aching, as these may radiate to a wide area, but on palpation it can readily be made out that certain places are often very painful on pressure'. Women were more affected than men and many were 'hopeless neurasthenics'. By 1913, the concept of fibrositis as proposed by Gowers and the pathology as described by Stockman were well known. Local pain as a result of pressure was accepted as a characteristic of the problem (Luff, 1913). In 1915, Llewellyn & Jones published their book entitled *Fibrositis* and cemented the name in the literature.

Although the 1920s saw little published on the topic of fibromyalgia, interest had not waned. In 1935, Telling emphasized the importance of fibrositis as a problem commonly addressed by private practitioners. He also pointed out the lack of physician unanimity on the subject and that 'in the minds of many, the nodules of fibrositis are only accessible to the finger of faith' (a statement frequently attributed to others). Other authors indicated that fatigue and nervous exhaustion were marked in patients with fibrositis, but 'notable for being decidedly out of proportion to disease' (Slocumb, 1936). It was pointed out that features of fibrositis such as 'chronic nervous exhaustion and fatigue' were almost always present and that the patient with fibrositis was often one who was referred to as having 'psychalgia'. The patient was unhappy, aching and annoyed at not having any objective findings. Nevertheless, a repetitive motif of complaints among patients was recognized and nodules continued to be considered a marker of fibrositis (Slocumb, 1936).

The discordant views held in the 1930s were most dramatically revealed in a symposium on fibrositis published in 1939. In the last article he was to write before his death, Stockman reiterated his claim that inflammatory hyperplasia of fibrous structures produced palpable thickenings and insisted that the pathology of fibrositis was both recognized and agreed upon (Stockman, 1939). Soon thereafter, Buckley took the opposite point of view, claiming signs of inflammation were absent (Buckley, 1940). Palpable nodules, when present, were no more common than in asymptomatic individuals and were frequently small fatty masses rather than inflammatory products. When present, nodules pressed 'firmly against underlying bone', produced pain, which would be expected 'even in normal people'. Others were even more to the point and indicated that those who suffer from fibrositis 'may show signs of fatigue from persistent pain', but they seldom appear ill and their appearance was often in 'marked contrast' to their 'miserable story' (Collins, 1940). In the same article, Collins intuitively recognized the difference between illness and disease by indicating that fibrositis was 'essentially a subjective phenomenon'. More importantly, he attempted to put to rest the idea that inflammation played a role in fibrositis. By examining some of Stockman's pathological material as well as his illustrations, Collins was more impressed with the negative findings of the biopsies and concluded that fibrositis was a subjective phenomenon with multiple etiological factors.

With 12% of all medical cases in England in the 1940s being diagnosed as fibrositis, a demand existed to understand the pathophysiology of this pain syndrome. Copeman and Ackerman were struck by lack of findings on the biopsy material of previously palpable nodules (Copeman & Ackerman, 1947). In an attempt to further understand low back pain, 'trigger points' were initially mapped out on their patients. Dissections of cadavers were then undertaken to evaluate the previously mapped out regions. The result was the finding of a 'basic fat pattern' where weak spots in fascia allowed potential herniation of fatty tissue. In further investigations, nodules were surgically exposed and found to be 'edematous' fat globules. It was concluded that inflammation was not present but, rather, an increase in fluid tension occurred for unknown reasons. When sufficient tension in an anatomically suitable area occurred, protrusion of fat, i.e., fat herniation, was possible. Treatment included injection or teasing of the nodule to disrupt it and reduce hydrostatic pressure. The question of nonsymptomatic nodules was not addressed, despite the fact that a contemporary study of 522 male army personnel found nodules not necessarily associated with any symptoms (Pugh & Christie, 1945).

Four diagnostic criteria for fibrositis were emphasized in the 1940s literature: local tenderness, reproduction of symptoms by pressure, presence of nodules and improvement with injection of procaine into tender areas. As these criteria were evolving, they were questioned as well (Elliot, 1944). Skeptics contended that tenderness was elicited in areas where counterpressure was encountered, i.e., over areas of bone or ligament that would be expected to be more sensitive. Palpation could not discriminate between superficial or deep tissue. Thus, a physician's bias could attribute tenderness to any tissue in which tenderness was expected (a problem that is unchanged over the decades). Anticipating today's evolving concepts, Elliot felt that tenderness implied an amplification of the pain threshold and the process of amplification could be found anywhere along the nervous system up to and including the spinal cord and thalamus.

Modern-day concepts of FMS date back to 1953 and the ability of Graham to synthesize disparate concepts and to chisel an amorphous set of ideas into a recognizable form (Graham, 1953). He pointed out the major manifestations of FMS: pain, stiffness, tenderness, and fatigue, without true constitutional findings in the presence of tenderness in the low back, gluteal, shoulder, neck and chest areas. He also noted its association with the weather and stress, as well as relief obtained with resolution of stress. He astutely indicated that FMS was a result of multiple factors, be they traumatic, emotional or other. Thus he emphasized that this was not a disease but rather a syndrome brought about by a variety of 'widely separate conditions'. This construct was advanced by Canadian researchers by mapping out the location of tender points, quantifying pain, introducing the concept of an abnormal sleep pattern and formalizing criteria for the diagnosis of FMS (Smythe & Moldofsky, 1977).

Definition

FMS is a chronic pain condition characterized by musculoskeletal aches, pains and stiffness and associated with exaggerated tenderness in multiple characteristic sites. In its study of FMS the American College of Rheumatology (ACR) found that a history of widespread pain combined with the presence of pain (defined as mild or greater) on digital palpation in 11 of 18 specific tender point sites provided the most accurate criteria for FMS (Wolfe et al., 1990). Specific stipulations for the examination included that palpation be done with an approximate force of 4 kg for a tender point to be positive. The subject had to indicate that palpation was painful, not just tender, as the criteria committee indicated that pain, not tenderness, should be the end-point of palpation. Definitions of tenderness (an abnormal sensitivity to touch or pressure, i.e., hyperalgesia) and pain (discomfort produced by irritation of nociceptors), however, were not provided. Thus, this fine discrimination was left up to the patient. Despite this distinction, a tender point was described as 'mild or greater tenderness' on palpation.

The core features of pain complaints and pain on palpation are invariably accompanied by numerous and characteristic features. These include disturbed sleep, typified by numerous awakenings and nonrestorative in its nature. A common complaint elicited from the patient is the feeling that 'I was run over by a truck'. Fatigue is almost always present, as is morning stiffness. Features less often present but still common include irritable bowel syndrome (IBS), headaches, subjective complaints of swelling and complaints of paresthesias. Modulation of symptoms by weather, stress, activity and rest are also present. The criteria committee did away with the concept of primary and secondary FMS as these entities were virtually indistinguishable and the diagnosis of FMS remained valid irrespective to any other diagnosis. It did recognize that the presence of other disorders could influence the expression and management of FMS. It did not address these disorders as being etiological in nature.

In 1993, an international meeting in Copenhagen adopted the ACR criteria but emphasized that the criteria were useful as research protocols (Consensus document, 1993). When it came to a 'pragmatic perspective' in the office, patients with typical historical features but fewer than 11 tender points could still be considered to have FMS. No exact number of tender points was suggested. The document proposed that the pain of FMS originated in muscle without valid or clear cut evidence to bolster that presumption.

Will the current diagnosis of FMS stand the test of time? Already there are calls for reassessing the present criteria (Wolfe, 1995). To some extent this questioning has been fueled by the litigation process and by the understanding that the lack of objective findings can be manipulated for secondary gain (Wolfe, 1993; Wolfe & The Special Report Committee, 1996).

Case presentation

A 48-year-old woman presented with generalized myalgias. Her history indicated that at age 43 years she was involved in a car accident. As a result, she suffered a whiplash injury leading to prolonged complaints of discomfort. Despite intensive physical therapy, neck pain persisted. Six months after her motor vehicle accident, she developed severe diarrhea associated with rectal bleeding. A diagnosis of ulcerative colitis was made and she was successfully treated with corticosteroid enemas. During this time, she noted increased neck discomfort and the onset of shoulder and low back discomfort. A rheumatology consultation was obtained. Tender points were noted and the diagnosis of fibromyalgia was made. She was able to cope with her musculoskeletal pains and continue her job in middle management of an insurance company. With downsizing of the company the job that she previously held was changed and she was placed into a more stressful situation. Whereas before she could manage 'to get by', in this new job she was overwhelmed. Demands were placed on her which she felt she was not able to meet. She found that she was having increased difficulty getting out of bed. Musculoskeletal pains became overwhelming and she complained of difficulty sleeping, continuous fatigue, stiffness in the morning and the onset of headaches. She also found that she had difficulty concentrating at work. She felt that her memory was becoming poor and that she was becoming both irritable, anxious and depressed. Her depression deepened and she eventually tried to commit suicide. She was placed on long-term disability. When seen for evaluation, she blamed her fibromyalgia for interfering with her abilities to handle the demands of work. She indicated that while out on disability her pains had lessened but she was anxious about returning to work feeling that her fibromyalgia would, once again, 'worsen'.

This case highlights many typical features found in the history of patients with fibromyalgia. Approximately one-third of patients date the onset of their FMS to a traumatic experience such as a motor vehicle accident or to an event such as an illness. Both an accident and an illness occurred to the patient in the illustrated case report. Nevertheless, she seemed to do well until a third major stressor finally produced full-blown fibromyalgia syndrome. This last stressor was a new position in her workplace for which she was not qualified and which overwhelmed her. Depression ensued and she became symptomatic. Although she blamed her disability on fibromyalgia, other interpretations can be made. Whereas this woman could previously cope, her new work demands overcame her coping mechanisms producing a situational depression. As a result, many typical depressive symptoms such as sleep disturbance, fatigue, difficulty concentrating and complaints of poor memory appeared. The clinical manifestations of FMS were exacerbated as well. Nevertheless, the ability to distinguish which process is responsible for which complaint is difficult. The intertwining of depression, stress and FMS in this patient makes it impossible to attribute her symptoms to any one specific cause.

Epidemiology

The prevalence of FMS has been studied in a number of settings including outpatients, private and hospital clinic populations, as well as community settings. The findings have varied depending on the definition and criteria used, methodology, setting and possibly ethnic background. In 1983, Campbell evaluated 596 patients in a hospital outpatient setting and found the prevalence of FMS to be approximately 6.3% (Campbell et al., 1983). In a similar setting Abeles found a nearly identical prevalence of 5.8% (Abeles et al., 1987). Not surprisingly when a rheumatology practice is surveyed the prevalence of FMS doubles (Wolfe et al., 1995). Community studies vary widely in their findings. Using unique criteria, a survey of a German community found FMS in 1.8% of the population surveyed (Raspe & Baumgartner, 1993), while a study in Norway noted a prevalence of 10.5% in women aged 20–49 years (Forseth & Gran, 1992).

The most thorough general population survey was conducted in Wichita, Kansas, where FMS was found in 3.4% of women and 0.5% of men (Wolfe et al., 1995). When controlled for age, a steady increase in prevalence rate with increasing age was noted. The highest prevalence of FMS was seen in the 70–79 year age group. In addition to being more common in the elderly, FMS was associated with anxiety, depression and somatization as well as a history of depression in the family. Thus, to a great extent, community FMS patients were similar to physician-treated ones.

In a different type of epidemiological study, a survey of low income minorities and their approaches to the relief of musculoskeletal pain was conducted. A total of 162 subjects from a low income minority community were interviewed. Subjects consequently underwent a rheumatological evaluation. All participants had self-perceived arthritis. Two-thirds of the sample were African-American and the rest Hispanic. Women comprised 80% of the group. Forty-two per cent of the Hispanic population had FMS. In contrast, only 3% of the African-American populations suffered from FMS (Bill-Harvey et al., 1989). It would thus seem that ethnic, cultural and familial factors all may play a role in FMS and have to be taken into account in any population survey.

Economic costs

Fibromyalgia syndrome (FMS) as a cause of disability is an increasingly important and contentious issue. The economic repercussions are enormous (Cameron, 1995). One estimate suggests that long-term disability payments for FMS in Canada may cost the insurance industry as much as $200 million per year (McCain et al., 1988). The enormity of the situation is underlined by a small British study indicating that 50% of FMS patients stopped working over a mean interval of four years (Ledingham et al., 1993). Although it is the physician's opinion which weighs most heavily in the disability rating, physicians are usually unable to assess disability (Wolfe & Potter, 1996). The problem is magnified in FMS where there are few if any validated tools to assess disability (White & Nielson, 1995), where there may be few physicians qualified to evaluate a chronic illness (Bennett, 1996), and where patient claims may be discordant to observed function capacity (Hidding et al., 1994). The conundrum is such that it has been suggested the physician substitute 'compassion and intelligence for medical truth' (Wolfe & Potter, 1996).

Confirmations

Psychological aspects

From the initial reports of Stockman in 1904, who considered some of his FMS patients to be 'hopeless neurasthenics', there has been recognition that psychological problems can be present in FMS patients. In the USA in the 1930s, patients with FMS were regarded as 'anxious unhappy patients' (Slocumb, 1936) and 'unhappy distraught individuals' (Halliday, 1941). Patients were thought, by some investigators, to have anxiety states and be more sensitive to stimuli than 'normal' individuals (Gordon, 1939). The term 'psychalgia' was used

(Slocumb, 1936) and there was a plea to evaluate the psychological status of patients as part of the work-up (Halliday, 1941). The first study of FMS and psychological disturbance suggested that 35 of 50 patients had significant psychological disorders (Ellman et al., 1942). Numerous potential underlying etiologies for FMS were thought to be present but it was felt that most cases were precipitated by a psychosomatic disorder and were greatly affected by emotional states (Graham, 1953). Patients with FMS were considered to have exaggerated responses to their 'ordinary trials of life' (Graham, 1953). Prior to 1975 the term fibrositis encompassed a cornucopia of entities and it is unclear how many of these patients fit present-day concepts of FMS.

Modern-day analysis of psychological disturbances in FMS dates back to the 1980s. In 1982, a study was done evaluating hospitalized FMS patients using the Minnesota Multiphasic Personality Inventory (MMPI) (Payne et al., 1982). A wide variety of psychological disturbances were noted. The conclusion of the authors was that psychological factors contributed significantly to physical complaints. Over the next decade and a half, numerous evaluations of the psychological status of patients with FMS were made. Studying outpatients rather than inpatients indicated that a third of individuals diagnosed with FMS patients were 'psychologically disturbed' (Wolfe et al., 1984). Many studies shared a high frequency of depressive disorders among FMS patients (Wolfe et al., 1984; Hudson & Pope, 1989; Burckhardt et al., 1993; Schuessler & Konermann, 1993; Vitanen et al., 1993; Martinez et al., 1995). In addition to current depression, patients with FMS were found to have a greater lifetime history of major depression and a significantly greater family history of major depression compared with control patients (Hudson & Pope, 1989). A dissenting voice argued that the lack of concordance in the timing of the onset of depression and fibromyalgia was inconsistent with a causal relationship (Goldenberg, 1989). This opinion, however, ignored a body of evidence that major depression leaves residual dysfunction even after the formerly depressed individual no longer meets criteria for depression (Lewinsohn et al., 1988), that recurrence rates of depression are high in numerous clinical samples (Surtees & Barkely, 1994), and that a nonspecific sense of distress persists in many individuals recovering after an episode of depression (Katon & Schulberg, 1992). The interrelationship between depression, distress and pain has been investigated. Clinical research studies indicate that depression influences musculoskeletal pain perception (Rajala et al., 1995). Some argue that FMS belongs to a group of disorders with high comorbidity with one another referred to as 'affective spectrum disorder' (Hudson & Pope, 1989). Empirical support for this construct was offered by the finding of combinations of somatization, depression and anxiety and a history of depression in the families of FMS patients investigated in a large community-based study (Wolfe et al., 1995).

Psychological stress also has been considered to play a role, as patients with FMS report more hassles than rheumatoid arthritis patients and normal controls (Darley et al., 1990). FMS patients concentrate on their pain and are more vocal in reporting their discomfort than patients with other chronic illnesses. Although given more 'practical help' by family and friends, FMS patients, nevertheless, are less satisfied by the attention given to them. They avoid common activities and argue that they are more limited in their daily activities (Gaston-Johansson et al., 1990). Patients with FMS claim their quality of life is poorer than patients with a primary diagnosis of rheumatoid arthritis, osteoarthritis, chronic obstructive pulmonary disease or insulin dependent diabetes (Burckhardt et al., 1993). When compared with rheumatoid patients, the FMS patients' intensity of pain and global discomfort are greater and stress factors in childhood more common than patients with rheumatoid arthritis (Schuessler & Konermann, 1993). Memory difficulty is a major complaint but, when tested, seems to be only a subjective process, possibly due to psychological stress (Kaplan et al., 1993). In addition to perceived memory difficulties, patients with FMS complain of decreased muscle strength and endurance but show no central or peripheral components of muscle fatigue (Mengshoel et al., 1995).

Contradictions

Neurohumoral abnormalities

In 1975, a research group from the University of Toronto, became aware that parachlorophenylalanine, an inhibitor of serotonin formation, could produce a pain syndrome when ingested (Moldofsky et al., 1975). They understood serotonergic function, recognized its role in pain and analgesia, regulation of sleep and affective states and hypothesized that a disorder of serotonin metabolism was responsible for the symptoms of fibrositis. In an uncontrolled study of poorly characterized patients he evaluated plasma tryptophan (the precursor of central nervous serotonin) and found an inverse relationship between the level of tryptophan and pain severity (Moldofsky & Warsh, 1978). Later studies addressed the same question. Discrepant findings, limited data analysis and methodological problems have interfered with the usefulness of the published literature. In one study low tryptophan levels were noted compared with controls, but numerous other amino acids were also significantly lower in FMS patients (Russell et al., 1992). The significance of this finding and the finding of a high incidence of depressive features in the FMS patients make it difficult to interpret the study especially since low tryptophan levels can be a marker of depression (Owens & Nemeroff, 1994). Other studies failed to show significant decreases of serum tryptophan in FMS but did show a reduced transport ratio of tryptophan into the central nervous system (Yunus et al., 1992*a*).

Platelets and serotonin-containing neurons show common similarities including [3H]-imipramine binding sites. The density of serotonin reuptake receptors on platelets was used to detect a deficiency of serotonin and patients with FMS were found to have higher densities of serotonin reuptake receptors on platelets (Russell et al., 1992). Other studies did not corroborate this finding and noted no alterations in platelet [3H]-imipramine binding in patients with FMS (Owens & Nemeroff, 1994).

Interest in other pain transmitters has included the evaluation of substance P, a neuropeptide, one of whose functions is to facilitate pain transmission in the central and peripheral nervous systems. Plasma levels of substance P were not elevated in patients with FMS (Reynolds et al., 1988). Cerebrospinal fluid (CSF) levels of substance P, on the other hand, were increased in FMS compared with control patients (Vaeroy et al., 1988; Russell et al., 1994). In these studies, the severity of pain inversely correlated with substance P levels in the CSF. Thus, whether CSF substance P plays any role in pain production in FMS remains unknown. Endorphins modulate pain and therefore are candidates for involvement in any pain modulation disorder. Studies indicate serum levels of β-endorphin to be similar in FMS and rheumatoid arthritis patients. When CSF β-endorphin levels in FMS and healthy controls were compared, no differences were noted (Vaeroy et al., 1988). Other studies indicate that when FMS and normal controls are compared there is no difference in plasma and urinary catecholamine concentration (Yunus, 1992*b*) nor interleukin 1 (Wallace et al., 1989) or interleukin 2 levels (Hader et al., 1991).

Stress and the possibility that FMS falls into the spectrum of stress-related illness has been suggested (Crofford, 1996). As a consequence of stress a variety of physiological changes occur including changes in the hypothalamic-pituitary-adrenal (HPA) axis and nervous system. The principal components of the general adaptation response involve the corticotropin-releasing hormone (CRH) and the autonomic nervous systems. In the presence of stress, CRH is released, leading to adrenocorticotropic hormone (ACTH) elevation and consequent glucorticoid release. There is an increase in epinephrine and norepinephrine production, but the growth and reproductive systems are inhibited. In some studies decreased cortisol levels after exercise and low 24-hour urine cortisol levels have been reported in FMS patients, which suggests possible dysregulation of the HPA axis; an increase in ACTH response to CRH is, paradoxically, associated with relative adrenal hyporesponsiveness (suggestive of a perturbed HPA axis) (Crofford, 1996). There have been variable findings in the dexamethasone suppression test (Ferraccioli et al., 1990). Insulin-like growth factor-I (somatomedin C) was found to be lower in FMS compared with controls by one group (Bennett et al., 1992). As somatomedin C is mostly produced in stage IV sleep, interference with its output was felt to be a corollary to a disturbed sleep pattern. It was claimed the result of this interference was to impact muscle and induce myalgia. Sleep disturbance and muscle homeostasis were thus linked (Bennett et al., 1992). Consequent investigations did not corroborate either the presence of low somatomedin C or the contention that it played a role in pain (Buchwald et al., 1996).

Muscle pathology

Numerous studies have been carried out with the assumption that FMS pain had an underlying muscle pathology (Kellegren, 1938*a,b*). One reason given for suggesting muscle involvement is that the patient complains of 'muscle' pain (Bennett et al., 1988). Studies of muscle have included those using light microscopy and histochemistry (Yunus & Kalyan-Raman, 1989), metabolic (Bengtsson & Henriksson, 1986), magnetic resonance (Sims, 1996), blood flow studies (Klemp et al., 1982), muscle strength testing (Sims, 1996), and electromyography (Durette et al., 1991). Findings of abnormalities have not been corroborated. At present, despite the persistent contentions of some, there are few data to indicate muscle pathology plays a role in the pain suffered by the FMS patient.

Alpha intrusions during delta sleep

An alteration in sleep physiology was hypothesized to be the underlying cause of FMS (Moldofsky et al., 1975). The discovery of the alpha electroencephalograph (EEG) nonrapid eye movement (NREM) sleep anomaly was a major step in the search for objective findings in FMS. In time, the alpha EEG sleep anomaly was shown to be nonspecific and yet it was claimed to be both a sensitive indicator as well as a core feature and biological marker of the syndrome (Moldofsky, 1989). More recent studies indicate the alpha NREM sleep anomaly is present in only a small proportion of patients with FMS (Carette et al., 1995), in proportionate number to controls (Drewes et al., 1993), or not found in FMS when patients with a chief complaint of fatigue are studied (Manu et al., 1994). When present, the alpha sleep anomaly does not correlate with pain severity or predict treatment response (Carette et al., 1995). The precise role of disturbed sleep in the pathophysiology of FMS remains unclear. Turning the theory of altered sleep upside down, the possibility that disturbed sleep is a manifestation, rather than a cause of FMS, has been raised (Clauw et al., 1994).

Pathogenic hypothesis

Diversity of opinion and disparate, contending and competing hypotheses regarding causation is prima facie evidence of how little is actually known about FMS. Persistent promulgation of pet theories does not necessarily reflect credibility. Phenomenon and epiphenomenon are often confused or ignored, conflicting findings discarded and competing thoughts disregarded. Muscle pathology continues to be evoked, although clearly not present. Serotonin deficiency and substance P elevation have not been thoroughly enough studied to indicate what role (if any) they play in the symptoms of FMS. Disordered sleep patterns and accompanying alpha EEG anomalies occur in FMS but are not universal and are also seen in a variety of other vague disorders of fatigue and even in normal individuals. Depression is not an uncommon finding in FMS patients but does not explain the etiology of FMS in those with normal psychological profiles. Stress intensifies symptoms in FMS but its etiological role and the role of any neurohumoral changes associated with stress in the relationship to FMS is purely conjectural. If the pain of FMS is referred from deep spinal structures, no formal investigation has been carried out to support this possibility. The babel of claims and counter claims makes it obvious that not only is the etiology of FMS obscure but that it is most likely multifactorial. Why generalized pain is the end result of multiple unrelated processes remains an enigma.

Diagnostic and treatment approaches

Diagnosis

The ACR criteria (Wolfe et al., 1990) established a frugal definition of FMS which included generalized pain above and below the waist and along the right and left sides of the body. In addition, axial skeletal pain had to be present in 11 of 18 (9 pairs) tender point sites on digital palpation. These sites included: (1) the occiput at the suboccipital muscle insertions, (2) low cervical region, (3) midpoint of the upper border of the trapezius, (4) at the supraspinatus origins near the medial border of the scapula, (5) at the second costochondral junctions, (6) 2 cm distal to the lateral epicondyles, (7) upper outer gluteal regions, (8) greater trochanters, and (9) medial fat pad of the knees. Symptoms had to be present for at least three months and digital pressure had to approximate to 4 kg. Although developed for research purposes, the ACR criteria had been widely used to aid clinical diagnosis. From a 'pragmatic perspective' the Copenhagen Declaration produced several noteworthy comments (Consensus document, 1993). These indicated that FMS is distinctive and could be diagnosed with 'clinical precision'. FMS could be confidently diagnosed in an individual with widespread musculoskeletal pain and numerous tender points. From a 'pragmatic perspective' the history was felt to be of great importance. Thus, when pain or aching were accompanied by fatigue, sleep disturbance and stiffness the possibility of FMS had to be strongly entertained. The finding of 11 tender points was not critical as it was felt some patients may have fewer than 11 tender points at the time of the examination. Indeed, since FMS seems to reflect a wide spectrum of pain (no different than blood pressure values), it has been suggested that FMS can be diagnosed with differing degrees of certainty from definite to probable and to possible FMS (Wolfe, 1993).

Pain is the reason patients seek medical care. In taking a history, the patient needs to be guided in providing specific information. Thus, the physician needs to direct questioning to where pain is located. Specific locations of pain involvement should be sought by asking about neck and low back pain, anterior chest wall, elbow region, trapezial and upper back regions, buttock, thigh and knee area pains. In addition, patients with true FMS invariably complain of fatigue, disturbed sleep pattern and morning stiffness. Without at least one of these symptoms being present FMS is unlikely. Symptoms suggestive of irritable bowel syndrome are common. Usual modulating factors include stress, anxiety and weather changes.

Once a diagnosis has been entertained, a tender point examination should be carried out. The most common mistake in the examination is the inability to judge how much force to use. The best approach is to use the thumb pad and increase force by 1 kg/s until 4 kg of pressure is achieved. A simple way to know that 4 kg of force has been achieved is to observe for whitening of the nail. Checking pressure on a pressure gauge can also be utilized to approximate 4 kg. A tender point is considered positive when the patient indicates it is painful. Although the ACR criteria committee evaluated control points (usually bony surfaces), it did not comment on how to interpret positive responses.

Psychological problems are common in FMS. If present, they undoubtedly play an important role in symptom expression and augmentation and have to be addressed. Laboratory abnormalities are not present in FMS. It is unusual to find other medical conditions that mimic FMS. Nevertheless, some problems that need to be at least considered, although not necessarily pursued, include hypothyroidism, widespread malignancy, polymyalgia rheumatica, osteomalacia, generalized osteoarthritis, early Parkinson's disease and the initial stages of connective tissue disease (Consensus document, 1993).

Treatment

Although many studies claim some success in the treatment of FMS, long-term assessments indicate that patients with a mean follow-up of up to 10.6 years do not do well, i.e., despite conventional treatments patients continue to suffer unaltered symptom severity (Wolfe & The Special Report Committee, 1996). Indeed, many seek alternative medicine (Balch & Balch, 1997). As we do not understand the causation of the syndrome, treatment approaches have remained symptomatic and heterogeneous, and are essentially based on the biases of the investigators.

Medications that have been tried are numerous. These include tricyclic compounds, muscle relaxers, analgesics, nonsteroidal anti-inflammatory medications, selective serotonin reuptake inhibitors, and others. Nonpharmacological approaches have included a variety of exercise programs, tender point injections, cognitive behavioral programs and occasionally others such as acupuncture and biofeedback. Long-term studies tend to be lacking. Most studies are short-term and therefore of questionable value as a treatment for chronic illness.

Presently, tricyclic antidepressants (TCA) are probably the most commonly used medications for patients with FMS. Amitriptyline is the one TCA that has been most extensively studied. Short-term studies indicate that it is beneficial in up to one-third of FMS patients (Carette et al., 1986; Goldenberg et al., 1986; Scudds et al., 1989). Long-term studies are less sanguine (Abeles et al., 1992). Prospective studies (Carette et al., 1994) did not show any prolonged beneficial effect of amitriptyline. Placebo seems to almost do as well. Dosing of amitriptyline is conservative. It is often initiated at 10 mg and slowly increased to 50 mg and taken an hour before sleep. Anticholinergic side-effects include drowsiness and dryness of the mouth. Similar effectiveness has been shown in a short-term trial for the antidepressant trazodone (Branco et al., 1996).

Muscle relaxers have been tried for no obvious reason (Bennett et al., 1988; Quimby et al., 1989) as EMG studies show no evidence of muscle spasm or any other abnormality (Moldolfsky et al., 1975). Short-term benefits have been claimed in both studies (Bennett et al., 1988; Quimby, 1989). Such conclusions are hampered by medication side-effects which inadvertently bias the studies (despite attempts at blinding) and make them the equivalent of open label investigations. When looked at long term, cyclobenzeprine did not show an advantage over placebo (Carrette et al., 1994). A limited, retrospective showed orphenadrine to be more useful than either amitriptyline or cyclobenzeprine (Abeles, 1992). Assessment measures of patients in some studies were unusual and unique and perhaps peculiar (Bennett et al., 1988).

The selective serotonin uptake inhibitors should, theoretically, be more useful than TCAs because of their greater potency in reducing serotonin uptake; however, study results are contradictory. Initial reports showed no improvement in symptoms (Wolfe et al., 1994). More recent investigations suggest that 20 mg of fluoxetine is similar in efficacy to 25 mg of amitriptyline. When these agents are combined, there is an additive effect with greater efficacy than with either medication alone (Goldenberg et al., 1996).

Non-steroidal anti-inflammatory drugs are of little help (Goldenberg et al., 1996). Studies of malic acid, alprazolam and clomipramine have suffered from a variety of technical defects including small subject numbers and have not been reproduced (Bibolotti et al., 1986; Russell et al., 1991, 1995). At this point there is little to recommend them.

Cardiovascular fitness training in the form of aerobic exercise is widely recommended, but the underlying assumption that justifies it has remained controversial (Mengshoel et al., 1995). This approach is based on the assumption that patients with FMS are not aerobically fit and lack of aerobic fitness is proposed to somehow contribute to pain. The concept that poor physical fitness and FMS are intertwined is attributable to a publication describing in anecdotal fashion the story of three aerobically fit individuals in whom FMS symptoms could not be produced despite stage IV sleep deprivation (Moldofsky et al., 1975). From this anecdote a hypothesis evolved asserting that a sedentary lifestyle results in consequent muscle deconditioning and a greater likelihood of being at risk of muscle microtrauma which in turn leads to increased pain (Bennett et al., 1988). The hypothesis was tested in a study that compared a flexibility exercise program to a cardiovascular fitness training program (McCain et al., 1988). No significant differences were found between groups with regard to pain intensity scores or the severity of sleep disturbance. Other studies note that physical training did not contribute significantly to reducing pain symptoms (Burckhardt et al., 1994), and did not change the severity of pain, psychological symptoms and functional disability (Nichols & Glenn, 1994). A combined cardiovascular fitness training and flexibility exercises, however, produced significant improvement in one study (Martin et al., 1996) that compared psychologically based muscle relaxation techniques that had shown promise in previous work (Kaplan et al., 1993).

The role of cognitive behavior therapy (CBT) programs remains unclear. Reports indicate that CBT may have a role in long-term treatment of FMS (White & Nielson, 1995) whereas others do not support this contention (Vlaeyen et al., 1996). Comprehensive multidisciplinary treatment of chronic pain has been recently used for patients with FMS (Bennett et al., 1996); an assessment of its efficacy must await controlled confirmatory studies.

Injections are used commonly for the treatment of a variety of musculoskeletal complaints. Injections are also commonly used for the treatment of FMS. The indication for and the role of injections in the treatment of FMS is unclear. A published survey of rheumatologists indicated an even division among those who felt injections were useful and those who did not (Abeles et al., 1995). The remaining rheumatologists were undecided. There was a wide discrepancy in beliefs and biases among those physicians who utilized injections for tender points with widely varying opinions on the length and gauge of needles and type of solute suitable for injection. To a great extent this reflects the literature concerning injections in soft tissue rheumatism. Injections of water as a local anesthetic for soft tissue 'rheumatism' were first proposed in 1885 (Halstad, 1885). Hypodermic injections of cocaine had been used either as monotherapy (Gowers, 1904) or in combination with injections of chromic acid (Stockman, 1904*b*). Little information was available concerning this form of treatment until 1938 when Kellgren published an account of his clinical experience with fibrositis (Kellgren, 1938*a*). The report indicated that injections into tender spots of a 1% solution of novocaine were extremely useful in the treatment of muscular pain. Others quickly concurred, advocating not only the use of novocaine, but also that of urea and quinine injections as well. The same year, Kellgren also published the first of his monumental studies on referred pain (Kellgren 1938*b*).

The use of injections in FMS is closely linked with the technique of dry-needling. This curious practice is based on Kellgren's view that the muscular pain in this condition was diffuse in nature and could be referred in a spinal segmental pattern; whether pain was local or segmental depended on the depth at which the tissue was located rather than upon its actual nature (Kellgren, 1938*b*). Later, clinical observations seemed to indicate that dry-needling localized and reproduced radiation of pain and that injection of local anesthetics such as procaine suppressed this process (Button, 1940; Steindler, 1940). Skeptics, on the other hand, claimed the use of injections in relieving pain was 'not so great as its enthusiastic advocates would wish their readers to believe' (Gordon, 1939). Others held the 'novocaine test' did not exclude other lesions and therefore was not diagnostic of anything specific (Elliot, 1944) and that injections were of no more use than they had been in the past for hysteria or melancholy (Halliday, 1942). It has also been pointed out that without the advantage of radiological guidance one could not be sure what tissue was being injected and one could not be certain as to what was the real source of the pain (Sinclair et al., 1948).

The discussion of the role of injections in FMS would be incomplete without a description of an alternative diagnosis, i.e., myofascial pain syndrome (Travell & Rinzler, 1952). Myofascial pain syndrome came to mean the presence of musculoskeletal pain associated with radiation of that pain in typical patterns that could be reproduced by palpation of trigger points. The utility of injections into tender areas of the body were studied for the most part in the context of this syndrome rather than FMS from the mid 1940s until the present. This construct recognized the obscure nature of myalgias and the fact that inflammatory findings were lacking in patients diagnosed with fibrositis (Travell et al., 1942). As manual pressure over 'tender zones' reproduced pain symptoms, injection of these tender zones were expected to abolish the pain. The proponents of this approach viewed the patients as having isolated pain syndromes and advocated a treatment program that involved a variety of measures but especially injections (physiological saline or procain) or dry-needling (Travell, 1955; Cooper, 1961). The empirical confirmation of these approaches is lacking and it is unclear what the myofascial pain syndrome actually represents. The primary care practitioner's decision to use or refer the patient for injection therapy will have to take into account the fact that when examining the same patient's myofascial pain experts disagree about physical findings, and that positive effects of these treatments are expected only in about one-third of cases, regardless of the type of injected solute or whether given by dry-needling alone (Abeles et al., 1997).

In summary, despite a rather gloomy outlook, treatment needs to be given. Multiple modalities are probably more worthwhile than one singular sequential approach. In this way small beneficial effects that otherwise might not be noted will be additive and possibly produce a noticeable response. Education, support and reassurance are important for the physician to offer during face-to-face encounters. The patient is educated about the syndrome, reassured about its benign albeit painful nature, made to understand its prevalence to dispel any sense of isolation, and offered ongoing emotional support. Antidepressants, muscle relaxers, analgesics and occasionally anxiolytics can all be tried. Aquatherapy programs, though not formally evaluated, anecdotally are enjoyed by patients. Other exercise, physical therapy and massage programs can be tried as can stress management and cognitive behavioral programs. Stressors need to be identified and addressed. Depression, dysthymia, anxiety and somatization may all need psychiatric or psychological intervention. Psychiatric intervention is especially important for those individuals in whom hopelessness has become embedded and who exhibit maladaptive pain behavior. For these individuals a psychiatric evaluation is especially important. The ultimate goal of therapy is for the patient to obtain enough insight to be able to assume much of the responsibility for her own pain management.

Conclusion

FMS represents a complex clinical picture in search of a distinguishing set of objective findings. If a syndrome is defined as a group of signs and symptoms that cluster together to form a recognizable entity, many would argue that FMS as presently constructed does provide an identifiable pattern meeting the definition of a syndrome. On the other hand, it can be argued that the brevity of its current definition allows it to be used almost indiscriminately by allowing additional attributions to be piled onto the point where the syndrome's characteristics are lost in an overwhelming mountain of complaints. Although theories on the etiology of FMS continue to be in a state of flux, the frequent symptomatic overlap with irritable bowel syndrome, chronic fatigue syndrome, migraine headache, temporomandibular joint dysfunction and major depression justifies its cautious integration into large constructs such as the 'affective spectrum disorder' (Hudson & Pope, 1989) and 'dysfunctional spectrum syndrome' (Yunus, 1994).

There is a variable spectrum of complaints and findings in patients with FMS. Mild FMS is found in the community in patients who do not feel the need to seek medical attention. At the opposite pole are patients offering numerous complaints and who are found to be tender everywhere they are touched. Experts state this latter group of patients are either nonclassifiable or in need of psychiatric intervention. Ironically, it may be this patient group that eventually may offer the clue to understanding FMS. As with any illness it is the most severe form that tends to shed light on etiology and lead to proper intervention.

The challenging nature of this syndrome is clearly related to the fact that the biomedical model of disease does not account for all the problems or complaints voiced by FMS patients. Following traditional methods of inquiry, researchers have been concerned with pathology and pathogenesis. The findings, however, did not account for how the patient experienced or reported the problem, i.e., the illness itself. To understand FMS, one needs to understand the social, cultural, psychological as well as biological aspects of the patient (Engel, 1977). Physicians treating FMS patients may be helped by the recognition that illness could occur in the absence of disease and that the course of an illness, at times, may be different than that of a disease (Kleinman et al., 1978). It is also useful to remember that factors which maintain functional disability may be different from those that initiated it (Abbey & Garfinkel, 1991). Without understanding the basis of the psychosocial model of illness, medical judgment can only be obfuscated. Suffering a painful condition is a private experience to which others have no access and one which drains energy and produces helplessness and hopelessness (Large, 1996). The challenge then is to pursue a compassionate and comprehensive treatment program for all aspects of the FMS patient's illness.

References

Abbey SG & Garfinkel PE (1991). Neurasthenia and chronic fatigue syndrome: the role of culture in the making of a diagnosis. *American Journal of Psychiatry*, **148**, 1638–46.

Abeles M (1992). The long-term effectiveness of orphenadrine citrate in the treatment of fibromyalgia. *Arthritis and Rheumatism*, **35**, (Suppl.), R40.

Abeles M, Garjian P & Marino C (1987). The primary fibrositis syndrome (PFS) – lack of dermal-epidermal junction immune deposition. *Arthritis and Rheumatism*, **30** (Suppl.), S8.

Abeles M, Busa J, Arguelles E & Urrows S (1991). Fibromyalgia syndrome in a medical outpatient population. *Arthritis and Rheumatism*, **34** (Suppl.), R39.

Abeles M, Manu P, Lane T & Matthews D (1992). Evaluation of musculoskeletal complaints in patients with the chronic fatigue syndrome. *Arthritis and Rheumatism*, **35** (Suppl.), R39.

Abeles M, Maestrello S & Waterman J (1995). A survey of rheumatologists use of tender point injections in fibromyalgia. *Arthritis and Rheumatism* **38** (Suppl.), R40.

Abeles M, Waterman J & Maestrello S (1997). Tender point injections in fibromyalgia. *Arthritis and Rheumatism*, **40** (Suppl.), S187.

Balch JF & Balch PA (1997). Prescription for nutritional healing. Garden City Park, NY: Avery Publishing Group.

Beard G (1869). Neurasthenia, or nervous exhaustion. *Boston Medical and Surgical Journal*, **3**, 217–21.

Beard GM & Rockwell AD (1900). *Sexual Neurasthenia (Nervous Exhaustion): Its Hygiene, Causes, Symptoms and Treatment*, 5th edn. New York: EB Treat & Co.

Bengtsson A & Henriksson KG (1986). Muscle biopsy in fibromyalgia: light microscopical and histochemical findings. *Scandanavian Journal of Rheumatology*, **15**, 1–6.

Bennett RM (1989). Physical fitness and muscle metabolism in the fibromyalgia syndrome: An overview. *Journal of Rheumatology*, **19**, 28–9.

Bennett RM (1996). Fibromyalgia and the disability dilemma. A new era in understanding a complex, multidimensional pain syndrome. *Arthritis and Rheumatism*, **39**, 1627–34.

Bennett RM, Gatter RA, Campbell SM, Andrews RP, Clark SR & Scarlo JA (1988). A comparison of cyclobenzaprine and placebo in the management of fibrositis. *Arthritis and Rheumatism*, **31**, 1535–42.

Bennett RM, Clark SR, Campbell SM & Burckhardt CS (1992). Low levels of somatomedin C in patients with the fibromyalgia syndrome: a possible link between sleep and muscle pain. *Arthritis and Rheumatism*, **35**, 1113–16.

Bennett RM, Burckhardt CS, Clark SR, O'Reilly CA, Wiens AN & Campbell SM (1996). Group treatment of fibromyalgia: a 6 month outpatient program. *Journal of Rheumatology*, **23**, 521–28.

Bibolotti E, Borghi C & Paculli E (1986). The management of fibrositis: a double-blind comparison of maprotiline, chlorimipramine, and placebo. *Clinical Trials Journal*, **23**, 269–80.

Bill-Harvey D, Rippey RM, Abeles M & Pfeiffer CA (1989). Methods used by urban, low-income minorities to care for their arthritis. *Arthritis Care and Research*, **2**, 60–4.

Branco JC, Martinini A & Palva T (1996). Treatment of sleep abnormalities and clinical complaints in fibromyalgia with trazadone. *Arthritis and Rheumatism*, **39** (Suppl.), S91.

Buckley CW (1940). Fibrositis: some old and new points of view. *Annals of Rheumatic Diseases*, **2**, 83–8.

Buchwald D, Umali J, Stene M (1996). Insulin-like growth factor-I (somatomedin C) levels in chronic fatigue syndrome and fibromyalgia. *Journal of Rheumatology*, **23**, 739–42.

Burckhardt CS, Clark SR & Bennett RS (1993). Fibromyalgia and quality of life: a comparative analysis. *Journal of Rheumatology*, **20**, 475–9.

Burckhardt CS, Mannerkorpi K, Hedenberg L, Bjelle A (1994). A randomized controlled clinical trial of education and physical training for women with fibromyalgia. *Journal of Rheumatology*, **20**, 475–9.

Button M (1940). Muscular rheumatism. Local injection treatment as a means of rapid restoration of function. *British Medical Journal*, **2**, 183–5.

Cameron RS (1995). The cost of long-term disability due to fibromyalgia, chronic fatigue syndrome and repetitive strain injury: the private insurance perspective. *Journal of Musculoskeletal Pain*, **3**, 1169–72.

Campbell SM, Clark S, Tindall EA, Forehand ME & Bennett RM (1983). Clinical characteristics of fibrositis. I. A 'blinded,' controlled study of symptoms and tender points. *Arthritis and Rheumatism*, **26**, 817–24.

Carette S, McCain GA, Bell DA & Fam AG (1986). Evaluation of amitriptyline in primary fibrositis: a double-blind, placebo-controlled study. *Arthritis and Rheumatism*, **29**, 655–9.

Carette S, Bell MJ, Reynolds WJ, Haraoui B, McCain GA, Bykerk VP, Edworthy SM, Baron M, Koehler BE, Fam AG, Bellamy N & Guimont C (1994). Comparison of amitriptyline, cyclobenzaprine and placebo in the treatment of fibromyalgia: a randomized, double-blind clinical trial. *Arthritis and Rheumatism*, **37**, 32–40.

Carette S, Oakson G, Guimont C & Steriade M (1995). Sleep and the clinical response to amitriptyline in patients with fibromyalgia. *Arthritis and Rheumatism*, **28**, 1211–17.

Clauw D, Blank C, Hiltz R, Katz P & Potolicchio L (1994). Polysomnography in fibromyalgia patients. *Arthritis and Rheumatism*, **37** (Suppl.), R19.

Collins DH (1940). Fibrositis and infection. *Annals of Rheumatic Diseases*, **2**, 144–6.

Consensus document on fibromyalgia: the Copenhagen declaration (1993).

Journal of Musculoskeletal Pain, **1**, 295–312.
Cooper AL (1961). Trigger point injection: its place in physical medicine. *Archives of Physical Medicine and Rehabilitation*, **42**, 704–9.
Copeman WSC & Ackerman WL (1947). Edema or herniations of fat globules as a cause of lumbar gluteal fibrositis. *Archives Internal Medicine*, **79**, 22–35.
Crofford LJ (1996). The hypothalamic-pituitary-adrenal stress axis in the fibromyalgia syndrome. *Journal of Musculoskeletal Pain*, **4**, 181–200.
Darley PA, Bishop GD, Russell IJ & Fletcher EM (1990). Psychological stress and the fibrositis/fibromyalgia syndrome. *Journal of Rheumatology*, **17**, 1380–5.
Drewes AM, Nielsen KD, Jennum P & Andreasen A (1993). Alpha intrusion in fibromyalgia. *Journal of Musculoskeletal Pain*, **1**, 233–8.
Durette MR, Rodriguez AA, Agre JC & Silverman JL (1991). Needle electromyographic evaluation of patients with myofascial or fibromyalgic pain. *American Journal of Physical and Medical Rehabilitation*, **70**, 154–6.
Elliot FA (1944). Apects of fibrositis. *Annals of Rheumatic Diseases*, **4**, 22–5.
Ellman P, Savage OA, Wittkower E & Rodgers TF (1942). Fibrositis. A biographical study of fifty civilian and military cases from the rheumatic unit, St. Stephens Hospital (London County Council), and a military hospital. *Annals of Rheumatic Diseases*, **3**, 56–76.
Engel GL (1977). The need for a new medical model: a challenge for modern medicine. *Science*, **196**, 129–35.
Ferraccioli G, Cavalieri F, Salaffi F, Fontana S, Scita F, Nolli M & Maestri D (1990). Neuroendocrinologic findings in primary fibromyalgia (soft tissue chronic pain syndrome) and in other rheumatic conditions (rheumatoid arthritis, low back pain). *Journal of Rheumatology*, **17**, 689–73.
Forseth KO & Gran JT (1992). The prevalence of fibromyalgia among women 20–29 years in Aarendal, Norway. *Scandinavian Journal of Rheumatology*, **21**, 74–8.
Gaston-Johansson F, Gustafsson M, Felldin R & Sanne H (1990). A comparative study of feelings, attitudes and behaviors of patients with fibromyalgia and rheumatoid arthritis. *Social Science and Medicine*, **31**, 941–7.
Goldenberg DL (1989). Psychiatric and psychologic aspects of fibromyalgia syndrome. *Rheumatic Disease Clinics of North America*, **15**, 105–14.
Goldenberg DL (1996). What is the future of fibromyalgia? *Rheumatic Disease Clinics of North America*, **22**, 393–406.
Goldenberg DL, Felson DT & Dinerman H (1986). A randomized, controlled trial of amitriptyline and naproxen in the treatment of patients with fibromyalgia. *Arthritis and Rheumatism*, **29**, 1371–7.
Goldenberg D, Mayskiy M, Mossey C, Ruthazer R & Schmid C (1996) A randomized, double-blind crossover trial of fluoxetine and amitriptyline in the treatment of fibromyalgia. *Arthritis and Rheumatism*, **39**, 1852–9.
Gordon RG (1939). The nature of fibrositis and the influences upon it. *Annals of Rheumatic Diseases*, **2**, 90–100.
Gowers WR (1904), Lumbago: its lessons and analogues. *British Medical Journal*, **1**, 117–24.
Graham W (1953). The fibrositis syndrome. *Bulletin of Rheumatic Diseases*, **3**, 51–2.
Hader N, Rimon D, Kinarty A & Lahat N (1991). Altered interleukin-2 secretion

in patients with primary fibromyalgia syndrome. *Arthritis and Rheumatism*, **34**, 866–77.

Halliday JL (1941). The concept of psychosomatic medicine. *Annals of Internal Medicine*, **15**, 666–77.

Halliday JL (1942). The obsession of fibrositis. *British Medical Journal*, **2**, 164.

Halstad WS (1885). Water as a local anesthetic. *NY Medical Journal*, **42**, 327.

Hidding A, van Santen M, De Klerk E, Gielen X, Boers M, Geenen R, Vlaeyen J, Kester A & van der Linden S (1994). Comparison between self-report measures and clinical observations of functional disability in ankylosing spondylitis, rheumatoid arthritis and fibromyalgia. *Journal of Rheumatology*, **21**, 818–23.

Hudson JI & Pope Jr HG (1989). Fibromyalgia and psychopathology: is fibromyalgia a form of 'affective spectrum disorder'? *Journal of Rheumatology*, **16** (Suppl. 19), 15–22.

Kaplan KH, Goldenberg DL & Galvin-Nadeau M (1993). The impact of a mediation-based stress reduction program on fibromyalgia. *General Hospital Psychiatry*, **15**, 284–9.

Katon W & Schulberg H (1992). Epidemiology and depression in primary care. *General Hospital Psychiatry*, **14**, 237–47.

Kellgren JH (1938*a*). A preliminary account of referred pains arising from muscle. *British Medical Journal*, **1**, 325–7.

Kellgren JH (1938*b*). Observations on referred pain arising from muscle. *Clinical Science*, **3**, 174–90.

Kleinman A, Eisenberg L & Good B (1978). Culture, illness, and care. Clinical lessons from anthropologic and cross-cultural research. *Annals of Internal Medicine*, **88**, 251–8.

Klemp P, Nielson H, Korsgard J & Crane P (1982). Blood flow in fibromyotic muscles. *Scandanavian Journal of Rehabilitation Medicine*, **14**, 81–2.

Large RG (1996). Psychological aspects of pain. *Annals of Rheumatic Diseases*, **55**, 340–5.

Ledingham J, Doherty S & Doherty M (1993). Primary fibromyalgia: an outcome study. *British Journal of Rheumatology*, **32**, 139–42.

Lewinsohn PM, Hoberman HM & Rosenbaum M (1988). A prospective study of risk factors for unipolar depression. *Journal of Abnormal Psychology*, **97**, 251–64.

Llewellyn LJ & Jones AB (1915). *Fibrositis*. London: Heinemann.

Luff AP (1913). The various forms of fibrositis and their treatment. *British Medical Journal*, **1**, 756–760.

Manu P, Lane T, Matthews DA, Castriotta RJ, Watson RK & Abeles M (1994). Alpha–delta sleep in patients with a chief complaint of chronic fatigue. *Southern Medical Journal*, **87**, 465–70.

Martin L, Nutting A, Macintosh BR, Edworthy SM, Butterwick D & Cook J (1996). An exercise program in the treatment of fibromyalgia. *Journal of Rheumatology*, **23**, 1050–3.

Martinez JE, Ferraz MB, Fontana AM & Atra E (1995). Psychological aspects of Brazilian woman with fibromyalgia. *Journal of Psychosomatic Research*, **39**, 167–74.

McCain GA, Bell DA, Mai F & Halliday PD (1988). A controlled study of the effects of a supervised cardiovascular fitness training program on the manifestations of the primary fibromyalgia syndrome. *Arthritis and Rheumatism*, **31**, 1135–41.

Mengshoel AM, Vollestad NK & Forre O (1995). Pain and fatigue induced by exercise in fibromyalgia patients and sedentary healthy subjects. *Clinical and Experimental Rheumatology*, **13**, 477–82.

Moldofsky H (1989). Sleep and the fibrositis syndrome. *Rheumatic Disease Clinics of North America*, **15**, 91–103.

Moldofsky H & Warsh JJ (1978). Plasma tryptophan in musculoskeletal pain in non-articular rheumatism (fibrositis syndrome). *Pain*, **5**, 65–71.

Moldofsky H, Scarisbrick P, England R & Smythe H (1975). Musculoskeletal symptoms and non-REM sleep disturbance in patients with 'fibrositis syndrome' and healthy subjects. *Psychosomatic Medicine*, **37**, 160–72.

Nichols DS & Glenn T (1994). Effects of aerobic exercise on pain perception, affect and level of disability in individuals with fibromyalgia. *Physical Therapy*, **74**, 327–32.

Owens J & Nemeroff CB (1994). Role of serotonin in the pathophysiology of depression: focus on the serotonin transporter. *Clinical Chemistry*, **40/2**, 288–95.

Payne TC, Leavitt F, Garron DC, Katz RS, Golden HE, Glickman PB & Vanderplate C (1982). Fibrositis and psychological disturbance. *Arthritis and Rheumatism*, **25**, 213–7.

Pugh LGC & Christie TA (1945). A study of rheumatism in a group of soldiers with reference to the incidence of trigger points and fibrositic nodules. *Annals of Rheumatic Diseases*, **5**, 8–10.

Quimby LG, Gratwick G, Whitney C & Block SR (1989). A randomized trial of cyclobenzaprine for the treatment of fibromyalgia. *Journal of Rheumatology*, **16** (Suppl.), 140–3.

Rajala V, Keinanen-Kivkaanniemi S, Vusimaki A & Kivela SK (1995). Musculoskeletal pains and depression in a middle-aged Finnish population. *Pain*, **61**, 451–7.

Raspe H & Baumgartner C (1993). The epidemiology of the fibromyalgia syndrome (FS): Different criteria different results. *Journal of Musculoskeletal Pain*, **1**, 149–52.

Reynolds WJ, Chiu B & Imman RD (1988). Plasma substance P levels in fibrositis. *Journal of Rheumatology*, **15**, 1802–3.

Russell IJ, Michalek JE, Vipraio GA, Fletcher E & Wall K (1989). Serum amino acids in fibrositis/fibromyalgia syndrome. *Journal of Rheumatology*, **16**, 1158–63.

Russell IJ, Fletcher EM, Michalek JE, McBroom PC & Hester GG (1991). Treatment of primary fibrositis/fibromyalgia syndrome with ibuprofen and alprazolam: a double-blind, placebo-controlled study. *Arthritis and Rheumatism*, **34**, 552–60.

Russell IJ, Vaeroy H, Javors M & Nyberg F (1992). Cerebrospinal fluid biogenic amine metabolities in fibromyalgia/fibrositis syndrome and rheumatoid arthritis. *Arthritis and Rheumatism*, **35**, 550–6.

Russell IJ, Orr D, Littman OB, Vipraio GA, Alboukrek D, Michalek JE, Lopez Y & MacKillip F (1994). Elevated cerebrospinal fluid levels of substance P in patients with fibromyalgia syndrome. *Arthritis and Rheumatism*, **37**, 1593–601.

Russell IJ, Michalek JE, Flechas JD & Abraham GE (1995). Treatment of fibromyalgia syndrome with super malic: a randomized double-blind, placebo-controlled, crossover pilot study. *Journal of Rheumatology*, **22**, 953–8.

Schuessler G & Konermann J (1993). Psychosomatic aspects of primary fibromyalgia syndrome. *Journal of Musculoskeletal Pain*, **1**, 229–36.

Scudds RA, McCain GA, Rollman GB & Harth M (1989). Improvements in pain responsiveness in patients with fibrositis after successful treatment with amitriptyline. *Journal of Rheumatology*, **16** (Suppl.), 998–103.

Sims RW (1996). Is there muscle pathology in fibromyalgia syndrome? *Rheumatic Disease Clinics of North America*, **22**, 245–66.

Sinclair DC, Feindel WH, Weddell G & Falconer A (1948). The intervertebral ligaments as a source of segmental pain. *Journal of Bone and Joint Surgery*, **30B**, 515–21.

Slocumb CH (1936). Differential diagnosis of periarticular fibrositis and arthritis. *Journal of Laboratory and Clinical Medicine*, **22**, 56–63.

Smythe H & Moldofsky H (1977). Two contributions to understanding of the 'fibrositis syndrome'. *Bulletin of Rheumatic Diseases*, **2228**, 928–31.

Steindler A (1940). The interpretation of sciatic radiation and the syndrome of low back pain. *Journal of Bone and Joint Surgery*, **22**, 28–34.

Stockman R (1904*a*). The causes, pathology and treatment of chronic rheumatism. *Edinburgh Medical Journal*, **15**, 107–16.

Stockman R (1904*b*). The causes, pathology, and treatment of chronic rheumatism. *Edinburgh Medical Journal*, **15**, 223–35.

Stockman R (1939). The treatment of sciatica, brachialgia and occipital headache. *Annals of Rheumatic Diseases*, **2**, 77–82.

Surtees PG & Barkley C (1994). Future imperfect: the long-term outcome of depression. *British Journal of Psychiatry*, **164**, 327–41.

Telling WH (1935). The clinical importance of fibrositis in general practice. *British Medical Journal*, **1**, 689–92.

Travell J (1955). Referred pain from skeletal muscle. *New York State Journal of Medicine*, **55**, 331–40.

Travell J & Rinzler SH (1952). The myofascial genesis of pain. *Postgraduate Medicine*, **11**, 425–34.

Travell J, Rinzler S & Herman M (1942). Pain and disability of the shoulder and arm. *Journal of the American Medical Association*, **120**, 417–22.

Vaeroy H, Helle R, Fore O, Kass E & Terenius L (1988). Elevated CSF levels of substance P and high incidence of Raynaud's phenomenon in patients with fibromyalgia: new features for diagnosis. *Pain*, **32**, 21–6.

Vitanen JV, Kautiainen H & Isomaki H (1993). Pain intensity in patients with fibromyalgia and rheumatoid arthritis. *Scandinavian Journal of Rheumatology*, **22**, 131–5.

Vlaeyan JWS, Teeken-Gruben NJG, Goossens EJB, Mölken R, Pelt R, van Eek PH & Herts P (1996). Cognitive-educational treatment of fibromyalgia: a randomized clinical trial. I. Clinical effects. *Journal of Rheumatology*, **23**, 1237–45.

Wallace DJ, Bowman RL, Wormsley SB & Peter JB (1989). Cytokines and immune regulation in patients with fibrositis. *Arthritis and Rheumatism*, **32**, 1334–5.

White KP & Nielson WR (1995). Cognitive-behavioral treatment of fibromyalgia syndrome: a follow-up assessment. *Journal of Rheumatology*, **22**, 717–21.

Wolfe F (1993). Fibromyalgia: on diagnosis and certainty. *Journal of Musculoskeletal Pain*, **1**, 17–35.

Wolfe F (1995). The future of fibromyalgia: some critical issues. In *Fibromyalgia, Chronic Fatigue Syndrome, and Repetitive Stress Injury*, ed. A. Chalmers, G.O. Littlejohn, I. Salit & F. Wolfe, pp. 3–15. New York: The Haworth Press.

Wolfe F & Potter J (1996). Fibromyalgia and work disability: Is fibromyalgia a disabling disorder? *Rheumatic Disease Clinics of North America*, **22**, 369–90.

Wolfe F & the Special Report Committee (1996). Special report: The F syndrome. A consensus report on fibromyalgia and disability. *Journal of Rheumatology*, **23**, 534–9.

Wolfe F, Cathey A, Kleinheksel S, Amos SP, Hoffman RG, Young DY & Hawley DJ (1984). Psychological status in primary fibrositis and fibrositis associated with rheumatoid arthritis. *Journal of Rheumatology*, **11**, 500–6.

Wolfe F, Smythe HA, Yunus B, Bennett R, Bombardier C, Goldenberg DL, Tugwell P, Campbell S, Abeles M, Clark P, Fam AG, Farber SJ, Fiechtner JJ, Franklin C, Gatter RA, Hamaty D, Lessard J, Lichtbroun AS, Masi AT, McCain GA, Reynolds WJ, Romano TJ, Russell IJ & Sheon RP (1990). The American College of Rheumatology 1990 criteria for the classification of fibromyalgia. Report of the multicenter criteria committee. *Arthritis and Rheumatism*, **33**, 160–72.

Wolfe F, Cathey A & Hawley DJ (1994). A double-blind placebo controlled trial of fluoxetine in fribromyalgia. Scandinavian Journal of Rheumatology, **23**, 255–9.

Wolfe F, Ross K, Anderson J, Russell I & Hebert LT (1995). Prevalence and characteristics of fibromyalgia in the general population. *Arthritis and Rheumatism*, **38**, 19–28.

Wolfe F, Bennett R, Caro X, Goldenberg DL, Russell IJ & Yunus MB (1996). Fibromyalgia symptom severity remains unaltered in long-term follow-up evaluations. *Arthritis and Rheumatism*, **39** (Suppl.), S277.

Yunus B (1994). Psychological aspects of fibromyalgia syndrome: a component of the dysfunctional spectrum syndrome. *Bailliéres Clinical Rheumatology*, **8**, 811–37.

Yunus B & Kalyan-Raman UP (1989). Muscle biopsy findings in primary fibromyalgia and other forms of nonarticular rheumatism. *Rheumatic Disease Clinics of North America*, **15**, 115–34.

Yunus B, Dailey JW, Aldag JC, Masi AF & Lobe PC (1992*a*). Plasma tryptphan and other amino acids in primary fibromyalgia: a controlled study. *Journal of Rheumatology*, **19**, 90–4.

Yunus B, Dailey JW, Aldag JC, Masi AF & Jobe PC (1992*b*). Plasma and urinary catecholamines in primary fibromyalgia: a controlled study. *Journal of Rheumatology*, **19**, 95–7.

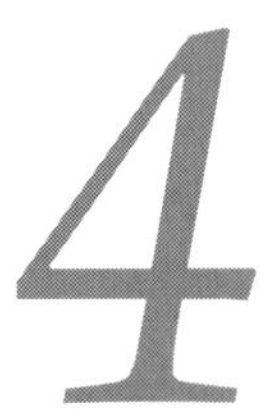

Irritable Bowel Syndrome

GEORGE F. LONGSTRETH

The functional gastrointestinal disorders, defined as a 'variable combination of chronic or recurrent gastrointestinal symptoms not explained by structural or biochemical abnormalities,' are categorized according to the part of the gastrointestinal tract to which the symptoms are attributed (Drossman et al., 1990, 1993). They are a common cause of patient visits to primary physicians and various specialists and result in high direct medical costs and indirect costs, such as work absenteeism. The irritable bowel syndrome (IBS) is the prototypic functional bowel disorder in terms of its heterogeneous nature, multifactorial pathogenesis and requirement for individualized diagnosis and treatment.

History

The concepts of IBS and its postulated pathogenesis have evolved since the earliest published descriptions of a disorder compatible with it in the nineteenth century (Drossman, 1994; Schuster, 1994). Initially, excessive colonic mucus production was emphasized as characteristic of IBS, giving rise to the name 'mucus colitis'. The early recognition of associated psychological factors was exemplified by Osler's emphasis on the patients' 'hysterical, hypochondriacal and neurasthenic personalities', characteristics which would now be applied to few IBS patients. Subsequent psychosomatic explanations of the disorder invoked psychoanalytical theory and biological predisposition. In the 1920s, IBS was described as a nervous response to stress, with emphasis on the etiological importance of colonic spasm, which was attributed to autonomic nerve dysfunction. Almy and others later showed that colonic contractions were increased by physical and psychological stress (Almy & Tulin, 1947; Deller & Wangel, 1965). Subsequent advances in research technology were accompanied by reports of large bowel myoelectrical and motility abnormalities, but these findings proved to be too variable and poorly reproducible for diagnostic use (Coremans et al., 1995). Recent research on the small bowel has identified that this part of the gastrointestinal tract is also important in the origin of symptoms (Kellow & Bennett, 1996). In addition, current investigation focuses on the role of increased intestinal smooth muscle reactivity (Lynn & Friedman, 1995) and visceral afferent mechanisms, including central nervous system processing of information (Silverman et al., 1997), in the pathogenesis of IBS symptoms.

Some clinicians realized long ago that IBS could mimic serious organic disease and that both pharmacological and psychological treatment should be considered according to the patient's needs (Ryle, 1928). The surge of scientific interest in IBS during the past two decades has brought increased awareness that both the traditional biomedical model of disease and a purely psychiatric explanation are inadequate keys to understanding and treating IBS (Drossman & Working Team Committee Chairmen, 1994). Instead, the ancient Greek concept of holism, in which the mind and body are inseparable, has re-emerged in the form of the biopsychosocial model popularized by Engel as the best conceptual framework (Drossman, 1996). This point of view regards IBS as a multifactorial disease in which biologically determined symptoms may be influenced by cultural, social, interpersonal and psychological factors.

In 1962, Chaudhary & Truelove performed a comprehensive clinical study of IBS and subdivided it into spastic colon (pain and bowel habit abnormality) and painless diarrhea. Of additional major importance to clinical practice was the report that certain symptoms distinguish IBS from organic disease (Manning et al., 1978). A rigorous multinational team consensus process developed the Rome diagnostic criteria from the Manning symptoms. The current definition of IBS requires pain (Thompson et al., 1992), which separates it from functional diarrhea and functional constipation.

Definition and symptoms

The Rome symptom-based diagnostic criteria (Table 4.1), which comprise pain, altered bowel habit and bloating, provide a standardized definition for IBS which has been used in many epidemiological surveys and treatment trials. The definition is also useful in conjunction with additional history, physical examination and further diagnostic evaluation in identifying IBS in clinical practice.

Table 4.1. *Symptom-based diagnostic criteria for irritable bowel syndrome*

At least three months of continuous or recurrent symptoms of:
(1) abdominal pain or discomfort that is:
  (a) relieved with defecation, and/or
  (b) associated with a change in frequency of stool, and/or
  (c) associated with a change in consistency of stool, and
(2) two or more of the following, at least on one-fourth of occasions or days:
  (a) altered stool frequency
  (b) altered stool form (lumpy/hard or loose/watery stool),
  (c) altered stool passage (straining, urgency, or feeling of incomplete evacuation),
  (d) passage of mucus, and/or
  (e) bloating or feeling of abdominal distension

Source: Adapted from Thompson et al. (1992).

The pain is variously described, such as dull, aching, sharp or cramping. It can be anywhere in the abdomen but is usually in the lower abdomen, and it tends to be diffuse rather than focal. It occasionally radiates to the lower back. Although it uncommonly awakens a patient from sleep, it may be experienced after the patient awakens for another reason. When most severe, it can simulate major organic disease and result in hospitalization (Doshi & Heaton, 1994) and inappropriate surgery.

The altered bowel habit includes changes in the frequency, form or passage of stool. Loose stools are small in volume and sometimes 'explosive' due to accompanying flatus. Diarrhea often occurs within minutes of eating and may be more common after meals in a restaurant than at home. It often begins shortly after arising before breakfast ('morning rush syndrome'). Urgency may be marked and incontinence may occur, especially in older patients. The altered form of solid stool may be described as pellet like (scybalous) or pencil like. The physician should realize that patients may regard 'diarrhea' as frequent passage of formed stools or less frequent liquid stools. 'Constipation' may mean infrequent stools or straining to defecate (dyschezia). Patients may have diarrhea-predominant or constipation-predominant IBS, suffer periods of both abnormalities, report that normal bowel habit alternates with periods of abnormality or state that stool is never normal. Sometimes the pattern changes. For example, an adult with diarrhea-predominant IBS may recall childhood constipation, perhaps even enema administration by his or her mother, which gradually evolved to diarrhea. Mucus may accompany the stool or be passed by itself and be mistaken by the patient for a 'worm'. A rare patient is so focused on the stool or mucus that she/he brings a sample of it to the physician or provides a photograph of it, an activity aptly named 'fecophotophilia' (Belsheim, 1981). The unsuccessful urge to pass stool may resemble the tenesmus of ulcerative proctitis. Bloating can be the most troublesome symptom and may be compared with being pregnant or blamed for poorly fitting clothing. It may be accompanied by flatus which is so embarrassing as to be socially disabling.

Women may locate the pain in the pelvis, seek gynecological consultation and be diagnosed as having chronic pelvic pain (Longstreth, 1994). Notably, surveys have revealed IBS in one-half or more of women with chronic pelvic pain, dyspareunia or dysmenorrhea (Prior et al., 1989; Walker et al., 1991; Crowell et al., 1994). The overlap of gynecological and gastrointestinal symptoms is further emphasized by the findings that menstruation exacerbates IBS symptoms (Whitehead et al., 1990*b*) and that IBS-type symptoms are associated with increased perimenstrual symptoms (Heitkemper & Jarrett, 1992).

Nongastrointestinal symptoms are common and increase in number as the severity of IBS increases (Guthrie et al., 1992; Longstreth & Wolde-Tsadik, 1993). Chronic fatigue, headache, urological symptoms and other multisystem complaints occur (Maxton et al., 1991*a*; Talley et al., 1991*a*) and fibromyalgia is especially common (Triadafilopoulos et al., 1991; Veale et al., 1991). Although there is disagreement as to whether various nongastrointestinal symptoms contribute to the diagnosis of IBS, it is clear that IBS is only one of multiple functional syndromes in many patients.

Case presentation

A 36-year-old woman was referred to a gastroenterologist because of lower abdominal pain, bloating, flatus and belching for many years. She reported constipation (small, hard, infrequent stools) alternating with diarrhea (small volume, loose, nonbloody stools 20 minutes after eating). The pain usually preceded bowel movements and was relieved by them.

Past history included hysterectomy and bilateral salpingo-ophorectomy one year before presentation; microscopic endometriosis was found. She complained of dyspareunia, but gynecological evaluation had revealed no cause. She also had chronic muscular aching.

Psychosocial history revealed that during childhood her brother had sexually molested her. She was a recovered alcoholic and had taken lithium for seven years to treat manic–depressive disorder.

Physical examination revealed a tender, rope-like sigmoid colon. A complete blood count was normal. Flexible sigmoidoscopy and barium enema were normal, but she had marked discomfort during both procedures.

The gastroenterologist explained IBS to her as a chronic, fluctuating but benign disorder related to a 'sensitive, poorly coordinated gastrointestinal tract'. He emphasized its association with her psychological problems by using simple terms such as 'stress' and 'colonic spasm'. A rheumatologist diagnosed fibromyalgia. Both her primary physician and psychiatrist saw her at periodic scheduled visits. A combination of increased dietary fiber and loperimide as needed improved her bowel habit irregularity. She seemed to cope better with her symptoms but continued to make episodic urgent requests for care.

Comment: This patient represents one extreme of the continuum of IBS severity in terms of the prominance of psychosocial factors, association with other functional somatic symptoms and refractoriness of symptoms.

Prevalence

Epidemiological surveys of various populations have found IBS to be quite common. For example, the disorder was found in 10–22% of Minnesota residents (Talley et al., 1991*b*), patients registered with British general practitioners (Jones & Lydeard, 1992), California health maintenance organization health examinees (Longstreth & Wolde-Tsadik, 1993) and US householders (Drossman et al., 1993). Most population studies have found the disorder to be two to three times as common in women as in men, especially constipation-predominant IBS, and it occurs throughout adult life (Talley et al., 1995*a*). It may be less common in Asian Americans than in other racial groups (Longstreth & Wolde-Tsadik, 1993), and its prevalence may be inversely related to household income (Drossman et al., 1993).

IBS is the seventh leading diagnosis among all physicians and the most common leading diagnosis among gastroenterologists. As in the population surveys, the ratio of women to men patients is about 3 : 1.

Economic costs

The cost in terms of both the direct medical expenses and indirect costs, such as work absenteeism, is considerable (Everhart &

Renault, 1991; Talley et al., 1995*b*). Although only one-fourth of people with IBS seek medical care (Talley et al., 1995*a*), there are between 2.4 and 3.5 million physician visits annually for IBS in the USA, during which 2.2 million prescriptions are written. In a national survey of US households, people with any functional gastrointestinal disorder were currently more likely to be too sick to work, had missed more days of work in the past year and had more physician visits for gut complaints and for nongastrointestinal complaints (Drossman et al., 1993). A survey of Minnesota residents, including calculation of their inpatient and outpatient health services charges exclusive of outpatient drug costs, revealed overall median charges incurred by subjects with IBS were $472 compared with $429 for controls (Talley et al., 1995*b*). It was estimated that IBS accounts for $8 billion of such medical charges annually in the white population of the USA. Unnecessary tests, inappropriate management, and even unnecessary surgery can increase the costs (Longstreth, 1995, 1997).

The impact of IBS on medical costs assumes even more significance when other aspects of the disorder are considered. IBS is a chronic, relapsing syndrome which may persist throughout adult life. There is considerable overlap of IBS with other functional gastrointestinal disorders and interchange with them over time (Drossman et al., 1993; Agreus et al., 1995).

Confirmations

Most researchers and clinicians accept the ability of the multinational Rome symptom criteria to identify IBS in epidemiological surveys and play a dominant diagnostic role in clinical practice. Their predictive value in distinguishing IBS from organic disease improves as the number of criteria increase (Manning et al., 1978; Talley et al., 1990; Poynard et al., 1992). The symptom criteria have been found to be similarly useful in men and women (Poynard et al., 1992; Taub et al., 1995); however, other researchers have reported them to be less accurate (Talley et al., 1990) and even useless (Smith et al., 1991) in men. Notably, the possible reduced accuracy of the criteria in men is mitigated by the preponderance of female patients. The concept of IBS as a distinct syndrome is further supported by the finding of clusters of all or most of the symptom criteria in community samples of women (Taub et al., 1995; Whitehead et al., 1990*a*). In addition, a diagnosis of IBS based predominantly on the symptom criteria holds up well over time. For example, no case of misdiagnosis occurred in patients diagnosed by symptom criteria, sigmoidoscopy and only basic laboratory tests during at least five years of follow-up (Harvey et al., 1987).

Excessive sensitivity to balloon distension in various parts of the gastrointestinal tract (visceral hyperalgesia) is characteristic of functional bowel disorders, including the colon of IBS patients, even though there may be higher tolerance to other stimuli such as cutaneous pain (Mayer & Raybould, 1990; Accarino et al., 1995). IBS patients also sense flatus and a defecation urge at lower volumes of rectal distension (Prior et al., 1990) and are more likely to sense physiological motility events in the duodenum (Kellow et al., 1991). There is a strong relationship between changes in rectal perception thresholds and symptom severity (Mertz et al., 1995).

Although major psychosocial factors are not associated with a diagnosis of IBS, they influence how symptoms are perceived and acted upon, and, therefore whether health care is sought. This finding at least partly explains why many people with IBS do not seek care (Drossman et al., 1995*a*; Talley et al., 1995*a*; Whitehead, 1996). The degree of psychosocial difficulty operant in an IBS patient's illness is often minor in patients with mild symptoms, but it tends to increase with worsening symptoms, becoming most prominent in patients with refractory symptoms. Of patients who have the most severe IBS, 40–60% have psychiatric disorders, especially depression and generalized anxiety disorder (Drossman et al., 1995*a*; Whitehead 1996). A history of sexual and physical abuse is a particularly important psychosocial factor, as initially emphasized by Drossman. Such a history increases with IBS severity and is correlated with multiple somatic complaints, psychiatric illness, physician visits and lifetime surgeries (Longstreth & Wolde-Tsadik, 1993; Drossman et al., 1995*b*, 1996; Walker et al., 1995). These measures of health status are affected independently by abuse and a functional as opposed to an organic diagnosis (Drossman et al., 1996). Furthermore, such psychological factors as anxiety, depression and somatization predispose patients to develop IBS after acute infectious diarrhea (Gwee et al., 1996).

Contradictions

A contrary opinion holds that the lack of specific psychopathology or pathophysiology calls into question the legitimacy of the symptom-based definition of IBS (Christensen, 1992). Such a view can allow the diagnosis of IBS only after exclusion of all organic diseases that are possible causes of a patient's symptoms. The requirement of a uniform cause for disease diagnosis would also call into question the classification of many other medical disorders. Physicians in other fields of medicine have also disagreed on whether knowledge of disease causation is necessary for a diagnosis and whether symptom patterns constitute adequate diagnostic guidelines (Scadding, 1996). Notably, the implication that many patients with symptoms typical of IBS require extensive diagnostic testing has major economic significance, especially in the present era of cost containment.

Healthy people often report that psychological stressors produce gastrointestinal symptoms. A survey of health examinees found that stress-induced abdominal pain and bowel habit change were more common in women than men and that such 'gut reactors' declined with age in each sex (Longstreth, 1993). Such stress effects were more common in subjects with IBS and increased in prevalence as the severity of IBS increased (Longstreth & Wolde-Tsadik, 1993). Stressful life events such as divorce and death of a loved one are also correlated with disability days and physician visits due to IBS symptoms (Creed et al., 1988; Whitehead et al., 1992). Various methodological problems complicate research on stress and IBS, however, leading some authorities to view such results with caution (Thompson & Gick, 1996).

Lactose malabsorption can cause abdominal discomfort, gas symptoms or diarrhea. Certain racial/ethnic groups, including African-Americans, Jews, Asians and people of Mediterranean descent, are predisposed to the disorder. The diagnosis of lactase deficiency in IBS patients infrequently results in symptom improvement (Newcomer & McGill, 1983; Tolliver et al., 1996). Lactase deficiency did not influence the development of IBS after infectious diarrhea (Gwee et al., 1996). Furthermore, there is a poor correlation among self-reported lactose intolerance, lactose malabsorption and symptoms actually produced by modest milk intake (Suarez et al., 1995).

Pathogenetic hypotheses

The mechanisms which lead to IBS are multifactorial and not mutually exclusive (Camilleri & Prather, 1992).

Abnormal motor function

The fluctuating nature of IBS complicates the interpretation of laboratory studies performed during a brief period of time when symptoms may be absent. Prolonged colonic contractions and an increase in myoelectrical slow waves were at one time suspected as specific for IBS. Further research revealed basal sigmoid motor activity varying from decreased to increased. Postprandial sigmoid motor activity has been found to be delayed in response, normal or increased in frequency, and both normal and increased myoelectrical slow wave activity have been reported. Furthermore, the abnormalities are poorly correlated with pain (Coremans et al., 1995).

Smooth muscle hyper-reactivity is reflected by the consistent finding that various acute stimuli such as eating, psychological stress, balloon distension and the injection of cholecystokinin cause an exaggerated motor response in the colon (Drossman et al., 1995*a*; Lynn & Friedman, 1995). Colonic transit measured by scintigraphy has revealed accelerated transit in patients with diarrhea-predominant IBS (Vassallo et al., 1992) and delayed transit in constipation (Stivland et al., 1991).

Recent attention has turned to ambulatory motility studies of the small bowel. Kellow and colleagues have described an increase in discrete, clustered contractions during phase II of the motility cycle in the waking state. Notably, the dysmotility is often coincident with symptoms (Kellow et al., 1990). In addition, high amplitude ileal contractions are associated with pain in IBS (Kellow & Phillips, 1987). Motor hyper-reactivity to balloon distension of the ileum occurs as in the colon (Kellow et al., 1988).

Visceral perception

The possible mechanisms responsible for visceral hyperalgesia include dysfunction of peripheral afferent nerves and/or central processing of afferent information. Hypotheses have been proposed for how psychological factors could alter pain sensitivity (Drossman et al., 1995*a*). In addition, disruption of the hypothalamic-pituitary-adrenal feedback loop (Mayer, 1996), autonomic dysfunction distinct for IBS symptom subgroups (Aggarwal et al., 1994), and aberrant brain activation with both anticipation and experience of visceral pain (Silverman et al., 1997) have been described.

Psychological distress

Notably, recent research has linked certain personality traits with jejunal sensorimotor dysfunction (Evans et al., 1996*a*). Such work suggests psychosocial factors contribute to excessive sympathetic response to stress, which in turn leads to small bowel sensorimotor disturbance.

Certain cognitive aspects may be important factors in IBS (Drossman et al., 1995*a*). For example, fear that a serious disease such as cancer has been overlooked can lead to heightened anxiety and emotional arousal which, in turn, amplify symptoms and cause further health care seeking. Such a pattern can be particularly important in patients who perceive their physician is uncertain about their diagnosis. Some patients regard a psychological explanation for their symptoms as a negative stigma and exhibit denial or hostility if they receive such an explanation. IBS patients tend to minimize psychological and stress-related factors in their lives.

Illness behavior 'refers to the ways people perceive, interpret and react to somatic sensations which may be related to disease or may be misinterpreted as symptoms of disease' (Drossman et al., 1995*a*). The multiple somatic complaints and resulting physician visits, disability days and increased surgery associated with IBS underscore the importance of illness behavior in adversely influencing quality of life and health care costs.

Luminal factors

Malabsorption of other sugars, such as fructose and sorbitol in fruit and 'sugar-free' candy, may also induce intestinal symptoms (Rumessen & Gudmand Høyer, 1988). Food sensitivity was incriminated as a common factor in one study in which dietary exclusion of at least one food, especially from the dairy or grain groups, was beneficial in one-half of IBS patients (Nanda et al., 1989). Bran is commonly used as a treatment for constipation, but some patients report that it worsens various symptoms (Francis & Whorwell, 1994). Food allergy only rarely plays a role (Zwetchkenbaum & Burakoff, 1988). Ileal sensitivity to bile acids may lead to diarrhea in some patients (Oddsson et al., 1978).

Bloating is sometimes a patient's dominant symptom, and it is often accompanied by the complaint of excessive flatus. Aerophagia causes belching and is a suspected contributor to bloating and flatus. A small volume of air is ingested with every swallow. As swallow frequency increases with anxiety, this psychological factor may contribute to gas symptoms (Drossman et al., 1995*a*). Although bloating may be associated with increasing abdominal girth throughout the day, it seems unrelated to increased abdominal gas, depression of the diaphragm, excess lumbar lordosis and voluntary protrusion; therefore, its pathogenesis in many patients remains unknown (Maxton et al., 1991*b*; Levitt et al., 1996). Rectal gas is increased by colonic fermentation of indigestible carbohydrates.

Guidelines for diagnostic work-up

Diagnosis from the symptom-based criteria is reliable when additional data from the history, physical examination and limited investigation are considered. The symptom criteria alone do not reliably distinguish IBS from inflammatory bowel disease (Thompson, 1984), and patients with ulcerative colitis in remission may have IBS symptoms (Isgar et al., 1983). The history can reveal whether the symptoms are due to drug use or ingestion of fructose or sorbitol (Lynn & Friedman, 1995). A long duration of symptoms favors IBS over organic disease (Kruis et al., 1984). Warning signs of an organic disease include bleeding, weight loss, fever and being awakened by symptoms. Hematochezia calls for diagnostic evaluation, but it is often caused only by coincidental hemorrhoids. Weight loss could be due to an organic medical disease or psychiatric comorbidity, such as major depression. In patients with refractory disease, it is particularly important to determine certain aspects of the patient's psychosocial status (Drossman, 1995). Physical examination helps to exclude organic disease and often offers an opportunity to the physician to demonstrate the origin of the pain by placing the patient's hand over a tender, rope-like sigmoid colon.

A limited laboratory and structural evaluation is all that is usually needed if the history reveals typical symptoms and no warning signs are detected by history or physical examination. A complete blood count should usually be carried out to check for anemia and leukocytosis which are never caused by IBS (Kruis et al., 1984); however, it is seldom abnormal in patients identified by symptom criteria (Tolliver et al., 1994). Other blood tests are generally unnecessary. If diarrhea is predominant or the history reveals potential exposure to *Giardia*, microscopical examination of fecal specimens may be indicated, but it is also rarely productive in patients with typical IBS (Tolliver et al., 1994). Although some authorities advise routine fecal occult blood testing (Schuster, 1993), the test seems optional if a structural colon examination is obtained when the clinical and laboratory features call for exclusion of carcinoma regardless of what the fecal occult blood test result would be. Routine abdominal ultrasound examination in confidently diagnosed patients may identify pathology, but it does not account for the symptoms (Francis et al., 1996). There is disagreement on the value of testing for lactase deficiency by laboratory methods or dietary lactose exclusion (Newcomer & McGill, 1983; Schuster, 1993; Suarez et al., 1995; Tolliver et al., 1996). It may be useful in some patients with predominant diarrhea. Large bowel motility studies are not useful (Coremans, 1995). A structural large bowel examination should be performed in most patients, but it usually can be limited to a flexible sigmoidoscopy. This procedure may be diagnostically useful because it often reveals hypersensitivity to pain (Cullingford et al., 1992). The induced discomfort may also help to convince the patient about the origin of her/his usual pain, and the normal findings may provide reassurance. Rectal biopsy is usually unnecessary (MacIntosh et al., 1992). Examination of the entire large bowel by barium radiography or colonoscopy may be indicated in older patients or those with a family history of colorectal neoplasia, a short symptom duration or atypical clinical or laboratory features for IBS. Once a confident diagnosis is made, repeat testing for a recurrence of similar symptoms which previously subsided is usually unnecessary.

Misdiagnosis can result in unnecessary surgery. There may be considerable overlap of gastrointestinal and gynecological symptoms (Longstreth, 1994). IBS predisposes women to undergo hysterectomy (Jones & Lydeard, 1992; Longstreth & Wolde-Tsadik, 1993; Longstreth, 1994) and other operations (Fielding, 1973; Burns, 1986; Creed et al., 1988; Longstreth & Wolde-Tsadik, 1993; Drossman et al., 1996). As one-fourth of women are not relieved of chronic pelvic pain by hysterectomy (Hillis et al., 1995) and IBS adversely influences the response of pain to the operation (Longstreth et al., 1990), collaboration with gynecologists may be needed to prevent unnecessary hysterectomy. Misdiagnosis by general surgeons can lead to unnecessary appendectomy and other operations (DeVaul & Faillace, 1978).

In summary, many patients with symptoms typical of IBS can be confidently diagnosed after the performance of flexible sigmoidoscopy and a complete blood count. Other tests can be carried out selectively. Importantly, tests of little or no value such as testing a fecal specimen obtained by digital rectal examination for occult blood (Gomez & Diehl, 1992) can lead to a 'cascade effect' of additional, fruitless testing which may be costly and hazardous (Mold & Stein, 1986) and make it more difficult to convince the patient about her/his diagnosis.

Treatment

A caring, knowledgeable doctor, usually a primary physician, is the most important element of therapy. The physician should listen actively and display appropriate empathy, validate the patient's concerns and the severity of symptoms, make an unequivocal diagnosis, and explain the disorder in simple physiological terms. Education and reassurance are crucial. Particularly useful sources of education are listed in Table 4.2. A strong physician–patient interaction is of major benefit, as was confirmed by the finding that notations in the medical record about psychosocial history, precipitating factors, and discussion of diagnosis and treatment with patients were associated with fewer return visits for IBS-related symptoms and fewer hospitalizations during a median follow-up of 29 years (Owens et al., 1995).

The performance of controlled treatment trials in IBS is complicated by its chronic nature, which diminishes the usefulness of short-term studies, and symptom variability. It is difficult to maintain 'blinding' in trials of fiber or pharmacological agents, as they often have characteristics or side-effects which make them identifiable to patients and physicians. Furthermore, a placebo response in short-term studies has usually occurred, sometimes in more than 70% of subjects. These

Table 4.2. *Sources of information on irritable bowel syndrome*

International Foundation for Functional Gastrointestinal Disorders, PO Box 17864, Milwaukee, WI 53217 IFFGD is a nonprofit educational and research organization for patients and physicians which addresses the issues surrounding life with functional bowel disorders and bowel incontinence. Members receive a quarterly newsletter and other publications
Thompson WG (1989). *Gut Reactions. Understanding Symptoms of the Digestive Tract.* New York: Plenum Press. This comprehensive book on IBS and other gastrointestinal disorders is pleasantly readable and accented with a touch of humor
Shimberg EF (1988). *Relief from IBS.* New York: Ballantine Books. This clearly written, brief book includes advice on diet, stress management and medications
What You Really Need To Know About Irritable Bowel Syndrome. Medical Audio Visual Communications, Inc., Niagara Falls, New York, 14305 (1-800-757-4868). This 40-minute videotape covers symptoms, diagnosis and treatment in a clear, factual manner

factors as well as various deficiencies in study methodology have led critical reviewers to conclude that no ideal study of fiber, drug or psychological therapy in IBS has been conducted (Klein, 1988; Pace et al., 1995; Talley et al., 1996). Considering these criticisms, no trial has proven conclusively that any therapy is effective; however, the usefulness of some treatments has been suggested by trial results and supported by clinical experience. A placebo effect may contribute to any treatment, although it may not be lasting. Therapy should be tailored to the individual patient, considering the type and severity of her/his symptoms and psychosocial factors (Drossman & Thompson, 1992; Drossman, 1995). Few patients are permanently cured. The emphasis is on helping patients to reduce symptoms and cope with them.

Abdominal pain

An anticholinergic agent such as dicyclomine, 10–20 mg before meals, can help some patients by reducing the meal-induced colonic motor response (Poynard et al., 1994). A tricyclic antidepressant drug can be effective, especially in patients with diarrhea-predominant IBS, by blocking afferent input and modifying small bowel motor function independent of its anticholinergic action (Greenbaum et al., 1987; Clouse et al., 1994; Gorard et al., 1994; Drossman et al., 1995*a*). Usually, only a low dose is needed, such as desipramine 25–50 mg at bedtime, and the analgesic effect may occur within days.

The greater anticholinergic effect of amitriptyline might make that drug more desirable when diarrhea is severe, especially in younger patients who are more tolerant to its side-effects. Insomnia sometimes responds to low-dose antidepressant therapy; depression usually requires a higher dose and a longer period of therapy before a response occurs. It is uncertain whether the newer, selective 5-hydroxytryptamine reuptake inhibitors, such as paroxetine, are as effective as the older, cheaper drugs. Their lack of anticholinergic effects might make them preferred in patients with constipation. Narcotic use should be avoided due to the risk of habituation. Patients with refractory symptoms require an especially detailed management plan, sometimes including referral for psychological treatment (Drossman, 1995). Rare patients should be referred to a comprehensive pain management center.

Diarrhea

Dietary exclusion of fructose, sorbitol or lactose can sometimes help (Rumessen & Gudmand-Høyer, 1988; Nanda et al., 1989). Loperamide in doses of 2–4 mg up to four times a day often stops diarrhea. Many patients take an inadequate dose and mistakenly use it only after diarrhea occurs. They should be taught that the drug is safe and often prevents postprandial diarrhea if it is taken before meals. It should also be taken prophylactically at other times if necessary, such as before leaving home. If a tricyclic drug is used for pain, associated diarrhea may improve. Occasional patients respond to a bile acid sequestrant such as cholestyramine (Oddsson et al., 1978).

Constipation

The use of medications associated with constipation should be reduced or stopped (Lynn & Friedman, 1995). If an antidepressant drug is used for pain, a drug which does not usually cause constipation should be used. Increasing dietary fiber is the mainstay of treatment, e.g., bran, one tablespoonful three times a day with meals; however, providing increased undigestible fiber with bran may be unpalatable to patients, and some report worsening of constipation, distension and pain (Francis & Whorwell, 1994). Other fiber supplements such as psyllium and methylcellulose may improve constipation, but they may also increase bloating in the absence of excessive gas production, presumably due to increased fecal mass (Levitt et al., 1996). Calcium polycarbophil, another bulking agent, may be particularly effective in patients with bloating (Toskes et al., 1993). Severe constipation often responds to lactulose therapy, but its use is limited by increased gas production (Levitt et al., 1996). If possible, stimulant laxatives should be avoided, as dependency may result.

Gas

When bloating is distressing to a patient, reassurance that no serious disorder is evident is important. Dietary change, such as a reduction in milk or wheat products, may be beneficial. Patients should be taught that flatus passage is normal. Flatus can be reduced by dietary exclusion of legumes or malabsorbed sugars.

Psychosocial factors

Patients suffering from such problems as stressful life events, depression and anxiety are most in need of a strong therapeutic relationship with a physician (Drossman & Thompson, 1992; Drossman, 1995). It is important to diagnose and treat major depression. Anxiety may require treatment, but chronic benzodiazepine-type anxiolytic drug therapy should generally be avoided. Although most patients do not require psychological referral, patients with depression or other severe psychological difficulties may benefit. As no trial of psychological therapy has met standards of methodological excellence (Talley et al., 1996), such treatment is empirical. Cognitive behavioral therapy, dynamic psychotherapy, hypnotherapy, relaxation training and biofeedback all have their proponents (Drossman et al., 1995*a*; Chang, 1996).

Investigational therapies (Chang, 1996)

The prokinetic agent, cisapride, may improve intractable constipation and reduce bloating. Serotonin-receptor antagonists and the somatostatin analogue octreotide are being evaluated regarding their ability to decrease rectal sensitivity. There is hopeful preliminary evidence that an opioid agonist specific for peripheral kappa receptors, fedotozine, reduces visceral pain (Junien & Riviere, 1995). The antispasmotic mebeverine is used outside of the USA (Evans et al., 1996*b*).

Conclusion

IBS is a common functional disorder which is best understood from the biopsychosocial concept of illness in which both biological and psychosocial factors influence symptom experience, behavior and outcome. It is a chronic, fluctuating disorder. Various associated nongastrointestinal symptoms are often present. The multiple pathogenetic factors include intestinal motor dysfunction, visceral hyperalgesia, psychological distress and luminal factors. Symptom-based diagnostic criteria are of primary importance, and IBS can usually be confidently diagnosed on the basis of a careful history, physical examination and limited diagnostic evaluation. Unnecessary testing is of economic concern, and misdiagnosis can result in inappropriate surgery. Treatment of the disorder should be individualized according to the pain, bowel habit abnormality, gas symptoms and psychosocial factors in each patient. The most important component of therapy is a good physician–patient relationship.

References

Accarino AM, Azpiroz F & Malagelada J-R (1995). Selective dysfunction of mechanosensitive intestinal afferents in irritable bowel syndrome. *Gastroenterology*, **108**, 636–43.

Aggarwal A, Cutts TF, Abell TL, Cardoso S, Familoni B, Bremer J & Karas J (1994). Predominant symptoms in irritable bowel syndrome correlate with specific autonomic nervous system abnormalities. *Gastroenterology*, **106**, 945–50.

Agréus L, Svärdsudd K, Nyrén O & Tibblin G (1995). Irritable bowel syndrome and dyspepsia in the general population: overlap and lack of stability over time. *Gastroenterology*, **109**, 671–80.

Almy TP & Tulin M (1947). Alterations in colonic function in man under stress: experimental production of changes simulating the 'irritable colon'. *Gastroenterology*, **8**, 616–26.

Belsheim MR (1981). A flash in the pan. *Canadian Medical Association Journal*, **125**, 819.

Burns DG (1986). The risk of abdominal surgery in irritable bowel syndrome. *South African Medical Journal*, **70**, 91.

Camilleri M & Prather CM (1992). The irritable bowel syndrome: mechanisms and a practical approach to management. *Annals of Internal Medicine*, **116**, 1001–8.

Chang L (1996). Evolving therapies for functional colonic disorders. *Current Opinions in Gastroenterology*, **12**, 32–8.

Chaudhary NA & Truelove SC (1962). The irritable colon syndrome. *Quarterly Journal of Medicine*, **31**, 307–22.

Christensen J (1992). Pathophysiology of the irritable bowel syndrome. *Lancet*, **340**, 1444–7.

Clouse RE, Lustman PJ, Geisman RA & Alpers DH (1994). Antidepressant therapy in 138 patients with irritable bowel syndrome: a five-year clinical experience. *Alimentary Pharmacology and Therapeutics*, **8**, 409–16.

Coremans G, Dapoigny M, Müller-Lissner S, Pace F, Smout A, Stockbrugger RW & Whorwell PJ (1995). Diagnostic procedures in irritable bowel syndrome. *Digestion*, **56**, 76–84.

Creed F, Craig T & Farmer R (1988) Functional abdominal pain, psychiatric illness, and life events. *Gut*, **29**, 235–42.

Crowell MD, Dubin NH, Robinson JC, Cheskin LJ, Schuster MM, Heller BR & Whitehead WE (1994). Functional bowel disorders in women with dysmenorrhea. *American Journal of Gastroenterology*, **89**, 1973–7.

Cullingford GL, Coffey JF & Carr-Locke DL (1992). Irritable bowel syndrome: can the patient's response to colonoscopy help with diagnosis? *Digestion*,

52, 209–13.

Deller DJ & Wangel AG (1965). Intestinal motility in man. 1. A study combining the use of intraluminal pressure recording and cineradiography. *Gastroenterology*, **48**, 45–57.

DeVaul RA & Faillace LA (1978). Persistent pain and illness insistence. A medical profile of proneness to surgery. *American Journal of Surgery*, **135**, 828–33.

Doshi M & Heaton KW (1994). Irritable bowel syndrome in patients discharged from surgical wards with non-specific abdominal pain. *British Journal of Surgery*, **81**, 1216–18.

Drossman DA (1994). Psychosocial and psychophysiologic mechanisms in GI illness. In *The Growth of Gastroenterologic Knowledge During the Twentieth Century*, ed. JB Kirsner, pp. 419–32. Philadelphia: Lea & Febiger.

Drossman DA (1995). Diagnosing and treating patients with refractory functional gastrointestinal disorders. *Annals of Internal Medicine*, **123**, 688–97.

Drossman DA (1996). Editorial: gastrointestinal illness and the biopsychosocial model. *Journal of Clinical Gastroenterology*, **22**, 252–4.

Drossman DA & Thompson WG (1992). The irritable bowel syndrome: review and a graduated multicomponent treatment approach. *Annals of Internal Medicine*, **116**, 1009–16.

Drossman DA & Working Team Committee Chairmen (1994). The functional gastrointestinal disorders and their diagnosis: a coming of age. In *The Functional Gastrointestinal Disorders*, ed. DA Drossman, pp. 1–23. Boston, MA: Little Brown.

Drossman DA, Funch-Jensen P, Janssens J, Talley NJ, Thompson WG & Whitehead WE (1990). Identification of subgroups of functional bowel disorders. *Gastroenterology International*, **3**, 159–72.

Drossman DA, Li Z, Andruzzi E, Temple RD, Talley NJ, Thompson WG, Whitehead WE, Janssens J, Funch-Jensen P, Corazziari E, Richter JE & Koch GG (1993). U.S. householder survey of functional gastrointestinal disorders. Prevalence, sociodemography, and health impact. *Digestive Diseases and Sciences*, **38**, 1569–80.

Drossman DA, Creed FH, Fava GA, Olden KW, Patrick DL, Toner BB & Whitehead WE (1995*a*). Psychosocial aspects of the functional gastrointestinal disorders. *Gastroenterology International*, **8**, 47–90.

Drossman DA, Talley NJ, Leserman, J, Olden KW & Barreiro MA (1995*b*). Sexual and physical abuse and gastrointestinal illness. Review and recommendations. *Annals of Internal Medicine*, **123**, 782–94.

Drossman DA, Li Z, Leserman J, Toomey TC & Hu YJB (1996). Health status by gastrointestinal diagnosis and abuse history. *Gastroenterology*, **110**, 999–1007.

Evans PR, Bennett EJ, Bak Y-T, Tennant CC & Kellow JE (1996*a*). Jejunal sensorimotor dysfunction in irritable bowel syndrome – clinical and psychosocial features. *Gastroenterology*, **110**, 393–404.

Evans PR, Bak Y-T & Kellow JE (1996*b*). Mebeverine alters small bowel motility in irritable bowel syndrome. *Alimentary Pharmacology and Therapeutics*, **10**, 787–94.

Everhart JE & Renault PF (1991). Irritable bowel syndrome in office-based practice in the United States. *Gastroenterology*, **100**, 998–1005.

Fielding JF (1973). Surgery and the irritable bowel syndrome: the singer as well as the song. *Irish Medical Journal*, **76**, 33–4.

Francis CY & Whorwell PJ (1994). Bran and irritable bowel syndrome: time for reappraisal. *Lancet*, **344**, 39–40.

Francis CY, Duffy JN, Whorwell PJ & Martin DF (1996). Does routine abdominal ultrasound enhance diagnostic accuracy in irritable bowel syndrome? *American Journal of Gastroenterology*, **91**, 1348–50.

Gomez JA & Diehl AK (1992). Admission stool guiac: use and impact on patient management. *American Journal of Medicine*, **92**, 603–6.

Gorard DA, Libby GW & Farthing MJG (1994). Influence of antidepressants on whole gut and orocaecal transit times in health and irritable bowel syndrome. *Alimentary Pharmacology and Therapeutics*, **8**, 159–66.

Greenbaum DS, Mayle JE, Vanegeren LE, Jerome JA, Mayor JW, Greenbaum RB, Matson RW, Stein GE, Dean HA, Halvorsen NA & Rosen LW (1987). Effects of desipramine on irritable bowel syndrome compared with atropine and placebo. *Digestive Diseases and Sciences*, **32**, 257–66.

Guthrie EA, Creed FH, Whorwell PJ & Tomenson B (1992). Outpatients with irritable bowel syndrome: a comparison of first time and chronic attenders. *Gut*, **33**, 361–3.

Gwee KA, Graham JC, McKendrick MW, Collins SM, Marshall JS, Walters SJ & Read NW (1996). Psychometric scores and persistence of irritable bowel after infectious diarrhea. *Lancet*, **347**, 150–3.

Harvey RF, Mauad EC & Brown AM (1987). Prognosis in the irritable bowel syndrome: a 5-year prospective study. *Lancet*, **1**, 963–5.

Heitkemper MM & Jarrett M (1992). Pattern of gastrointestinal and somatic symptoms across the menstrual cycle. *Gastroenterology*, **102**, 504–13.

Hillis SD, Marchbanks PA & Peterson HB (1995). The effectiveness of hysterectomy for chronic pelvic pain. *Obstetrics and Gynecology*, **86**, 941–5.

Isgar B, Harman M, Kaye MD & Whorwell PJ (1983). Symptoms of irritable bowel syndrome in ulcerative colitis in remission. *Gut*, **24**, 190–2.

Jones R & Lydeard S (1992). Irritable bowel syndrome in the general population. *British Medical Journal*, **304**, 87–90.

Junien JL & Riviere P (1995). Review article: the hypersensitive gut: peripheral kappa agonists as a new pharmacological approach. *Alimentary Pharmacology and Therapeutics*, **9**, 117–26.

Kellow JE & Bennett E (1996). Functional disorders of the small intestine. *Seminars in Gastrointestinal Diseases*, **7**, 208–16.

Kellow JE & Phillips SF (1987). Altered small bowel motility in irritable bowel syndrome is correlated with symptoms. *Gastroenterology*, **92**, 1885–93.

Kellow JE, Phillips SF, Miller LJ & Zinmeister AR (1988). Dysmotility of the small intestine in irritable bowel syndrome. *Gut*, **29**, 1236–43.

Kellow JE, Gill RC & Wingate DL (1990). Prolonged ambulant recordings of small bowel motility demonstrate abnormalities in the irritable bowel syndrome. *Gastroenterology*, **98**, 1208–18.

Kellow JE, Eckersley CM & Jones MP (1991). Enhanced perception of physiological intestinal motility in the irritable bowel syndrome. *Gastroenter-*

ology, **101**, 1621–7.

Klein KB (1988). Controlled treatment trials in the irritable bowel syndrome: a critique. *Gastroenterology*, **95**, 232–41.

Kruis W, Thieme CH, Weinzierl M, Schussler P, Holl J & Paulus W (1984). A diagnostic score for the irritable bowel syndrome. Its value in the exclusion of organic disease. *Gastroenterology*, **87**, 1–7.

Levitt MD, Furne J & Olsson S (1996). The relation of passage of gas and abdominal bloating to colonic gas production. *Annals of Internal Medicine*, **124**, 422–4.

Longstreth GF (1993). Bowel patterns and anxiety. Demographic factors. *Journal of Clinical Gastroenterology*, **17**, 128–32.

Longstreth GF (1994). Irritable bowel syndrome and chronic pelvic pain. *Obstetrical and Gynecological Survey*, **49**, 505–7.

Longstreth GF (1995). Irritable bowel syndrome: a multimillion-dollar problem. *Gastroenterology*, **109**, 2029–42.

Longstreth GF (1997). Irritable bowel syndrome. Diagnosis in the managed care era. *Digestive Diseases and Sciences*, **42**, 1105–11.

Longstreth GF & Wolde-Tsadik G (1993). Irritable bowel-type symptoms in HMO examinees. Prevalence, demographics, and clinical correlates. *Digestive Diseases and Sciences*, **38**, 1581–9.

Longstreth GF, Preskill DB & Youkeles L (1990). Irritable bowel syndrome in women having diagnostic laparoscopy or hysterectomy. Relations to gynecologic features and outcome. *Digestive Diseases and Sciences*, **35**, 1285–90.

Lynn RB & Friedman LS (1995). Irritable bowel syndrome. Managing the patient with abdominal pain and altered bowel habits. *Medical Clinics of North America*, **79**, 373–90.

MacIntosh DG, Thompson WG, Patel DG, Barr R & Guindi M (1992). Is rectal biopsy necessary in irritable bowel syndrome? *American Journal of Gastroenterology*, **87**, 1407–9.

Manning, AP, Thompson WG, Heaton KW & Morris AF (1978). Towards positive diagnosis of the irritable bowel. *British Medical Journal*, **2**, 653–4.

Maxton DG, Morris J & Whorwell PJ (1991*a*). More accurate diagnosis of irritable bowel syndrome by the use of 'non-colonic' symptomatology. *Gut*, **32**, 784–6.

Maxton DG, Martin DF, Whorwell PJ & Godfrey M (1991*b*). Abdominal distension in female patients with irritable bowel syndrome: exploration of possible mechanisms. *Gut*, **32**, 662–4.

Mayer EA (1996). Breaking down the functional and organic paradigm. *Current Opinions in Gastroenterology*, **12**, 3–7.

Mayer EA & Raybould HE (1990). Role of visceral afferent mechanisms in functional bowel disorders. *Gastroenterology*, **99**, 1688–704.

Mertz H, Naliboff B, Munakata J, Niazi N & Mayer EA (1995). Altered rectal perception is a biological marker of patients with irritable bowel syndrome. *Gastroenterology*, **109**, 40–52.

Mold JW & Stein HF (1986). The cascade effect in the clinical care of patients. *New England Journal of Medicine*, **314**, 512–14.

Nanda R, James R, Smith H, Dudley CRK & Jewell DP (1989). Food intolerance and the irritable bowel syndrome. *Gut*, **30**, 1099–104.

Newcomer AD & McGill DB (1983). Irritable bowel syndrome. Role of lactase deficiency. *Mayo Clinic Proceedings*, **58**, 339–41.

Oddsson E, Rask-Madsen J & Krag E (1978). A secretory epithelium of the small intestine with increased sensitivity to bile acids in irritable bowel syndrome associated with diarrhoea. *Scandinavian Journal of Gastroenterology*, **13**, 409–16.

Owens DM, Nelson DK & Talley NJ (1995). The irritable bowel syndrome: long-term prognosis and the physician–patient interaction. *Annals of Internal Medicine*, **122**, 107–12.

Pace F, Coremans G, Dapoigny M, Müller-Lissner SA, Smout A, Stockbruegger RW & Whorwell PJ (1995). Therapy of irritable bowel syndrome: an overview. *Digestion*, **56**, 433–42.

Poynard T, Coutourier D, Frexinos J, Bommelaer G, Hernandez M, Dapoigny M, Buscail L, Benand-Agostini H, Chaput JC, Rheims N & the French Cooperative Study Group (1992). French experience of Manning's criteria in the irritable bowel syndrome. *European Journal of Gastroenterology and Hepatology*, **4**, 747–52.

Poynard T, Naveau S, Mory B & Chaput JC (1994). Meta-analysis of smooth muscle relaxants in the treatment of irritable bowel syndrome. *Alimentary Pharmacology and Therapeutics*, **8**, 499–510.

Prior A, Wilson K, Whorwell PJ & Faragher EB (1989). Irritable bowel syndrome in the gynecological clinic. Survey of 798 new referrals. *Digestive Diseases and Sciences*, **34**, 1820–4.

Prior A, Maxton DG & Whorwell PJ (1990). Anorectal manometry in irritable bowel syndrome: differences between diarrhoea and constipation predominant subjects. *Gut*, **31**, 458–62.

Rumessen JJ & Gudmand-Høyer E (1988). Functional bowel disease: malabsorption and abdominal distress after ingestion of fructose, sorbitol, and fructose-sorbitol mixtures. *Gastroenterology*, **95**, 694–7.

Ryle JA (1928). An address on the chronic spasmodic affections of the colon and the diseases which they simulate. *Lancet*, **2**, 111–19.

Scadding JG (1996). Essentialism and nominalism in medicine: logic of diagnosis in disease terminology. *Lancet*, **348**, 594–6.

Schuster MM (1993). Irritable bowel syndrome. In *Gastrointestinal Disease. Pathophysiology/Diagnosis/Management*, ed. MH Sleisenger & JS Fordtran, pp. 917–33. Philadelphia: WB Saunders.

Schuster MM (1994). Irritable bowel syndrome. In *The Growth of Gastroenterologic Knowledge During the Twentieth Century*, ed. JB Kirsner, pp. 211–19. Philadelphia: Lea & Febiger.

Silverman DHS, Munakata JA, Ennes H, Mandelkern MA, Hoh CK & Mayer EA (1997). Regional cerebral activity in normal and pathological perception of visceral pain. *Gastroenterology*, **112**, 64–72.

Smith RC, Greenbaum DS, Vancouver JB, Henry RC, Reinhart MA, Greenbaum RB, Dean HA & Mayle JE (1991). Gender differences in Manning criteria in the irritable bowel syndrome. *Gastroenterology*, **100**, 591–5.

Stivland T, Camilleri M, Vassallo M, Proana M, Rath D, Brown M, Thomford G,

Pemberton J & Phillips S (1991). Scintigraphic measurement of regional gut transit in idiopathic constipation. *Gastroenterology*, **101**, 107–15.

Suarez FL, Savaiano DA & Levitt MD (1995). A comparison of symptoms after the consumption of milk or lactose-hydrolyzed milk by people with self-reported severe lactose intolerance. *New England Journal of Medicine*, **333**, 1–4.

Talley NJ, Phillips SF, Melton LJ, Mulvihill C, Wiltgen C & Zinmeister AR (1990). Diagnostic value of the Manning criteria in irritable bowel syndrome. *Gut*, **31**, 77–81.

Talley NJ, Phillips SF, Bruce B, Zinmeister AR, Wiltgen C & Melton LJ (1991*a*). Multisystem complaints in patients with the irritable bowel syndrome and functional dyspepsia. *European Journal of Gastroenterology and Hepatology*, **3**, 71–7.

Talley NJ, Zinmeister AR, Van Dyke C & Melton LJ III (1991*b*). Epidemiology of colonic symptoms and the irritable bowel syndrome. *Gastroenterology*, **101**, 927–34.

Talley NJ, Zinmeister AR & Melton LJ III (1995*a*). Irritable bowel syndrome in a community: symptom subgroups, risk factors and health care utilization. *American Journal of Epidemiology*, **142**, 76–83.

Talley NJ, Gabriel SE, Harmsen WS, Zinmeister AR & Evans RW (1995*b*). Medical costs in community subjects with irritable bowel syndrome. *Gastroenterology*, **109**, 1736–41.

Talley NJ, Owen BK, Boyce P & Paterson K (1996). Psychological treatments for irritable bowel syndrome: a critique of controlled treatment trials. *American Journal of Gastroenterology*, **91**, 277–86.

Taub E, Cuevas JL, Cook EW, Crowell M & Whitehead WE (1995). Irritable bowel syndrome defined by factor analysis. Gender and race comparisons. *Digestive Diseases and Sciences*, **40**, 2647–55.

Thompson WG (1984). Gastrointestinal symptoms in the irritable bowel compared with peptic ulcer and inflammatory bowel disease. *Gut*, **25**, 1089–92.

Thompson WG & Gick M (1996). Irritable bowel syndrome. *Seminars in Gastrointestinal Diseases*, **7**, 217–29.

Thompson WG, Creed F, Drossman DA, Heaton KW & Mazzacca G (1992). Functional bowel disease and functional abdominal pain. *Gastroenterology International*, **5**, 75–91.

Tolliver BA, Herrera JL & DiPalma JA (1994). Evaluation of patients who meet clinical criteria for irritable bowel syndrome. *American Journal of Gastroenterology*, **89**, 176–8.

Tolliver BA, Jackson MS, Jackson KL, Barnett ED, Chastang JF & DiPalma JA (1996). Does lactose maldigestion really play a role in the irritable bowel? *Journal of Clinical Gastroenterology*, **23**, 15–17.

Toskes PP, Connery KL & Ritchey TW (1993). Calcium polycarbophil compared with placebo in irritable bowel syndrome. *Alimentary Pharmacology and Therapeutics*, **7**, 87–92.

Triadafilopoulos G, Simms RW & Goldenberg DL (1991). Bowel dysfunction in fibromyalgia syndrome. *Digestive Diseases and Sciences*, **36**, 59–64.

Vassallo M, Camilleri M, Phillips SF, Brown ML, Chapman NJ & Thomforde

GM (1992). Transit through the proximal colon influences stool weight in irritable bowel syndrome. *Gastroenterology*, **102**, 102–8.

Veale D, Kavanagh G, Fielding JF & Fitzgerald O (1991). Primary fibromyalgia and the irritable bowel syndrome: different expressions of a common pathogenetic process. *British Journal of Rheumatology*, **30**, 220–2.

Walker EA, Gelfand AN, Gelfand MD, Koss MP & Katon WJ (1995). Medical and psychiatric symptoms in female gastroenterology clinic patients with histories of sexual victimization. *General Hospital Psychiatry*, **17**, 85–92.

Walker EA, Katon WJ, Jemelka R, Alfrey H, Bowers M & Stenchever MA (1991). The prevalence of chronic pelvic pain and irritable bowel syndrome in two university clinics. *Journal of Psychosomatic Obstetrics and Gynecology*, **12** (Suppl.), 65–75.

Whitehead WE, Crowell MD, Bosmajian L, Zonderman A, Costa PT Jr, Benjamin C, Robinson JC, Heller BR & Schuster MM (1990*a*). Existence of irritable bowel syndrome supported by factor analysis of symptoms in two community samples. *Gastroenterology*, **98**, 336–40.

Whitehead WE, Cheskin LJ, Heller BR, Robinson JC, Crowell MD, Benjamin C & Schuster MM (1990*b*). Evidence for exacerbation of irritable bowel syndrome during menses. *Gastroenterology*, **98**, 1485–9.

Whitehead WE, Crowell MD, Robinson JC, Heller BR & Schuster MM (1992). Effects of stressful life events on bowel symptoms: subjects with irritable bowel syndrome compared with subjects without bowel dysfunction. *Gut*, **33**, 825–30.

Whitehead WE (1996). Psychosocial aspects of functional gastrointestinal disorders. *Gastroenterology Clinics of North America*, **25**, 21–34.

Zwetchkenbaum JF & Burakoff R (1988). Food allergy and the irritable bowel syndrome. *American Journal of Gastroenterology*, **83**, 901–4.

5

Premenstrual Syndrome

TERI PEARLSTEIN

Premenstrual symptoms in women are a common phenomenon, and the clinician must perform a careful medical and psychological screening to evaluate the severity of the symptoms as well as to rule out comorbid psychiatric and medical disorders. Progress in defining the premenstrual syndrome (PMS) in the past two decades has allowed recent studies to begin to elucidate the etiology and treatment of premenstrual symptoms. This chapter reviews the diagnostic issues, epidemiological variables, pathogenetic hypotheses and the treatment options now available to treat PMS.

History

The term 'premenstrual tension' was coined by Frank 70 years ago (Frank et al., 1937), but descriptions of emotional symptoms being related to menstruation date back to antiquity (Severino & Moline, 1989). In the past two decades, progress has been made in defining premenstrual symptoms, assessing prevalence and predictors, searching for etiologies and assessing the efficacy of pharmacological and nonpharmacological treatments. Research criteria for definitions of severe premenstrual symptoms have existed in the two most recent editions of the *Diagnostic and Statistical Manual of Mental Disorders*, DSM-III-R (1987) and DSM-IV (American Psychiatric Association, 1994). Although some authors question the validity of disturbing premenstrual symptoms as constituting an 'illness' (Gurevich, 1995; Richardson, 1995), the existence of research diagnostic criteria has expanded the knowledge about the etiology and treatment of premenstrual symptoms.

Definition

PMS can be defined as emotional, behavioral and physical symptoms that occur in the luteal phase of the menstrual cycle of women, with resolution of the symptoms following the menses. Symptoms can occur for a few days prior to menses in mild cases or for the two weeks between ovulation and menses for more severe cases. Over 100 premenstrual symptoms have been described (Severino & Moline, 1989). Common symptoms are irritability, mood swings, anxiety, feeling out-of-control, feeling overwhelmed, food cravings for sugar or salty foods, increased appetite, fatigue, breast tenderness and abdominal bloating. Other common symptoms include difficulty concentrating, lowered motor coordination, avoidance of social activities, lowered efficiency, insomnia and headaches. A small number of women report premenstrual increases in energy and efficiency.

The definition of PMS is generally confirmed by daily prospective charting of symptoms over one or two menstrual cycles. Several rating forms exist for women to use which are most commonly visual analog scales or lists of symptoms that women might rate from '1' (not present) to '6' (severe), as an example. The rating methods vary somewhat in the number of symptoms assessed and the 'percent premenstrual increase' in severity required, but the most common PMS symptoms are included in most currently used daily rating forms. The many methodological problems involved with how daily ratings lead to a diagnosis have been reviewed (Schnurr et al., 1994). The purpose of the daily ratings is to confirm the timing of the symptoms with the luteal phase of the menstrual cycle and to assess the degree of chronic symptomatology in the follicular phase. A substantial proportion of women seeking treatment for PMS will not have symptoms confined to the luteal phase with an absence of symptoms during the follicular phase. The women who fail to meet criteria for PMS after prospective daily symptom charting will often have underlying depressive or anxiety disorders that are premenstrually exacerbated (DeJong et al., 1985).

Case presentation

Mrs Y was a 36-year-old married woman who contacted a PMS clinic in her area after referral from her gynecologist. Although Mrs Y had noted a few days of irritability, fatigue and food cravings in the week preceding her period since college years, her symptoms had become much more intense and persistent following the weaning of her third child six months previously. Obvious to Mrs Y, her husband and her older two children, the ten days preceding menses each month were notable for out-of-control feelings, mood swings, lack of patience and angry outbursts, feeling overwhelmed, fatigue, social isolation and insomnia. Mrs Y rated her ten most troublesome symptoms from 0 ('not present') to 3 ('severe') on a daily basis for two menstrual cycles. A clinician in the PMS clinic reviewed the daily ratings and interviewed Mrs Y at both the follicular and luteal phases of one menstrual cycle. The clinical interview during the follicular phase confirmed the absence of major depression, dysthymia, bipolar disorder, panic disorder, generalized anxiety disorder, somatization disorder, bulimia or a substance use disorder. The physical and pelvic examinations by a gynecologist were unremarkable and thyroid function tests were normal. There were no symptoms of endometriosis or dysmenorrhea. It was confirmed that Mrs Y had moderately severe PMS with the absence of follicular symptoms. Mrs Y opted to try for one month the lifestyle modifications that were taught in a group education format weekly. Mrs Y achieved partial resolution of her PMS after following recommendations for changes in her diet, increasing exercise and relaxation. Mrs Y then elected a trial of an antidepressant drug during her two luteal weeks each cycle which brought about complete improvement in her symptoms of PMS.

Prevalence

Premenstrual symptoms occur on a continuum, with approximately 20% of women experiencing no premenstrual difficulties, approximately 75% of women experiencing mild to moderate emotional, behavioral and physical premenstrual symptoms, and approximately 5% of women experiencing severe premenstrual symptoms that impact on functioning and cause role impairment. Premenstrual dysphoric disorder (PMDD) is the diagnosis in the DSM-IV (see Table 5.1) that describes the severest form of PMS in 5% of menstruating women. The PMDD criteria require confirmation of the diagnosis by daily symptom charting for two cycles (at least 5 out of 11 symptoms must be present), the absence of follicular psychological symptoms and significant premenstrual symptom severity.

The only epidemiological variable consistently associated with PMDD is a relationship with depression. The presence of PMDD has been associated with increased rates of prior major depression (Har-

Table 5.1. *Research criteria for premenstrual dysphoric disorder*

(A) In most menstrual cycles during the past year, five (or more) of the following symptoms were present for most of the time during the last week of the luteal phase, began to remit within a few days after the onset of the follicular phase, and were absent in the week postmenses, with at least one of the symptoms being either (1), (2), (3) or (4):

(1) markedly depressed mood, feelings of hopelessness, or self-deprecating thoughts;
(2) marked anxiety, tension, feelings of being 'keyed up', or 'on edge';
(3) marked affective lability (e.g., feeling suddenly sad or tearful or increased sensitivity to rejection);
(4) persistent and marked anger or irritability or increased interpersonal conflicts;
(5) decreased interest in usual activities (e.g., work, school, friends, hobbies);
(6) subjective sense of difficulty in concentrating;
(7) lethargy, easy fatigability or marked lack of energy;
(8) marked change in appetite, overeating or specific food cravings;
(9) hypersomnia or insomnia;
(10) a subjective sense of being overwhelmed or out-of-control;
(11) other physical symptoms, such as breast tenderness or swelling, headaches, joint or muscle pain, a sensation of 'bloating', weight gain

(B) The disturbance markedly interferes with work or school or with usual social activities and relationships with others (e.g. avoidance of social activities, decreased productivity and efficiency at work or school)

(C) The disturbance is not merely an exacerbation of the symptoms of another disorder, such as Major Depressive Disorder, Panic Disorder, Dysthymic Disorder or a Personality Disorder (although it may be superimposed on any of these disorders)

(D) Criteria A, B and C must be confirmed by prospective daily ratings during at least two consecutive symptomatic cycles. (The diagnosis may be made provisionally prior to this confirmation)

Source: based on information from the *Diagnostic and Statistical Manual of Mental Disorders*, Washington, DC. Copyright 1994 American Psychiatric Association, pp. 717–18.

rison et al., 1989*b*; Severino et al., 1989; Pearlstein et al., 1990), and prior postpartum depression may also be increased in women with PMDD (Chuong & Burgos, 1995; Pearlstein et al., 1990). Studies of women with PMDD do not report increased rates of personality disorder diagnoses, but a study of personality traits suggested similarity to women with depressive disorders (Parry et al., 1996). Epidemiological studies of women with PMS or PMDD examining age, menstrual cycle characteristics, socioeconomic variables, lifestyle variables or cognitive attributions fail to show a consistent association with PMS.

Economic costs

The economic costs of premenstrual syndrome have not been well studied, a regrettable fact given the large number of women affected, the relatively high cost of pharmacological treatment and the impact of inevitable absenteeism on wages and employment opportunities.

Confirmations

Studies in populations of menstruating women confirm the common presence of psychological, behavioral and physical changes prior to menstruation. Premenstrual symptoms have been reported in women in many cultures. It is difficult to delineate where 'normal' premenstrual symptoms end and a clinically significant premenstrual disorder begins. Women with PMS are likely to be a heterogeneous group and there is no specific laboratory test or physical sign to help diagnosis. The existence of research criteria for PMDD has helped to define the syndrome in women with the severest symptoms and studies with well-defined samples now offer some pathogenetic hypotheses and suggest several promising medication options.

Recent studies have compared neurotransmitter function in women with PMS to control subjects. Several studies suggest altered serotonin function in women with well-defined PMS or PMDD. These studies include measurement of whole blood serotonin, serotonin platelet uptake, platelet tritiated imipramine binding, and challenge tests with tryptophan, fenfluramine and buspirone (for reviews, see Severino, 1994; Pearlstein, 1995; Halbreich, 1996). The exacerbation of premenstrual symptoms after tryptophan depletion in women with PMS is another indicator of serotonin dysregulation in this disorder (Menkes et al., 1994). A recent report did not replicate a serotonin abnormality after fenfluramine challenge (Bancroft & Cook, 1995). In some studies, the serotonin abnormality appeared in the follicular phase, making serotonin dysfunction a possible trait rather than a state marker.

Abnormalities of the noradrenergic system in women with PMS have been suggested in some studies, and women with PMS show an increased sensitivity to panicogenic agents (Halbreich, 1995). A recent study suggests that gamma-aminobutyric acid (GABA) function may be decreased in women with PMDD (Halbreich et al., 1996). This author suggests that the anxiogenic and anxiolytic effects of progesterone and its metabolites may be modulated through their influence on the GABA-A receptor (Halbreich, 1996).

Contradictions

Most authors agree that premenstrual psychological and behavioral changes are common, but some authors feel more needs to be scientifically known about PMS before a 'syndrome' should be identified. Identifying premenstrual symptoms as a 'syndrome' gives it an 'illness' label (Gurevich, 1995) and may portray symptoms that are a normal part of women's experience as being 'pathological' (Richardson, 1995). A woman's experience of the menstrual cycle is influenced by expectations, attributions, stressors, biological factors and psychological symptoms. There is concern that the existence of PMS as a 'diagnosis' will contribute to women's negative expectations about the experience of the menstrual cycle. PMS may also be a misused label such as when a woman attributes the symptoms of an underlying psychiatric or medical disorder to be only 'PMS'. Although the PMDD criteria in DSM-IV require the absence of symptoms in the follicular phase, the stipulation that PMDD 'may be superimposed on another disorder' makes diagnosis unclear in some cases.

Although the symptoms of PMS clearly vary with the phases of the menstrual cycle, studies of the hypothalamic-pituitary-gonadal (HPG) axis in women with PMS have not yet consistently shown a specific abnormality or a definite relationship with symptoms. Most studies have failed to show consistent abnormalities of gonadotropins, ovarian steroids or their metabolites in women with PMS or PMDD (Halbreich et al., 1986; Rubinow et al., 1988; Schmidt et al., 1994). One study of pulsatile luteinizing hormone (LH) secretion reported altered LH secretion in women with PMS compared with controls (Facchinetti et al., 1993), but two studies reported no alteration of LH secretion in women with PMS compared with controls (Reame et al., 1992; Lewis et al., 1995). A placebo-controlled trial of a progesterone receptor blocker, mifepristone, indicated that 'PMS' could occur in the absence of the luteal phase and with low levels of estrogen and progesterone (Schmidt et al., 1991). Thus, there is no current evidence that specific HPG axis abnormality leads to PMS.

Pathogenetic hypotheses

Multiple biological etiologies for PMS have been proposed in the past several decades. As mentioned in the previous section, studies of the HPG axis have not suggested a specific abnormality. As recently reviewed (Rubinow & Schmidt, 1995), neuroendocrinology studies have also not shown consistent abnormalities in the hypothalamic-pituitary-adrenal or hypothalamic-pituitary-thyroid axes. Thyroid disorders do not seem to be increased in women with PMS, but a subset of women with PMS may have abnormal subclinical baseline thyroid function or abnormalities to thyroid-releasing hormone stimulation (Girdler et al., 1995; Korzekwa et al., 1996).

As mentioned above, several studies suggest altered serotonin function in women with PMS and abnormalities in the noradrenergic and GABA systems have been suggested. As recently reviewed (Parry, 1994), altered sleep, decreased melatonin levels and decreased luteal beta-endorphin levels are reported in women with PMS, while abnormalities in glucose, cortisol and prolactin have not been consistently reported. Older studies have investigated the possible pathogenetic role of mineralocorticoids, prostaglandins, vitamins and minerals without clear associations in women with PMS (for a review, see Severino & Moline, 1989, pp. 94–141). One of the pathogenetic abnormalities in PMS may be dysregulated monoamine neurotransmitter function which leads to a vulnerability to the gonadal hormone fluctuations of the menstrual cycle which then trigger mood and anxiety symptoms. If such a link between gonadal hormones and the neurotransmitters involved in mood and anxiety regulation could be delineated, more could potentially be learned about other mood disorders linked to women (e.g. seasonal affective disorder, rapid-cycling bipolar disorder, postpartum depression). Treatment can be directed to either eliminating the trigger (e.g., ovarian suppression) or correcting the 'vulnerability' (e.g., serotonergic antidepressants) (Rubinow & Schmidt, 1995). It is likely, however, that there are other pathogenetic mechanisms besides the interaction between gonadal hormones and monoamine neurotransmitters that will explain the heterogeneity of symptoms reported in women with PMS.

Diagnostic and treatment approaches

Diagnosis

As mentioned above, daily symptom charting for two menstrual cycles is necessary for the diagnosis of PMS. The ratings identify the symptoms, their timing with the menstrual cycle, their severity and their presence or absence during the follicular phase. Other psychiatric and medical disorders should be ruled out. It is important to assess for the presence of depressive disorders, bipolar disorder, anxiety disorders, somatoform disorders, eating disorders, substance use disorders, seizures, chronic fatigue syndrome, thyroid disorder, endometriosis, dysmenorrhea and other medical conditions. A physical examination and pelvic examination are advised, and thyroid function tests should be obtained if indicated.

Treatment

The multiple proposed etiologies of PMS have led to studies examining the efficacy of a multitude of treatments for PMS. The older studies involved women without prospective confirmation of the diagnosis of PMS, making the results of these studies difficult to interpret due to the probable mixed diagnoses of the women studied. Many of the well-designed recent studies have involved women with PMDD and the results of these studies have suggested several promising treatments for PMDD. It is assumed that these treatments would also be beneficial for the much larger number of women with PMS, but this remains to be studied. It is also unknown whether these treatments would also be beneficial for the large group of women whose premenstrual symptoms are exacerbations of chronic psychological or medical problems. The treatment studies reviewed here will include antidepressant medications, other psychotropic medications, hormonal medications, nonpharmacological strategies and miscellaneous treatments.

Most clinicians now consider serotonergic antidepressants the first line treatment for PMS because of studies confirming their efficacy and tolerability. Large multisite double-blind trials with fluoxetine (Steiner et al., 1995) and sertraline (Yonkers et al., 1997) have established the efficacy of selective serotonin reuptake inhibitors (SSRIs) for the treatment of PMDD. Smaller double-blind trials report efficacy with fluoxetine (Stone et al., 1991; Menkes et al., 1992; Wood et al., 1992; Ozeren et al., 1997; Su et al., 1997), paroxetine (Eriksson et al., 1995) and clomipramine (Sundblad et al., 1991). Recent open trials suggest efficacy with sertraline (Freeman et al., 1996*b*), paroxetine (Yonkers et al., 1996) and fluvoxamine (Freeman et al., 1996*a*). The efficacy of other antidepressants has been less studied. An open trial has suggested efficacy for nefazodone (Freeman et al., 1994). Studies of tricyclic antidepressants (not placebo controlled) have yielded mixed results (Harrison et al., 1989*a*; Taghavi et al., 1995; Freeman et al., 1996*b*). Two recent placebo-controlled trials have compared an SSRI to a nonserotonergic antidepressant. Paroxetine was reported to be superior to both maprotiline and placebo (Eriksson et al., 1995) and fluoxetine was superior to both bupropion and placebo (Pearlstein et al., 1997). Efficacy with the SSRIs in PMDD has been achieved with doses similar to those used in the treatment of major depression (i.e. fluoxetine 20 mg daily, sertraline 100–150 mg daily and paroxetine 20–30 mg daily), whereas efficacy with clomipramine was achieved with lower doses (25–75 mg daily) than is used for other disorders. Most of the studies of SSRI treatment have reported that efficacy was achieved with daily dosing of the medication. Recently administration of sertraline during just the two weeks of the luteal phase was reported to be helpful (Halbreich &

Smoller, 1997). Specific recommendations for length of treatment do not exist but premenstrual symptoms have been reported to recur in women after effective medication is discontinued even after one year (Pearlstein & Stone, 1994).

Most psychiatric syndromes respond to antidepressants in a non-specific way, and the selective efficacy of serotonergic antidepressants for PMDD is noteworthy. It is possible that the antidepressant is correcting the proposed dysregulation of serotonin in women with PMS, and that the enhancement of serotonin is beneficial in a shorter amount of time than in the traditional antidepressant response (at least four weeks). It was noted in both of the multisite studies cited above that relief of premenstrual symptoms with the SSRI occurred in the first menstrual cycle (Steiner et al., 1995; Yonkers et al., 1997). Efficacy has been reported in a placebo-controlled trial of clomipramine administered in the luteal phase only (Sundblad et al., 1993) and a report suggests efficacy of SSRIs administered in the luteal phase only (Halbreich & Smoller, 1997). Thus, serotonergic antidepressants are selectively effective for PMDD and demonstrate a short onset of action. It is assumed that SSRIs would also be uniquely beneficial for women with PMS (not PMDD) and a multisite study of an SSRI in PMS is currently in progress.

Other psychotropic medications that have been studied in women with PMS or PMDD include alprazolam, buspirone, fenfluramine and lithium. Five placebo-controlled studies have examined the efficacy of alprazolam administered in the luteal phase only. Doses did not exceed 0.25 mg three times a day in most of these studies. Four of these studies suggested efficacy for alprazolam (Smith et al., 1987; Harrison et al., 1990; Berger & Presser, 1994; Freeman et al., 1995), while one did not (Schmidt et al., 1993). One of the studies showed a selective efficacy of alprazolam for women with PMDD whereas women with premenstrual exacerbation of chronic symptoms did not respond (Berger & Presser, 1994). Buspirone may provide efficacy (Rickels et al., 1989; Brown et al., 1990) but deserves more study. An initial report suggested efficacy of fenfluramine for some premenstrual symptoms (Brzezinski et al., 1990) but this medication also needs further study. Older studies with lithium have methodological problems, but the results do not indicate efficacy for treatment of PMS.

Hormonal strategies for the treatment of PMS and PMDD have been fairly extensively studied. Hormonal strategies include medications that suppress ovulation and hormonal supplements during the luteal phase. Gonadotropin-releasing hormone (GnRH) agonists act by initially stimulating the pituitary to produce follicle-stimulating hormone (FSH) and LH, then subsequently causing downregulation of GnRH receptors. This downregulation leads to decreased FSH and LH secretion, cessation of ovulation and cyclic estrogen and progesterone release. Several double-blind studies have reported the efficacy of GnRH agonists in the treatment of PMS and PMDD (Muse et al., 1984; Bancroft et al., 1987; Hammarback & Backstrom, 1988; Hussain et al., 1992; Brown et al., 1994; Rubinow & Schmidt, 1995; Studd & Leather, 1996), although negative studies exist (Helvacioglu et al., 1993). One study suggested that GnRH agonists are less effective in women with premenstrual exacerbation of depression (Freeman et al., 1993), while another study reported less efficacy with moderate to severe premenstrual depression (Brown et al., 1994). Limitations of GnRH agonist treatment include the need for parenteral administration and the long-term risks of cardiac disease and osteoporosis due to prolonged anovulation and decreased estrogen levels. Add-back regimens of replacement estrogen and progesterone have been suggested to reduce the health risks of long-term GnRH agonist use. Some women, however, report the return of typical symptoms of PMS with the add-back regimen (Mortola et al., 1991; Rubinow & Schmidt, 1995; Studd & Leather 1996) that may be reduced by less frequent administration of the progesterone (Mezrow et al., 1994).

Other methods of ovulation suppression that have been studied include danazol, estrogen, long-acting progestins and oral contraceptives (OCs). Older studies with danazol, a synthetic derivative of ethisterone, have suggested efficacy (for a review, see Muse, 1993). Recent placebo-controlled, crossover trials of women with PMS have reported efficacy with danazol (Deeny et al., 1991; Hahn et al., 1995). It has been suggested that the benefit of danazol is secondary to the induction of anovulation (Halbreich et al., 1991). Side-effects, particularly depression, may limit the usefulness of danazol (Muse, 1993). Reviews of the older studies of OCs suggest equivocal results (Muse, 1993; Severino & Moline, 1989, pp. 181–4). Recent controlled studies failed to show efficacy of a triphasic OC compared with placebo (Graham & Sherwin, 1992) or of a triphasic OC compared with a monophasic OC after four cycles (Backstrom et al., 1992). One study reported that OCs prolonged or delayed premenstrual dysphoria (Bancroft & Rennie, 1993). Both estrogen implants and transdermal patches have been reported to decrease premenstrual symptoms but the cyclic addition of an oral progestin to decrease endometrial hyperplasia can cause undesirable psychological effects (Watson & Studd, 1993). A recent study of transdermal estrogen in women with PMS (follicular symptoms were not commented on) reported that lower doses were better tolerated than higher doses, although both were effective in reducing symptoms (Smith et al., 1995). There are as yet no published controlled trials of long-acting progestins, such as medroxyprogesterone acetate (Depo-Provera) or levonorgestral (Norplant) in PMS.

Studies of the results of hysterectomy on PMS has been reviewed and the relief of PMS cannot be predicted with certainty (Metcalf et al., 1992). A recent study comparing women's perceptions of PMS before and after hysterectomy suggested a decrease following surgery, but there was no confirmation of the PMS (Braiden & Metcalf, 1995). Ovariectomy with hysterectomy is considered to be one of the last treatment considerations, and should not be pursued unless PMS is very difficult to control. Most clinicians suggest suppression of ovulation by pharmacological agents as the preferred option.

The administration of progesterone during the luteal phase is probably one of the oldest and most studied treatments for PMS. Reviews of the double-blind, placebo-controlled studies of progesterone have been reviewed and they do not suggest any efficacy (Freeman, 1993; Rivera-Tovar et al., 1994). Studies have examined progesterone vaginal suppositories or oral micronized progesterone. The largest placebo-controlled trial of progesterone suppositories failed to show efficacy for progesterone (Freeman et al., 1990) and a large recent comparison of oral micronized progesterone, alprazolam and placebo reported efficacy for alprazolam only (Freeman et al., 1995). A small recent comparison of oral progesterone, vaginal progesterone and placebo did not find significant differences between the treatments and there was a 40% placebo response (Vanselow et al., 1996) and a recent small placebo-controlled trial reported a decrease in nervous symptoms on only one of many assessment measures (Baker et al., 1995). A recent placebo-controlled trial did report progesterone to be superior to placebo (Magill, 1995). Reviews of studies of the synthetic progesterone dydrogesterone have also had largely negative results (Freeman, 1993; Rivera-Tovar et al., 1994). Although premenstrual progesterone use continues as a treatment for PMS, it has minimal support from the research literature.

Other somatic treatments have had initial promising reports in well-designed studies and deserve further research. These include calcium (Thys-Jacobs et al., 1989), magnesium (Facchinetti et al., 1991), vitamin E (London et al., 1987), mefenamic acid (Mira et al., 1986), naltrexone (Chuong et al., 1988), spironolactone (Hellberg et al., 1991; Wang et al., 1995) and doxycycline (Toth et al., 1988). Light therapy (Cerda & Parry, 1994) and sleep deprivation (Parry et al., 1995) also deserve further study. Nonpharmacological treatments that include dietary changes, exercise, cognitive-behavioral treatment, relaxation and group treatment have been reviewed recently (Pearlstein, 1996). Dietary recommendations of increased complex carbohydrate consumption and frequent meals may alleviate symptoms by providing more tryptophan for serotonin synthesis, and exercise may improve mood by increasing beta-endorphin levels. Dietary treatment recommendations need controlled studies. A small number of controlled studies do suggest efficacy for aerobic exercise, cognitive-behavioral techniques and relaxation (Rivera-Tovar et al., 1994; Pearlstein, 1996).

Conclusion

Studies conducted in the past decade have helped to define the most common symptoms of PMS and have helped to identify the subset of women with PMS who have the severest symptoms. Although specific etiologies have not been identified, it is expected that women with PMS have a vulnerability to express symptoms following the changes in gonadal hormones at each cycle. Other than previous depression, predictors of PMS or PMDD are not clear.

The clinician has several treatment options for a woman with PMS. Positive efficacy is most impressive with SSRIs and GnRH agonists, the former medications having the advantages of oral administration and fewer long-term health risks. Many of the treatment studies discussed in this chapter were conducted with women with the severe form of PMS, PMDD, and it can only be assumed at this point that the results are generalizable to the much larger group of women with PMS. SSRIs may also be a treatment option for women with premenstrual exacerbation of chronic underlying mood and anxiety symptoms. Many other pharmacological and nonpharmacological treatments deserve further study.

References

American Psychiatric Association (1994). *Diagnostic and Statistical Manual for Mental Disorders*, 4th edn. (DSM-IV). Washington, DC: American Psychiatric Press.

Backstrom T, Hansson-Malmstrom Y, Lindhe B, Cavalli-Bjorkman B & Nordernstrom S (1992). Oral contraceptives in premenstrual syndrome: a randomized comparison of triphasic and monophasic preparations. *Contraception*, **46**, 253–68.

Baker ER, Best RG, Manfredi RL, Demers LM & Wolf GC (1995). Efficacy of progesterone vaginal suppositories in alleviation of nervous symptoms in patients with premenstrual syndrome. *Journal of Assisted Reproduction and Genetics*, **12**, 205–9.

Bancroft J, Boyle H, Warner P & Fraser HM (1987). The use of an LHRH agonist, buserelin, in the long-term management of premenstrual syndromes. *Clinical Endocrinology*, **27**, 171–82.

Bancroft J & Cook A (1995). The neuroendrocrine response to *d*-fenfluramine in women with premenstrual depression. *Journal of Affective Disorders*, **36**, 57–64.

Bancroft J & Rennie D (1993). The impact of oral contraceptives on the experience of perimenstrual mood, clumsiness, food craving and other symptoms. *Journal of Psychosomatic Research*, **37**, 195–202.

Berger CP & Presser B (1994). Alprazolam in the treatment of two subsamples of patients with late luteal phase dysphoric disorder: a double-blind, placebo-controlled crossover study. *Obstetrics and Gynecology*, **84**, 379–85.

Braiden V & Metcalf G (1995). Premenstrual tension among hysterectomized women. *Journal of Psychosomatic Obstetrics and Gynecology*, **16**, 145–51.

Brown CS, Ling FW, Farmer RG & Sone BF (1990). Buspirone in the treatment of premenstrual syndrome. *Drug Therapy Supplement*, 112–20.

Brown CS, Ling FW, Andersen RN, Farmer RG & Arheart KL (1994). Efficacy of depot leuprolide in premenstrual syndrome: effect of symptom severity and type in a controlled trial. *Obstetrics and Gynecology*, **84**, 779–86.

Brzezinski AA, Wurtman JJ, Wurtman RJ, Gleason R, Greenfield J & Nader T (1990). d-Fenfluramine suppresses the increased calorie and carbohydrate intakes and improves the mood of women with premenstrual depression. *Obstetrics and Gynecology*, **76**, 296–301.

Cerda GM & Parry BL (1994). The effects of bright light therapy on symptoms of depression, anxiety and hibernation in patients with premenstrual syndrome. *Journal of Women's Health*, **3**, 5–15.

Chuong CJ & Burgos DM (1995). Medical history in women with premenstrual syndrome. *Journal of Psychosomatic Obstetrics and Gynecology*, **16**, 21–27.

Chuong, CJ, Coulam CB, Bergstralh EJ, O'Fallon WM & Steinmetz GI (1988). Clinical trial of naltrexone in premenstrual syndrome. *Obstetrics and Gynecology*, **72**, 332–6.

Deeny M, Hawthorn R & McKay Hart D (1991). Low dose danazol in the treatment of the premenstrual syndrome. *Postgraduate Medical Journal*, **67**, 450–4.

DeJong R, Rubinow DR, Roy-Byrne P, Hoban MC, Grover GN & Post RM (1985). Premenstrual mood disorder and psychiatric illness. *American Journal of Psychiatry*, **142**, 1359–61.

Eriksson E, Hedberg MA, Andersch B & Sundblad C (1995). The serotonin reuptake inhibitor paroxetin is superior to the noradrenaline reuptake inhibitor maprotiline in the treatment of premenstrual syndrome. *Neuropsychopharmacology*, **12**, 167–76.

Facchinetti F, Borella P, Sances G, Fioroni L, Nappi RE & Genazzani AR (1991). Oral magnesium successfully relieves premenstrual mood changes. *Obstetrics and Gynecology*, **78**, 177–81.

Facchinetti F, Genazzani AD, Martignoni E, Fioroni L, Nappi G & Genazzani AR (1993). Neuroendocrine changes in luteal function in patients with premenstrual syndrome. *Journal of Clinical Endocrinology and Metabolism*, **76**, 1123–7.

Frank RT, Goldberger MA, Salmon UJ & Felshin G (1937). Amenorrhea: its causation and treatment. *Journal of the American Medical Association*, **109**, 1863–9.

Freeman EW (1993). Progesterone therapy for premenstrual syndrome. In *Modern Management of Premenstrual Syndrome*, ed. S. Smith & I. Schiff, pp. 152–60. New York: Norton.

Freeman EW, Rickels K, Sondheimer SJ & Polansky M (1990). Ineffectiveness of progesterone suppository treatment for premenstrual syndrome. *Journal of the American Medical Association*, **264**, 349–53.

Freeman EW, Rickels K, Sondheimer SJ, Denis A, Pfeifer S & Weil S (1994). Nefazodone in the treatment of premenstrual syndrome: a preliminary study. *Journal of Clinical Psychopharmacology*, **14**, 180–6.

Freeman EW, Rickels K, Sondheimer SJ & Polansky M (1995). A double-blind trial of oral progesterone, alprazolam and placebo in treatment of severe premenstrual syndrome. *Journal of the American Medical Association*, **274**, 51–7.

Freeman EW, Rickels K & Sondheimer SJ (1996*a*). Fluvoxamine for premenstrual dysphoric disorder: a pilot study. *Journal of Clinical Psychiatry*, **57** (Suppl. 8), 56–60.

Freeman EW, Rickels K, Sondheimer SJ & Wittmaack FM (1996*b*). Sertraline versus desipramine in the treatment of premenstrual syndrome: an open-label trial. *Journal of Clinical Psychiatry*, **57**, 7–11.

Freeman EW, Sondheimer SJ, Rickels K & Albert J (1993). Gonadotropin-releasing hormone agonist in treatment of premenstrual symptoms with and without comorbidity of depression: a pilot study. *Journal of Clinical Psychiatry*, **54**, 192–5.

Girdler SS, Pedersen CA & Light KC (1995). Thyroid axis function during the menstrual cycle in women with premenstrual syndrome. *Psychoneuroendocrinology*, **20**, 395–403.

Graham CA & Sherwin BB (1992). A prospective treatment study of premenstrual symptoms using a triphasic oral contraceptive. *Journal of Psychosomatic Research*, **36**, 257–66.

Gurevich M (1995). Rethinking the label: who benefits from the PMS construct? *Women and Health*, **23**, 67–98.

Hahn PM, Van Vugt DA & Reid RL (1995). A randomized, placebo-controlled, crossover trial of danazol for the treatment of premenstrual syndrome. *Psychoneuroendocrinology*, **20**, 193–209.

Halbreich U (1995). Premenstrual dysphoric disorders, anxiety, and depressions: vulnerability traits or comorbidity. *Archives of General Psychiatry*, **52**, 606.

Halbreich U (1996). Pre-menstrual syndromes. In *Psychiatric Issues in Women (Clinical Psychiatry Series)*, ed. U. Halbreich, pp. 667–86. London: Bailliére's.

Halbreich U & Smoller JW (1997). Intermittent luteal phase sertraline treatment of dysphoric premenstrual syndrome. *Journal of Clinical Psychiatry*, **58**, 399–402.

Halbreich U, Endicott J, Goldstein S & Nee J (1986). Premenstrual changes and changes in gonadal hormones. *Acta Psychiatrica Scandinavica*, **74**, 576–86.

Halbreich U, Petty F, Yonkers K, Kramer GL, Rush AJ & Bibi KW (1996). Low plasma γ-aminobutyric acid levels during the late luteal phase of women with premenstrual dysphoric disorder. *American Journal of Psychiatry*, **153**, 718–20.

Halbreich U, Rojansky N & Palter S (1991). Elimination of ovulation and menstrual cyclicity (with danazol) improves dysphoric premenstrual syndromes. *Fertility and Sterility*, **56**, 1066–9.

Hammarback S & Backstrom T (1988). Induced anovulation as treatment of premenstrual tension syndrome. *Acta Obstetricia et Gynecologica Scandinavica*, **67**, 159–66.

Harrison WM, Endicott J & Nee J (1989*a*). Treatment of premenstrual depression with nortriptyline: a pilot study. *Journal of Clinical Psychiatry*, **50**, 136–9.

Harrison WM, Endicott J, Nee J, Glick H & Rabkin JG (1989*b*). Characteristics of women seeking treatment for 'Premenstrual syndrome'. *Psychosomatics*, **30**, 405–11.

Harrison WM, Endicott J & Nee J (1990). Treatment of premenstrual dysphoria with alprazolam. *Archives of General Psychiatry*, **47**, 270–5.

Hellberg D, Claesson B & Nilsson S (1991). Premenstrual tension: a placebo-controlled efficacy study with spironolactone and medroxyprogesterone acetate. *International Journal of Gynecology and Obstetrics*, **34**, 243–8.

Helvacioglu A, Yeoman RR, Hazelton JM & Aksel S (1993). Premenstrual syndrome and related hormonal changes: long-acting gonadotropin releasing hormone agonist treatment. *Journal of Reproductive Medicine*, **38**, 864–70.

Hussain SY, Massil JH, Matta WH, Shaw RW & O'Brien PMS (1992). Buserelin in premenstrual syndrome. *Gynecological Endocrinology*, **6**, 57–64.

Korzekwa MI, Lamont JA & Steiner M (1996). Late luteal phase dysphoric disorder and the thyroid axis revisited. *Journal of Clinical Endocrinology and Metabolism*, **81**, 2280–4.

Lewis, LL, Greenblatt EM, Rittenhouse CA, Veldhuis JD & Jaffe RB (1995). Pulsatile release patterns of luteinizing hormone and progesterone in relation to symptom onset in women with premenstrual syndrome. *Fertility and Sterility*, **64**, 288–92.

London RS, Murphy L, Kitlowski KE & Reynolds MA (1987). Efficacy of alpha-tocopherol in the treatment of premenstrual syndrome. *Journal of Reproductive Medicine*, **32**, 400–4.

Magill PJ (1995). Investigation of the efficacy of progesterone pessaries in the relief of symptoms of premenstrual syndrome. *British Journal of General Practice*, **45**, 589–93.

Menkes DB, Taghavi E, Mason PA, Spears GFS & Howard RC (1992). Fluoxetine treatment of severe premenstrual syndrome. *British Medical Journal*, **305**, 346–7.

Menkes DB, Coates DC & Fawcett JP (1994). Acute tryptophan depletion aggravates premenstrual syndrome. *Journal of Affective Disorders*, **32**, 37–44.

Metcalf MG, Braiden V, Livesey JH & Wells JE (1992). The premenstrual syndrome: amelioration of symptoms after hysterectomy. *Journal of Psychosomatic Research*, **36**, 569–84.

Mezrow G, Shoupe D, Spicer D, Lobo R, Leung B & Pike M (1994). Depot leuprolide acetate with estrogen and progestin add-back for long-term treatment of premenstrual syndrome. *Fertility and Sterility*, **62**, 932–7.

Mira M, McNeil D, Fraser IS, Vizzard J & Abraham S (1986). Mefenamic acid in the treatment of premenstrual syndrome. *Obstetrics and Gynecology*, **68**, 395–8.

Mortola JF, Girton L & Fischer U (1991). Successful treatment of severe premenstrual syndrome by combined use of gonadotropin-releasing hormone agonist and estrogen/progestin. *Journal of Clinical Endocrinology and Metabolism*, **71**, 252A–252F.

Muse K (1993). Treatment of premenstrual syndrome with ovulation suppression. In *Modern Management of Premenstrual Syndrome*, ed. S. Smith & I. Schiff, pp. 128–36. New York: Norton.

Muse KN, Cetel NS, Futterman LA & Yen SSC (1984). The premenstrual syndrome: effects of 'medical ovariectomy'. *New England Journal of Medicine*, **311**, 1345–9.

Ozeren S, Corakci A, Yucesoy I, Mercan R & Erhan G (1997). Fluoxetine in the treatment of premenstrual syndrome. *European Journal of Obstetrics and Gynecology*, **73**, 167–70.

Parry BL (1994). Biological correlates of premenstrual complaints. In *Premenstrual Dysphorias: Myths and Realities*, ed. J. H. Gold & S. K. Severino, pp. 47–66. Washington, DC: American Psychiatric Press.

Parry BL, Cover H, Mostofi N, LeVeau B, Sependa PA, Resnick A & Gillin JC (1995). Early versus late partial sleep deprivation in patients with premenstrual dysphoric disorder and normal comparison subjects. *American Journal of Psychiatry*, **152**, 404–12.

Parry BL, Ehlers CL, Mostofi N & Phillips E (1996). Personality traits in LLPDD and normal controls during follicular and luteal menstrual-cycle phases. *Psychological Medicine*, **26**, 197–202.

Pearlstein TB (1995). Hormones and depression: what are the facts about premenstrual syndrome, menopause and hormone replacement therapy? *American Journal of Obstetrics and Gynecology*, **173**, 646–53.

Pearlstein T (1996). Nonpharmacologic treatment of premenstrual syndrome. *Psychiatric Annals*, **26**, 590–4.

Pearlstein TB & Stone AB (1994). Long-term fluoxetine treatment of late luteal phase dysphoric disorder. *Journal of Clinical Psychiatry*, **55**, 332–5.

Pearlstein TB, Frank E, Rivera-Tovar A, Thoft JS, Jacobs E & Mieczkowski TA (1990). Prevalence of axis I and axis II disorders in women with late luteal phase dysphoric disorder. *Journal of Affective Disorders*, **20**, 129–34.

Pearlstein TB, Stone AB, Lund SA, Scheft H, Zlotnick C & Brown WA (1997). Comparison of fluoxetine, bupropion, and placebo in the treatment of premenstrual dysphoric disorder. *Journal of Clinical Psychopharmacology*, **17**, 261–6.

Reame NE, Marshall JC & Kelch RP (1992). Pulsatile LH secretion in women with premenstrual syndrome (PMS): evidence for normal neuroregulation of the menstrual cycle. *Psychoneuroendocrinology*, **17**, 205–13.

Richardson JTE (1995). The premenstrual syndrome: a brief history. *Social Science and Medicine*, **41**, 761–7.

Rickels K, Freeman E & Sondheimer S (1989). Buspirone in treatment of premenstrual syndrome. *Lancet*, **1**, 777.

Rivera-Tovar A, Rhodes R, Pearlstein TB & Frank E (1994). Treatment efficacy. In *Premenstrual Dysphorias: Myths and Realities*, ed. J. H. Gold & S. K. Severino, pp. 99–148. Washington, DC: American Psychiatric Press.

Rubinow, DR & Schmidt PJ (1995). The neuroendocrinology of menstrual cycle mood disorders. *Annals of the New York Academy of Sciences*, **771**, 648–659.

Rubinow DR, Hoban MC, Grover GN, Galloway DS, Roy-Byrne P, Andersen R & Merriam GR (1988). Changes in plasma hormones across the menstrual cycle in patients with menstrually related mood disorder and in control subjects. *American Journal of Obstetrics and Gynecology*, **158**, 5–11.

Schmidt PJ, Grover GN & Rubinow DR (1993). Alprazolam in the treatment of premenstrual syndrome. *Archives of General Psychiatry*, **50**, 467–73.

Schmidt PJ, Nieman LK, Grover GN, Muller KL, Merriam GR & Rubinow DR (1991). Lack of effect of induced menses on symptoms in women with premenstrual syndrome. *New England Journal of Medicine*, **324**, 1174–9.

Schmidt PJ, Purdy RH, Moore PH, Paul SM & Rubinow DR (1994). Circulating levels of anxiolytic steroids in the luteal phase in women with premenstrual syndrome and in control subjects. *Journal of Clinical Endocrinology and Metabolism*, **79**, 1256–60.

Schnurr PP, Hurt SW & Stout AL (1994). Consequences of methodological decisions in the diagnosis of late luteal phase dysphoric disorder. In *Premenstrual Dysphorias: Myths and Realities*, ed. J. H. Gold & S. K. Severino, pp. 19–46. Washington, DC: American Psychiatric Press.

Severino SK (1994). A focus on 5-hydroytryptamine (serotonin) and psychopathology. In *Premenstrual Dysphorias: Myths and Realities*, ed. J. H. Gold & S. K. Severino, pp. 67–98. Washington, DC: American Psychiatric Press.

Severino SK & Moline ML (1989). *Premenstrual Syndrome: A Clinician's Guide*. New York: Guilford Press.

Severino SK, Hurt SW & Shindledecker RD (1989). Late luteal phase dysphoric disorder: special analysis of cyclic symptoms. *American Journal of Psychiatry*, **146**, 1155–60.

Smith RNJ, Studd JWW, Zamblera D & Holland EFN (1995). A randomized comparison over 8 months of 100 μg and 200 μg twice weekly doses of transdermal oestradiol in the treatment of severe premenstrual syndrome. *British Journal of Obstetrics and Gynaecology*, **102**, 475–84.

Smith S, Rinehart JS, Ruddock VE & Schiff I (1987). Treatment of premenstrual syndrome with alprazolam: results of a double-blind, placebo-controlled, randomized crossover clinical trial. *Obstetrics and Gynecology*, **70**, 37–43.

Steiner M, Steinberg S, Stewart D, Carter D, Berger C, Reid R, Grover D & Streiner D (1995). Fluoxetine in the treatment of premenstrual dysphoria. *New England Journal of Medicine*, **332**, 1529–34.

Stone AB, Pearlstein TB & Brown WA (1991). Fluoxetine in the treatment of late luteal phase dysphoric disorder. *Journal of Clinical Psychiatry*, **52**, 290–3.

Studd J & Leather AT (1996). The need for add-back with gonadotrophin-releasing hormone agonist therapy. *British Journal of Obstetrics and Gynaecology*, **103** (Suppl. 14), 1–4.

Su TP, Schmidt PJ, Danaceau MA, Tobin MB, Rosenstein DL, Murphy DL & Rubinow DR (1997). Fluoxetine in the treatment of premenstrual dysphoria. *Neuropsychopharmacology*, **16**, 346–56.

Sundblad C, Hedberg MA & Eriksson E (1993). Clomipramine administered during the luteal phase reduces the symptoms of premenstrual syndrome: a placebo-controlled trial. *Neuropsychopharmacology*, **9**, 133–45.

Sundblad C, Modigh K, Andersch B & Eriksson E (1991). Clomipramine effectively reduces premenstrual irritability and dysphoria: a placebo-controlled trial. *Acta Psychiatrica Scandinavica*, **85**, 39–47.

Taghavi E, Menkes DB, Howard RC, Mason PA, Shaw JP & Spears GFS (1995). Premenstrual syndrome: a double-blind controlled trial of desipramine and methylscopolamine. *International Clinical Psychopharmacology*, **10**, 119–22.

Thys-Jacobs S, Ceccarelli S, Bierman A, Weisman H, Cohen M & Alvir J (1989). Calcium supplementation in premenstrual syndrome: a randomized crossover trial. *Journal of General Internal Medicine*, **4**, 183–9.

Toth A, Lesser ML, Naus G, Brooks C & Adams D (1988). Effect of doxycycline on pre-menstrual syndrome: a double-blind randomized clinical trial. *Journal of International Medical Research*, **16**, 270–9.

Vanselow W, Dennerstein L, Greenwood KM & deLignieres B (1996). Effect of progesterone and its 5α and 5β metabolites on symptoms of premenstrual syndrome according to route of administration. *Journal of Psychosomatic Obstetrics and Gynecology*, **17**, 29–38.

Wang M, Hammarback S, Lindhe BA & Backstrom T (1995). Treatment of premenstrual syndrome by spironolactone: a double-blind, placebo-controlled study. *Acta Obstetricia et Gynecologica Scandinavica*, **74**, 803–8.

Watson NR & Studd JWW (1993). The use of estrogen in the treatment of premenstrual syndrome. In *Modern Management of Premenstrual Syndrome*, ed. S. Smith & I. Schiff, pp. 137–51. New York: Norton.

Wood SH, Mortola JF, Chan YF, Moossazadeh F & Yen SSC (1992). Treatment of premenstrual syndrome with fluoxetine: a double-blind, placebo-controlled, crossover study. *Obstetrics and Gynecology*, **80**, 339–44.

Yonkers KA, Gullion C, Williams A, Novak K & Rush AJ (1996). Paroxetine as a treatment for premenstrual dysphoric disorder. *Journal of Clinical Psychopharmacology*, **16**, 3–8.

Yonkers KA, Halbreich U, Freeman E, Brown C, Endicott J, Frank E, Parry B, Pearlstein T, Severino S, Stout A, Stone A & Harrison W (1997). Symptomatic improvement of premenstrual dysphoric disorder with sertraline treatment: a randomized controlled trial. *Journal of the American Medical Association*, **278**, 983–8.

6

Interstitial Cystitis

NGOC HO, JAMES A. KOZIOL AND
C. LOWELL PARSONS

Interstitial cystitis (IC) is a chronic debilitating disorder affecting primarily females. It is characterized by pain in the region of the bladder and pelvic musculature, and variable motor and sensory dysfunctions of the bladder. There is currently no consensus regarding the unique clinical, endoscopic or histological features of IC. Diagnosis is typically based on the patients' symptomatology, urological evaluation, including cystoscopy and histopathological findings, and the exclusion of other recognizable bladder diseases. The most prevalent symptoms of IC are urinary frequency, urgency, and suprapubic, pelvic or perineal pain. Although the etiology of this disease remains obscure, putative causative agents include infection, vascular or lymphatic obstruction, neurogenic, endocrinological or inflammatory causation, autoimmune reactions, dysfunction of the bladder mucus and the presence of toxic substances in the urine. As it is a syndrome, perhaps several etiologies are operating. The wide range of treatment modalities also reflects this lack of etiological clarity. The majority of patients can expect relief of their symptoms to varying degrees, even though treatment is frequently nonspecific and noncurative.

The direct medical costs for diagnosis and treatment, as well as the indirect costs due to significant work disability and other limitations of patient functional status, are potentially large. Yet no systematic studies of the costs of illness for interstitial cystitis have been published.

History

Inflammations present in the bladder wall of female patients were depicted as transmural or 'interstitial' cystitis (IC) by Skene (1878) in a monograph on female bladder and urethral disease. This was later described by Nitze (1907) as 'cystitis parenchymatosa', an uncommon lesion of the urinary bladder. Subsequently, it was popularized by Hunner (1915), who called it 'a rare type of bladder ulcer', and later, the 'elusive' Hunner's ulcer (1918). In his initial report, Hunner described eight patients with inflammations in the bladder wall and symptoms of frequency, nocturia, urgency and perineurial pain. Cystoscopic examination demonstrated small ulcers or areas of dead white scar tissues with surrounding hyperemia which bled upon contact, a sign of ulceration. The cause of the lesion was unknown in all cases. Unfortunately, these findings of ulceration by Hunner have led to the underdiagnosis of IC, because it was later learned that only 5–10% (Sant, 1991) of IC patients actually have ulcers.

Messing & Stamey (1978) first described the 'nonulcer' variety of IC and emphasized its prevalence. The lack of ulceration in the majority of patients was in direct conflict with previous descriptions of IC. This led to a more frequent diagnosis of IC and the realization that there were two subtypes of the disease: the uncommon Hunner's ulcer disease, and the more common 'early' or 'nonulcer' variety. Messing & Stamey also established the presence of 'mucosal glomerulations' as the endoscopic hallmark of the condition.

In 1984, an advocacy group, The Interstitial Cystitis Association (ICA), was formed in the USA. Its goals are focused on education, research and patient support. In 1987–88, two multidisciplinary workshops on IC were held by the National Institute of Arthritis, Diabetes, Digestive and Kidney Diseases (NIDDK), a branch from the National Institutes of Health, to review knowledge regarding the syndrome, to identify areas for future research and to establish guidelines for diagnosis. The latter has relied heavily upon physicians' interpretation of the disorder and is based mainly on the exclusion of other recognizable bladder diseases. Two ground-breaking projects were funded by the NIDDK during this period. One examined the activities of the mucosal lining of the bladder and its involvement in the symptoms of IC. The other examined the effect of a synthetic sulfated polysaccharide, Elmiron®, on the mucosal lining to alleviate symptoms of IC. In addition, another project, partially funded by the ICA, examined the role of the mast cell and IC (Slade, 1989).

Since 1987, the NIDDK contribution toward IC research has consistently grown. In 1990, they spent $1.6 million on seven projects. In 1991, through the persistency of the ICA, they granted $2.5 million of additional funding. In 1993, $4 million was given for research (Ratner et al., 1994). This growing investment reflects a rise in awareness and concern for a cryptic syndrome with no known cause and increasing incidence. Since 1992 in the USA the NIDDK has implemented a nationwide IC data base. Nine clinical centers and one data coordinating center are involved in the collection of data on more than 1300 people with mild, moderate or severe symptoms. It is expected that this project will provide more insight on the development, course and treatment of IC (Hanno, 1994).

Definition

Interstitial cystitis is a syndrome characterized by variable motor and sensory dysfunctions of the bladder. The most prevalent symptoms of IC are urinary frequency, urgency and suprapubic, pelvic or perineal pain. Frequency at night is especially indicative of IC, because patients suffering from other voiding dysfunctions typically do not complain of nightly voiding. Pathological features include inflammation, edema and vasodilation of the submucosa and detrusor layers of the bladder wall (Hunner, 1915; Messing & Stamey, 1978; Holm-Bentzen et al., 1985; Johansson & Fall, 1989). This can result in scarring and stiffening of the bladder, diminution in bladder capacity and glomerulations (petechial hemorrhages). In rare cases, ulcers in the bladder lining can occur.

IC can be classified into the two categories of Hunner's ulcer (classic) and nonulcer (early), based on cystoscopic findings. The cystoscopic appearance of the ulcerative or 'classic' type was described by Johansson & Fall (1989):

> It displays single or multiple patches of reddened bladder mucosa. The redness, on careful examination, is shown to be caused by erythema of the mucosa with small vessels radiating to a central, pale scar, fibrin deposit or coagulum. Central rupture at this site occurs during bladder distension with the patient under general or spinal anesthesia, at a hydrostatic pressure of 70 to 80 cm water. After mucosal rupture, oozing of blood from the mucosal margins and the ulcer bottom occurs, and this is the so-called elusive ulcer of Hunner. After a second distension petechial hemorrhages frequently are seen in areas next to the ulcer but also frequently in areas distant from the ulcer. Another characteristic, postdistension finding is mild or occasionally marked bullous swelling.

Another distinction is that granulation tissue was present in 94% of the ulcerative cases. The remaining 6% had moderate symptoms and only limited biopsy tissues were available for examination. In contrast, no granulation tissue was found in nonulcerative IC patients (Jokinen et al., 1972).

The nonulcerative or 'early' type of IC does not display circumscript lesions, only hemorrhages that are commonly referred to as glomerulations. This occasionally is seen during the first filling, but usually appears on redistention throughout the vesical mucosa. Occasionally, stellate scars that crack and bleed, or mucosal fissures, may be seen (Messing & Stamey, 1978; Hanno & Wein, 1987*a,b*; Johansson & Fall, 1989).

Koziol et al. (1995) investigated whether the classification of 565 cases of IC into ulcer and nonulcer categories from cystoscopic findings could be corroborated with epidemiological data relating to demographics, risk factors, symptoms, pain and psychosocial factors. In an initial univariate analysis of the epidemiological data, they identified ten noninvasive variables (hematuria, pain centered at right, lower abdomen, standing relieves pain, sharp pain, weight change or eating disorder, irritable bowel syndrome, dull aching pain, dyspareunia, and efficacy of urination) to be significantly associated with the presence of Hunner's ulcers. None of the ten variables could individually discriminate ulcer from nonulcer patients with a high degree of accuracy, i.e., individually among these ten variables, the correct classification rates of the IC patients into the ulcer and nonulcer categories ranged from 57% to 71%. Hence, no one variable could adequately discriminate between the two categories with high sensitivity and high specificity. On the other hand, they found that reasonable accuracy in classifying ulcer versus nonulcer patients was obtainable from statistical methodologies that combine the ten variables into multivariate classification rules, with overall misclassification rates of 20% or smaller. Their findings suggest the two categories of IC might well represent different manifestations of the underlying disease pathophysiology.

Koziol et al. (1994, 1995, and unpublished results) recently reported that 10–20% of IC patients suffer from the classic type. This is more than a previous estimate by Sant (1991) of 5–10%. It should be noted, however, that the cohort of IC patients studied by Koziol et al., from tertiary care centers, is likely to be more representative of moderate to severe IC, with very few early onset patients. The bladder capacity is found to be more reduced in the classic type of IC. Messing & Stamey (1978) reported cystoscopy findings in 16 patients (nine early and seven classic) under anesthesia. They found all but one patient to have a bladder capacity less than 450 ml in the classic IC type, and all of the early IC types to have capacity more than 450 ml. Johansson & Fall (1989) found the mean capacity to be 453 ml (range 75–1100 ml) in patients with classical IC, compared with 816 ml (range 450–1250 ml) in patients with early IC. Another revealing distinction between the two types is the concentration of mononuclear cells present in the mucosa. Of the patients with classic IC, 91% had an extensive inflammatory response (2+ or 3+), which was in stark contrast to the early IC patients, of whom only 20% had + or 2+ degree of mononuclear inflammatory infiltrate (Johansson & Fall, 1989). Erickson et al. (1994) found that patients with severe inflammation (100 or more mononuclear cells/high power field or lymphoid aggregates) experienced better symptom relief after cystoscopy with bladder distention under anesthesia than patients with milder inflammation (less than 100 mononuclear cells/high power field).

Case presentations

Case 1

A 19-year-old patient was referred from the Student Health Center with history of recurrent urinary tract infection. In the past seven months she had been diagnosed with 'six urinary tract infections'. On each occasion she had a culture performed at the health center which was available for review. On the very first visit she had one culture positive for *E. coli* and, subsequent to that, she had five cultures showing no infection. Prior to this, she was treated with multiple courses of antibiotic therapy and then referred to Urology. She gave a seven month history of pain during sex (and for several days thereafter) and 'infections associated with sex'. For evaluation she had urine culture performed by catheterization which showed no infection. A urodynamic evaluation demonstrated a bladder capacity of 220 ml (normal 450 ml) and sensory urgency to void at 70 ml (normal 150 ml). She also kept a voiding log for three days and averaged ten voids per day, 45 ml per void. She previously had an intravenous pyelogram which showed normal upper urinary tract and no significant bladder pathology.

The working diagnosis was interstitial cystitis. She was treated with a bladder dilatation and had dramatic relief of her symptoms. Pain with sexual intercourse completely resolved. She has remained asymptomatic for the past two years and has not been seen since she graduated from the university.

Case 2

A 45-year-old female was referred with a chronic history of interstitial cystitis. Her symptoms of urinary urgency/frequency date back 20 years, perhaps longer, when she noted she was a more frequent voider than other individuals. Currently she states she voids about 16 times a day and one to three times at night. She had adjusted her life style around the urgency/frequency somewhat successfully. Approximately six years ago she started to experience great discomfort and/or pain associated with her bladder, which steadily progressed. She noted that the pain became worse just before her menstrual cycle and was aggravated by sexual intercourse both during and for several days after.

She first consulted a physician for complaints associated with her bladder perhaps 15 years ago. At this time she was told she had a 'bladder infection'. The patient stated she had had a large number of 'infections' over the years which were treated with antibiotics. It was about six years ago that she first saw a urologist for the pain associated with her bladder and he told her she had trigonitis. This resulted in therapy which was initially a urethral dilation which did little to relieve her symptoms. Subsequently, approximately four years ago, she underwent a course of dimethylsulfoxide treatment at which point she experienced significant remission of her symptoms for six to eight months. Then the symptom of pain began to reappear and she had a cystoscopy and dilatation of her bladder performed under anesthesia about three years ago and had relief of symptoms for perhaps six to ten months. The patient has been on a number of medications including antidepressants, antibiotics and anticholinergic therapy, none of which specifically relieved her symptoms.

On urodynamic evaluation she was noted to have a bladder capacity of approximately 240 ml (normal 450 ml) and first sensation to void at 75 ml. The patient kept a voiding log and she averaged 70 ml per void and voided 14 times per day and two times at night. While she does have adequate bladder function, she has a low urine flow rate compared with normals. Urinary culture and cytology were normal and urinalysis showed no hematuria.

A course of intravesical heparin therapy was initiated and she self-administered the drug once per day. After approximately six to eight months, she had significant relief of her symptoms and has been maintained on this therapy three times per week and has been in remission for almost 1.5 years.

These two patients represent typical presentations for the IC syndrome. The younger patient represents what the older patient probably had at a similar age and stage of disease, but the disease usually has a significant delay in diagnosis because it is misdiagnosed as recurrent 'bladder infections'. Any woman who is chronically treated with antibiotics after sexual intercourse and who is treated for repeated infections during the course of a year, in all likelihood, has IC, in a mild, moderate or severe form. The problem with correctly diagnosing the 19-year-old is related both to her age and to severity of her symptoms.

As urinary tract infection (UTI) has similar symptoms and is easier to treat (antibiotics), this is the usual diagnosis made. Compounding this error is the fact that in the early stages, IC flares with sexual intercourse and the menstrual cycle for only several days and appears to respond well to antibiotic therapy. When the IC symptoms resolve, the antibiotic is given credit for the improvement.

Most physicians have a bias that the disease has to be more severe and present in older females. It is important to recognize IC in the younger age group because it can be treated relatively easily and one can induce remissions that last for a long period of time. Otherwise, the disease tends to incubate slowly with the symptoms gradually progressing and the bladder becoming more and more dysfunctional and difficult to treat. The younger patient represents a typical response in a milder patient in that a minimal dilatation procedure resulted in prolonged remission.

The second patient represents a more typical patient who is more likely to be diagnosed with IC. The former was diagnosed only because she happened to present to our clinic. Many urologists would have concurred with the UTI diagnosis and evaluated as such with perhaps radiographs and cystoscopy. In all likelihood, the younger patient would have taken 10–12 years of symptoms before she would have been classified as IC. The latter patient, initially classified as trigonitis, has a more typical history for the advanced case. It usually begins with urgency/frequency and only after years does the pain begin to appear. The patient is more likely to seek urological care because of the increasing discomfort associated with her bladder. This is the patient who will eventually be diagnosed as IC, although initially she may be told she has urinary tract infections and then other diagnoses like trigonitis. Basically it is the same disease process for both patients and one should use the term IC for all diagnoses as these patients, for the most part, represent the same patient population with varying degrees of severity.

Prevalence, incidence and epidemiological factors

Prevalence

Oravisto (1975) estimated the prevalence of IC for Helsinki, Finland, and in the surrounding area to be 10.6 patients per 100 000 inhabitants for the total population. The female prevalence was 18.1 per 100 000 women of all ages.

An epidemiology study by Held et al. (1990) used three methods to estimate the prevalence of IC in the USA from information supplied in a random survey of 127 board certified urologists. The three estimated values were 16.3 per 100 000; 25.1 per 100 000; and 76.3 per 100 000, the average being 36.6 per 100 000.

Bade et al. (1995), on the basis of a urologist-based questionnaire study, estimated the prevalence of IC in the Netherlands to be 8–16 cases per 100 000 female patients, in close agreement with Oravisto's estimate. On the other hand, a recent population-based survey (Jones et al., 1994) suggested that the prevalence of IC in the USA might well exceed 0.51% among adults, an order of magnitude higher than any previous finding (although the methodology of Jones et al. has yet to be validated).

Incidence

Between 1962 and 1972, Oravisto (1975) observed a minimal annual incidence rate of 0.66 cases of IC per 100 000 inhabitants in the city of Helsinki and surrounding area. The yearly estimated female incidence rate during the same period was 1.2 cases per 100 000 women. Held et al. (1990) estimated an incidence rate for the USA to be 2.6 per 100 000, a figure four times higher than the estimate reported by Oravisto.

Several possibilities for the incongruities in incidence and prevalence rates between the two studies were postulated by Held et al.: (1) extrapolation of Oravisto's estimates from Finland in 1975 to the USA in 1987 may not be valid; (2) there may be a nonresponse bias from the 1987 survey, as the response rate from urologists asked to participate in the survey was only 26%; and (3) the population may not be the same for these two studies, as there were no uniform or established diagnostic criteria for IC applied in both studies.

Epidemiological factors

Koziol et al. (1994) examined epidemiological evidence relating to: (1) demography, (2) medical history, (3) type and severity of symptoms, (4) location, frequency and intensity of pain, (5) duration of symptoms, (6) behaviors that exacerbate or curtail symptoms, and (7) psychosocial factors, in 565 IC patients. Patients were classified into three severity groups based on treatment histories and physiological findings relating to IC. This classification scheme was used subsequently to ascertain whether variables such as risk factors, duration of disease, symptoms and psychosocial factors were related to disease history and severity. Category 3 included 111 patients (19.7%) with severe symptoms whose urologist had found a Hunner's ulcer (classic IC). Category 2 included 403 patients (71.3%) with severe symptoms who had documented abnormal bladder biopsies and urodynamic and endoscopic findings excluding neurological causes of frequency/urgency.

Category 1 included 51 patients (9.0%) with severe symptoms who had documented abnormal bladder biopsies but lacked reports of other supportive endoscopic and urodynamic findings. Patients were also classified into four subgroups with respect to the number of years with symptoms, the purpose here being to ascertain whether any survey response variables tend to increase or decrease among patients as the number of years with symptoms increases. A brief discussion of these findings is given next.

Demography

Patients were primarily Caucasian (94.3%) and female (88.8%). Patients suffering from the classic syndrome were significantly older than other IC patients. The mean age reported for these patients was 57.9 years; the mean age reported for early IC patients was 50.1 years. (In a recent study, Close et al. (1996) identified the occurrence of IC in a small group of children. The significance of IC symptoms in this cohort will be better understood when more knowledge on the etiology and natural history of IC is acquired. Patients suffering from the classic syndrome experienced first symptoms at a later date than early IC patients. Oravisto (1980) reported that the symptoms associated with IC generally progress rapidly to a final state, with little worsening thereafter. Koziol et al. noted similarly that symptoms typically plateau within five years of onset, and that onset of IC is not homogenous over time. Overall, patients with symptoms for longer periods of time tended to be older than patients with symptoms for shorter periods.

Risk factors

Sixty-four percent of IC patients and only 23% of controls had one or more risk factors from the grouping hysterectomy, abdominal cramping, irritable bowel syndrome, spastic colon and a cluster of factors with a possible psychosomatic component ($p < 0.00001$). Overall, 72% of patients and 50% of controls had one or more risk factors from the grouping consisting of sensitivity or allergic reaction to medication, rheumatoid arthritis, sinusitis, food allergy, hay fever, asthma and a cluster of immunopathological abnormalities associated with an autoimmune component ($p < 0.00001$). Other investigators have also reported a high frequency of allergy among IC patients: Messing & Stamey (1978), 25%; Oravisto et al. (1970), 26%; Holm-Bentzen et al. (1987), 34%; Hand (1949), 15% in IC patients versus 8.5% in controls. As a large number of IC patients undergo surgical, gynecological and obstetric procedures, Hollander (1994) suggested that an allergy to silk sutures remaining in the urogenital region might cause the symptoms of IC in some susceptible individuals. Silk had also been reported to cause symptoms of pneumonitis, pulmonary fibrosis, postoperative 'pyoderma gangrenosum' and asthma (Nagazawa & Umegae 1990; Wen et al., 1990; Uragoda et al., 1991; Long et al., 1992). Oravisto et al. (1970) observed that in two of their patients, symptoms began abruptly after a gynecological operation. In contrast, Koziol found no significant relation between asthma and symptoms of IC ($p = 0.153$).

Few studies have investigated any genetic or ethnic associations with IC. Oravisto (1980) reported IC developing in a set of monozygotic twins and in a mother and daughter. From the sample obtained by Koziol (1994), two sets of sisters, including one set of monozygotic twins, were found with formally diagnosed IC. One cannot therefore dismiss a genetic component to the origin of IC. Held et al. (1990) had reported 14% (126 of 902) of one sample of IC patients to be of Jewish origin compared with 3% (3 of 119) of a general population sample. In comparison, 15.3% (20 of 131) of the sample in Koziol's study are of Jewish origin, a higher-than-expected proportion under a nonassociation model. This suggestion of an excess risk of IC among individuals of Jewish origin would not be unique to IC, for example ulcerative colitis is two to four times more frequent in individuals of Jewish origin than in nonJews. There is also the possibility that IC may be diagnosed more quickly and, therefore, more frequently within this population owing to easier access to high quality health care.

Symptoms of interstitial cystitis

Substantial proportions of patients reported symptoms of urgency (91.9%), frequency (91.2%), pelvic pain (69.9%), pelvic pressure (63.3%), dysuria (60.5%), pain during intercourse (55.2%), burning (55.1%), awakened at night by pain (50.8%), pain for days after intercourse (36.7%) and hematuria (21.6%). In addition, patients with bladder ulcers tended to report greater frequency (increased number of voids per 24-hour period, shorter intervals between nighttime voids) than other IC patients; they also reported blood in their urine more often and were more likely to be awakened at night by IC pain. Frequency, bladder spasms and efficacy of urinating were found to increase significantly as duration of symptoms increased.

Pain

Over 55% of patients reported daily or constant pain and nearly 57% characterized their pain as severe or excruciating. Frequency and intensity did not seem to vary across severity groups, nor did frequency, intensity and type of pain vary with duration of symptoms. Patients with the classic syndrome tended to report less dull, aching pain, but more spasms and sharp or hot, stabbing pain in the right lower abdomen compared with the other IC patients. Urinating was quite effective in relieving IC pain, particularly for Hunner's ulcer patients. Medication was also somewhat effective, but behaviors such as hot baths, heating pad, activity or diversion from the pain, lying down (stretched out), lying down (curled up), sitting and standing seemed ineffective. Stress increased IC pain in 61% of patients. Pain during sexual intercourse was reported by 50% of respondents. Acidic, alcoholic or carbonated beverages and spicy foods tended to increase IC pain for more patients with the classic syndrome compared with other IC patients. Patients tended to become increasingly intolerant of the listed beverage and food types as the number of years with symptoms increased, although the trends usually were not statistically significant.

Psychosocial factors

Overall, a substantial number of patients reported psychological or related symptoms such as: an inability to enjoy their usual activities, 68% (only 5.7% of patients found travel not to be difficult or impossible, 10.3% leisure activities and 11.6% sleep); tiredness, 63.6%; depression, 56.4%; inability to concentrate, 50%; insomnia or excessive daytime sleepiness, 49.7%; weight change or eating disorder, 36.4%; feelings of worthlessness, 30.8%; experience of phobias, anxiety or panic attacks, 27.3%; a nervous breakdown or undergoing psychiatric care, 16.7%. There were insignificant differences in the prevalence of symptoms when patients' reports were classified either by severity or by duration. Difficulties in performing everyday tasks were experienced at equivalent rates by patients in each severity group regardless of duration of symptoms, with the exception that there was less job satisfaction in terms of positions matching qualifications among the long-term (ten or more years with symptoms) IC patients than among those with fewer than ten years with symptoms. Family relationships and responsibilities were adversely affected in 70% of the patients.

Economic costs

The economic costs of IC can be profound. Held and colleagues provided economic findings from a 1987 epidemiological investigation of IC (these estimates might be viewed as provisional, as few details concerning the conduct, reliability or validity of this study were provided). Held et al. (1990) divided the costs of IC into two components: (1) medical care, which includes the cost of hospitalizations, doctors and therapy; and (2) losses due to the inability to work, and emotional and physical suffering. In 1987, the average annual medical cost per IC patient was estimated to be $3870. This leads to a total estimated annual cost in the USA of $170.3 million (using an estimated prevalence in 1987 of 44 000 female IC patients). This estimate, however, includes medical costs in the absence of IC. The estimated incremental medical cost attributable to IC is $116.6 million per year.

In terms of indirect costs, Held et al. (1987) estimated that 24.9% of female IC patients were less likely to be working full-time compared with a normal female population (matched for age, sex and education). This loss in income was partially compensated by a 4.1% increase in part-time work, again compared with a matched sample. IC patients were also reported to receive on the average $3.41 less per hour than did a matched sample. Using the national average wage rate for all females, the lost income per year would amount to $4039 per patient, not including any wage reduction for those IC patients who were able to work. The inclusion of the IC wage reduction would increase the amount to $7084 per year. The total lost incomes in 1987 would amount to $177.7 million or $311.7 million with the wage reduction.

Confirmations

Unanimity of views has not been obtained on any of the major research findings relating to IC. We outline, in the following sections, research contradictions regarding IC, along with research findings relating to the therapeutic effectiveness of various treatment modalities in IC.

Contradictions

Dysfunctional bladder epithelium

The bladder mucosa is lined by a layer of sulfonate glycosaminoglycans (GAGs): hyaluronic acid, heparin, chondroitin, sulfates, dermatin sulfate and keratin sulfate. Lilly & Parsons (1990) suggested that the bladder surface GAG is the principal mechanism by which the epithelium maintains this permeability barrier between the bladder wall and urine. A defective GAG layer would subject the bladder cells to harmful solutes. The bladder surface GAG contains negatively charged sulfated polysaccharide groups that have a high affinity for binding water molecules. As a result of this, the hydrated surface layer forms an underlying barrier between the bladder wall tissues and the urine. This barrier prevents the urinary solutes (such as urea and calcium) from damaging the bladder cells.

Lilly & Parsons (1990) examined the ability of surface GAG to prevent a small molecule, urea, from moving across the epithelium in humans. They conducted a three-stage study: stage 1, urea instillation;

stage 2, treatment of the bladder with protamine sulfate, 5 mg/ml (100 ml total volume), for 15 minutes followed by urea; and stage 3, 2000 units/ml (100 ml total volume) of heparin for 15 minutes, followed by urea. At the end of each stage, the urea content was measured. A control group of 27 volunteers had 100 ml of a 200 g/l urea solution placed into their bladders for 45 minutes. The net flow of urea from the bladder lumen was 5.1%. From this initial group, 19 individuals who were capable of completing the study proceeded to stage 2. These volunteers had protamine sulfate (5 mg/ml) instilled in the bladder for 15 minutes, then removed and a second urea analysis done. Urea loss was significantly higher at 22% ($p < 0.02$ by Student's t-test). In stage three, a solution of heparin (1000 units per ml) was instilled for 15 minutes followed by a third urea analysis; urea loss was reversed to 9%. All volunteers experienced significant urinary urgency and discomfort after protamine treatment. These symptoms were relieved by the instillation of heparin. One might conclude from this study that the most important permeability defense mechanism of the epithelium is the surface GAG, which prevents the small molecule urea from leaking across it. This defense mechanism can be impaired by a quaternary amine, such as protamine sulfate, and can be restored by a sulfated polysaccharide (heparin) when placed into the bladder. This in turn suggests that the polysaccharide on the surface of the bladder is an effective permeability barrier. Intact polysaccharide appears to be a broad spectrum, cell surface defense mechanism. A deficiency of this layer, either by poor quality or quantity or by the presence of urinary quaternary amines (similar to protamine), may be an important initiator of the disease. The overall importance of understanding the role of urinary GAG is further illustrated by the therapeutic value of using exogenous polysaccharide to treat urinary tract disease, a therapy based on the augmentation of natural defense mechanisms or the inactivation of urinary polysaccharide.

Chelsky et al. (1994) argued that the 'epithelial leak' theory may not be valid. They determined bladder permeability in a more direct fashion by measuring the actual transvesical migration of the radioisotope ^{99m}technetium-diethylenetriaminepentaacetic acid (^{99m}Tc-DTPA) into the systemic circulation in ten IC patients and nine sex-matched normal controls. ^{99m}Tc-DTPA is somewhat larger in size than urea, a test compound that is often used by Parsons et al. (1987, 1990, 1991), but it is still a relatively small molecule as evidenced by its ability to undergo glomerular filtration. Presumably, the permeability of ^{99m}Tc-DTPA should be similar to that of urea. Chelsky et al. (1994) found considerable variability in the absorption of this acid within the two groups of patients and controls; differences between the two groups were not statistically significant. This implies that although some IC patients have a more permeable bladder than others, the same is true for normal, symptom-free volunteers. Thus, the concept of increased bladder permeability in IC was not supported by this examination of bladder permeability using ^{99m}Tc-DTPA as a test compound.

Mast cells

The mast cell is a potential pathogenetic effector mechanism in IC. The mast cell is a tissue cell of loose connective tissue which contains water-soluble metachromatic-staining cytoplasmic granules. The cells are most prominent in the perivascular areas. Their origin is not known. Mast cells are more numerous where the local nutrition of the connective tissue is enhanced, as in hyperemia or lymph stasis. As healing progresses and the fibrous tissue becomes less cellular, the local mast cell population may decline; when nothing remains but dense scar tissue, the mast cell may be absent. Simmons & Bunce (1958) reported mast cells in the wall of the normal bladder, with these cells secreting histamines. Riley & West (1953) found the amount of histamine in various tissues to be proportional to the mast cell content. Histamine release causes pain, fibrosis and hyperemia, notable features of IC. One might conjecture that many of the pathological changes in the bladder wall occurring in IC may be secondary to the presence of mast cells and the local release of histamine.

Some investigators have attempted to quantify the presence of mast cells with respect to symptoms. Holm-Bentzen et al. (1987) attempted to elucidate differences in symptoms, cystoscopy and cytometric findings in 115 patients with a painful bladder with and without detrusor mastocytosis. On the basis of mast cell counts in the bladder biopsies of the detrusor muscle, the patients were divided into two groups: those with more than 28 mast cells per mm^2 and those with fewer than 28. Patients with more than 28 mast cells per mm^2 had hematuria more often than the other patients (23% versus 13%). The former had a significantly more damaged bladder than the other painful bladder patients, as half of these patients had redness, scarring and increased vascularization of the bladder mucosa at cystoscopy before bladder distension. The bladder capacity also was significantly reduced in these patients. Petechial bleeding was found in 60–75% of the patients in both groups, not a significant difference. The patients without detrusor mastocytosis had a vulnerable mucosa after bladder distension (petechial bleeding), but there was no chronic contracted bladder. Holm-Bentzen et al. concluded that if patients with chronic abacterial cystitis of unknown etiology are divided into two groups on the basis of less or more than 28 mast cells per mm^2, certain differences in the clinical findings between the groups can be ruled out; however, as the groups largely overlapped, mast cells cannot be the only factor responsible for the symptoms.

Johansson & Fall (1989) suggested that only patients with classic IC have elevated mast cells counts. They conducted a detailed histopathological analysis of the lesions seen in patients with classic and early IC. Mast cell counts were determined in 47 classic and 30 early IC patients, and 14 controls. The data showed that mast cells were significantly increased in the patients with the classic syndrome only; in particular, mast cells were increased in the lamina propria as well as in the detrusor muscle. The mucosal mast cells were seen in the urothelium of all patients except two with the classic syndrome, but they were not detected in any patients with the early syndrome. Mast cell density was markedly increased in patients with classic IC, especially in the lamina propria. There was no significant difference in mast cell numbers in the detrusor muscle or lamina propria between the early IC patients and the controls, but numbers differed significantly between these two groups and the classic IC patients ($p < 0.05$).

Hanno et al. (1990) evaluated 55 patients with IC and compared them with a control group of 21 patients who had voiding dysfunction conclusively proved to be other than IC on evaluation. The latter group included patients being screened for bladder and prostate cancer, and those with hyperactive bladder dysfunction and voiding dysfunctions other than IC. Of the patients diagnosed as having IC, 64% had detrusor mastocytosis compared with 80% of non-IC patients. Mean detrusor mast cell counts were not statistically different between the two groups.

From these various findings, it is apparent that although detrusor mastocytosis might be an important mediator of the disease, it cannot be used to confirm the diagnosis of IC.

In contrast, the many reports of the success of synthetic polysaccharides in the treatment of IC cannot be discounted. Such successes support the concept that some patients with the IC syndrome do indeed have a leaky epithelium.

In a clinical study of IC, Parsons et al. (1987) used a dose of 100 mg of sodium pentosanpolysulfate (PPS) three times daily for a minimum of four months, which was continued for longer than 18 months in some individuals. A total of 62 IC patients were evaluated at two different medical centers. Subjective improvements were greater in all parameters when the drug was compared with placebo therapy, with significant improvement in pain, urgency, frequency and nocturia. Objective improvement in average voided volumes was greater with the drug than with placebo ($p = 0.009$).

Parsons et al. (1993) conducted a randomized, prospective, double-blind, placebo-controlled study at seven clinical centers on 148 IC patients. Patients received orally either 100 mg PPS or a placebo three times daily. Of the patients on drug therapy, 32% showed significant improvement compared with 16% of those on placebo ($p = 0.01$).

Patients on drug therapy experienced a significant diminution in pain and urgency ($p = 0.04$ and 0.01, respectively) on analogue scales. In addition, more drug patients showed an average increment of more than 20 ml voided volume than did placebo patients ($p = 0.02$). In a later study, Parsons et al. (1994) reported that, in over half of a cohort of 48 IC patients, intravesical heparin controlled the symptoms of IC with continued improvement even after one year of therapy.

Mulholland et al. (1990) compared PPS with placebo for the symptomatic therapy of IC in a double-blind, multicenter study. A total of 110 patients were enrolled and treated for three months. Overall improvement of greater than 25% was reported by 28% of the PPS-treated patients and by only 13% of the placebo-treated patients ($p = 0.03$). The investigators' overall evaluation provided similar results, 26% versus 11% in favor of PPS ($p = 0.07$).

Fritjofsson et al. (1987) studied 87 patients with IC symptoms in a two-year protocol at 17 centers in Finland and Sweden. The medication (400 mg of PPS daily in two oral doses) was discontinued after six months. The responses were evaluated every four weeks during treatment and every three months thereafter for two years. Most patients responded favorably, many experiencing a decrease in pain as early as four weeks from the start of treatment. Pain reduction was typically sustained at each three-month follow-up period.

Kalota et al. (1992) demonstrated in two in vivo models and an in vitro model the ability of PPS to reduce toxic effects of acrolein (the active metabolite of cyclophosphamide, capable of damaging the transitional epithelium of the bladder). In the in vivo models (adult female rats), they showed that PPS can improve the functional properties of the GAG layer of the intact bladder (relative to adherence and permeability). Although PPS does not appear to have a complete protective effect against acrolein-induced tissue damage, it does prevent a significant amount of damage from cyclophosphamide's metabolite acrolein when given intravesically for 15 minutes prior to the instillation of acrolein. In the in-vitro model, there was an increased survival of cell tissues following the use of PPS pretreatment with various concentrations of acrolein.

J.A. Koziol et al. (unpublished results) examined the effect of sulfated polysaccharide therapy in IC patients classified into three severity levels of IC: mild, moderate and severe. These levels were determined based on patients' symptoms, in particular, pain, urgency and nocturia scores. They found no apparent improvement in symptoms during polysaccharide therapy among those patients in the mild group, a slight improvement among the moderate group and a dramatic improvement among those patients in the severe group. In general, pain and urgency scores tended to decline throughout the therapeutic interval, whereas nocturia seemed to plateau after 12–24 months on therapy. Pain and urgency seemed relatively more affected by polysaccharide therapy than nocturia.

Based on these findings, it is plausible that a defect or absence of the surface GAG layer is involved in the pathogenesis of IC. It is suggested that this mucous barrier functions abnormally in a subset of individuals with IC. Hence, synthetic polysaccharides will help only these individuals. It is estimated that more than 70% of IC patients will benefit from this treatment regimen (Parsons & Walker, 1996).

Pathogenetic hypothesis

The lack of specific pathognomonic markers for the diagnosis of IC has resulted in a host of plausible hypotheses for its etiology. Among these are bacterial, fungal and viral infections, lymphovascular obstruction, autoimmunity, mast cells, dysfunctional bladder epithelium, neurological, endocrinological and psychoneurotic disorders. Among these, dysfunctional bladder epithelium and mast cells are currently areas of extensive research activity relating to causative factors of IC.

IC is a condition in which few specific diagnostic criteria have been established. It is widely believed that the etiology of IC is multifactorial. From the brief review given above of dysfunctional bladder epithelium and mast cell correlates of IC, one might reasonably conclude that IC is multiply pathogenic, with different avenues leading to the same symptoms.

Lilly & Parsons (1990) described a subset of IC patients with a 'leaky' epithelium, whose IC symptoms could be alleviated by synthetic polysaccharide therapy. An experimental study conducted on humans demonstrated that when the bladder surface glycosaminoglycans are impaired by a quaternary amine, their ability to prevent exogenous molecules from moving across the epithelium is compromised. This transepithelial 'leak' may be reversed by treatment with sulfated polysaccharides. The success of this type of therapy is found, on average, in over 50% of IC patients (Parsons & Mulholland 1987; Lilly & Parsons 1990; Mulholland et al., 1990; Parsons et al., 1991, 1993, 1994; Kalota et al., 1992).

Mast cells are often found in increased numbers in IC patients relative to normal controls. As with autoimmune antibodies, this measure is also found with other urological disorders. There is a significant increase of mast cells in patients with classic IC compared with early IC, but no difference in mast cell level between early IC patients and a group of normal controls (Johansson & Fall, 1989).

Hence, mastocytosis may be an important mediator in patients with classic IC, but it cannot be used to confirm the diagnosis of IC.

So far, it appears that no single treatment prescribed in accordance with a hypothesized etiology will benefit all patients with IC. Each treatment, nonetheless, will probably benefit a select subset of IC patients. If, in fact, the etiology of IC is multifactorial, it is critical to identify distinct subgroups of these patients: such subdivision of this ill-defined syndrome will allow for more effective treatment programs by identifying a treatment of choice appropriate for each particular subgroup.

Diagnostic and treatment approaches

Diagnosis

Without any specific pathognomonic marker, diagnosis of IC can be difficult. Diagnostic guidelines were established in workshops held in August 1987 and November 1988 in the USA by the National Institute of Arthritis, Diabetes, Digestive and Kidney diseases (NIDDK) (Hanno, 1994). These guidelines were established primarily to ensure that the groups of patients studied would be relatively uniform. They are not meant to define the condition. The following is an outline of exclusionary rules established from the NIDDK workshops on the diagnosis of IC. One should be wary of making a positive diagnosis of IC in the presence of any of these factors, although its absence does not eliminate the possibility of IC:

(1) Capacity of greater than 350 cc on awake cystometry using either a gas or liquid filling medium.
(2) Absence of an intense urge to void with the bladder filled to 100 cc of gas or 150 ml of water during cystometry, using a fill rate of 30–100 cc/min.
(3) The demonstration of phasic involuntary bladder contractions on cystometry using the fill rate described above.
(4) Duration of symptoms of less than nine months.
(5) Absence of nocturia.
(6) Symptoms relieved by antimicrobials, urinary antiseptics, anticholergics or antispasmodics.
(7) A frequency of urination, while awake, of less than eight times per day.
(8) Diagnosis of bacterial cystitis or prostatitis within a three-month period.
(9) Bladder or ureteral calculi.
(10) Active genital herpes.

(11) Uterine, cervical, vaginal or urethral cancer.
(12) Urethral diverticulum.
(13) Cyclophosphamide or any type of chemical cystitis.
(14) Tuberculous cystitis.
(15) Radiation cystitis.
(16) Benign or malignant bladder tumors.
(17) Vaginitis.
(18) Age less than 18 years.

To be diagnosed with IC, patients must undergo cystoscopic examination under general anesthesia with hydrodistention of the bladder and bladder biopsy. Typical cystoscopic features of IC are rarely seen under local anesthesia. Adequate distention of the bladder is necessary to reveal glomerulations, an endoscopic hallmark of the disease. Glomerulations, however, can also occur in other bladder disorders (e.g., radiation cystitis, carcinoma in situ); hence, their appearance must be evaluated in conjunction with other manifestations of the syndrome to confirm a diagnosis of IC. Glomerulations may be focal or patchy, or numerous and diffuse. They usually occur in areas just lateral to the urethral orifices and bladder neck. More diffuse hemorrhages will occur in the posterior bladder wall and dome. Bladder capacity upon distention is determined at a hydrostatic pressure of 70–100 cm water for 1–3 minutes, the endpoint reached when fluid begins to leak around the cystoscope sheath or starts to flow backward into the container. Blood in the draining fluid after hydrodistention and the presence of glomerulations upon redistention are typical features of IC. In a large number of cases, glomerulations and bleeding will not be significant until the bladder is filled for a second time. In a small number of cases, bladder distention will initiate cracks and grooves in the mucous membrane, and occasionally one encounters the occurrence of a true Hunner's ulcer. If glomerulation, scars or ulcers are confined to areas subjected to direct trauma from the cystoscope, previous biopsy or transurethral resection sites, the diagnosis of IC should not be made. Bladder biopsy and urodynamic evaluation are necessary to rule out cancer and other pathological conditions (Sant, 1991). To date, there are still no specific pathological findings for IC; however, Balagani et al. (1991) have successfully induced cystoscopic changes seen in the bladders of IC patients in the bladders of rabbits by exposure to IC urine. They suggest that the urine in IC patients may have some toxin (molecular weight greater than 10 000 s) that can set up the inflammatory condition of IC. The definition of IC and, subsequently, its diagnosis are still evolving and thus further changes can be anticipated.

Treatment

The two case presentations represent the typical person with IC undergoing treatments that controlled their disease. There are a number of available treatment options for mild, moderate and severe patients. These treatment plans have to encompass other patient problems such as allergies or chronic depression associated with the disease. Several treatment options will be reviewed that are quite successful at managing the IC syndrome.

Antihistamines

Antihistamines are critical to managing IC in people with hay fever, sinusitis or food allergies. Antihistamines have been tried in IC but without controlled studies. Antihistamines were chosen because of the possible role of mast cells (Simmons 1961; Bohne et al., 1962; Smith & Dehner, 1972; Larsen et al., 1982).

While most patients may not respond to antihistamines, subsets of patients seem to derive major benefit, especially when antihistamines are combined with other therapy. Allergic people in particular will benefit from chronic therapy with hydroxyzine 25–50 mg at bedtime (Theoharides, 1994). The side-effect of fatigue will go away after four weeks. This is an extremely effective way to manage allergies when the medication is used chronically, but if used sporadically most of its effect is lost. Beneficial effects appear two to three months after the start of treatment and patients are urged to stay on medication for at least three months to determine its effectiveness. If helpful, hydroxyzine should be continued indefinitely.

Heparinoid therapy

One major breakthrough in therapy is the use of heparin-like drugs (heparin, PPS-Elmiron®). When effective, they reverse the course of the disease and patients rarely become resistant to their use.

Heparin

Heparin, when given by injection, has been reported to alleviate the symptoms of IC (Lose et al., 1983). Again this was not in a controlled study. Long-term systemic heparin therapy should not be employed in most individuals as it may result in osteoporosis in patients who use it for 26 weeks or more.

In our experience, intravesical heparin has significant activity in approximately 50% of patients (Parsons et al., 1994). Here, too, the data were obtained in an uncontrolled investigation. Previous controlled studies by the author demonstrated a placebo effect of approximately 20%, suggesting possible activity for heparin (Parsons & Mulholland, 1987).

We frequently start all patients with moderate to severe symptoms on a combination of oral Elmiron® and intravesical heparin, with a goal of gradually tapering the heparin once remission occurs. The technique uses 10 000 units of heparin in 10 ml of saline. This solution is instilled intravesically initially daily, then after three to four months reduced gradually, if the patient improves, to three to four times per week. If there is no effect after three months, increase to daily instillation of 20 000 units. This treatment can be carried on indefinitely.

It takes two to four months to begin to see improvements, but encourage therapy for at least six months before abandoning it in severe patients. The best improvements are noted after one to two years. Long-term therapy is recommended for patients with moderate or worse disease who respond to its use. Serum prothrombin (PT) and prothrombin time (PTT) are monitored for several weeks after therapy begins to rule out the formation of an unusual antibody to heparin or systemic absorption (heparin should not be absorbed across the bladder mucosa). Patients may be instructed in self-catheterization so this therapy can be performed at home.

Pentosanpolysulfate

Parsons et al. (1987, 1990) first reported pentosanpolysulfate (PPS, Elmiron®) as active at ameliorating the symptoms of IC. As PPS is a sulfated polysaccharide, theoretically it may augment the bladder surface defense mechanism or detoxify agents in urine which have a capacity to attack the bladder surface (e.g., quaternary amines).

In a controlled clinical study, 42% of patients with IC were shown to have their symptoms controlled with PPS versus 20% for placebo (Parsons & Mulholland, 1987). This has been borne out in several subsequent studies including a five-center trial where 28% of patients improved versus 13% on placebo (Mulholland et al., 1990) and in a seven-center study of 150 patients where 32% of patients improved on drug versus 15% on placebo (Parsons et al., 1993). Additionally, an English–Danish study found a significant reduction of pain in patients on PPS compared with placebo (Holm-Bentzen et al., 1987).

PPS is employed in an oral dose of 100–200 mg three times per day. In patients with moderate disease, it appears to be about 40–50% effective. In the controlled clinical trials carried out with patients with severe disease, activity was lower. Response to therapy is first seen after 6–10 weeks. Patients do better after 6–12 months of therapy.

Continued use of PPS for several years leads to long-term disease control in most patients whose IC responds to the drug initially. This has not been previously found with any other therapy except heparin.

Dimethylsulfoxide

Dimethylsulfoxide (DMSO) was approved for use in IC in 1977 (Stewart et al., 1968). While no controlled clinical trials were ever conducted with DMSO, it does appear to induce remission in 34–40% of patients with IC. The difficulty with DMSO is that it may induce an excellent remission in the first one to three cycles of therapy, but as an individual relapses and requires subsequent treatment, progressive resistance to its beneficial effects is seen in almost all patients.

For treatment of IC, instill 50 ml of 50% DMSO into the bladder for 5–10 minutes. Longer periods are unnecessary as DMSO is rapidly absorbed into the bloodstream. Instillations are performed on an outpatient basis or the patient can be taught to perform it at home.

The author recommends that patients receive six to eight weekly DMSO treatments to determine whether a therapeutic response is achieved. If the patient has moderate to severe symptoms, therapy should be continued for an additional four to six months once every other week. Remember, once you stop DMSO therapy, the patient is likely to become resistant to its use.

Some patients will experience a flare of symptoms when DMSO is placed into the bladder. This phenomenon may be related to the ability of DMSO to degranulate mast cells and may occur primarily in patients who have significant bladder mastocytosis. Nonetheless, DMSO may be very effective at treating these patients.

Should the patient experience pain with DMSO, give 10 ml of 2% viscous lidocaine (Xylocaine) jelly intravesically 15 minutes before instilling DMSO. If this is not successful, use an injectable narcotic or ketoralac (Toradol®) 60 mg intramuscularly before the intravesical instillation. The flare of symptoms associated with DMSO usually disappears over 24 hours. As patients receive subsequent treatments, the pain tends to diminish.

Patients may receive DMSO therapy indefinitely. As originally reported by Stewart et al. (1968), patients have used DMSO weekly for several years without problems. DMSO has been reported to be associated with cataracts in animals; however, this complication has not been reported in humans. Nonetheless, if your patient is receiving long-term DMSO therapy, he or she should have a slit lamp evaluation at three to six months.

Hydrodistention of the bladder under anesthesia

The report by Bumpus in 1930 of bladder hydrodistention improving the symptoms of IC resulted in this procedure being a mainstay of therapy (Bumpus, 1930). Few would question the activity of hydrodistention in ameliorating the symptoms in 60% of IC patients.

Hydrodistention must be performed under anesthesia as it is not possible to dilate a painful bladder without anesthesia. Pressure dilatation of the bladder using a syringe should not be carried out as it can result in rupture of these atrophic bladders; a maximum of 80–100 cm of water pressure is recommended.

The mechanism by which hydrodistention improves symptoms is unknown; several theories have been postulated. Neuropraxis induced by mechanical trauma may occur in some individuals; however, few patients awaken with decreased pain which support the neuropraxis concept. Rather, about 90% awaken from anesthesia with significantly worse pain that slowly improves over two to three weeks. This pain usually requires narcotic analgesia. Remission will occur over several weeks.

As a result of the increased pain, it is recommended that all patients receive belladonna and opium rectal suppositories immediately in the recovery room. Better yet, instill 10 ml of 2% viscous Xylocaine® into the bladder at the end of hydrodistention. The patient should be discharged with a narcotic to control the increased pain.

As most patient's symptoms are exacerbated by hydrodistention, we believe that this is due to epithelial damage from the mechanical trauma. The disruption in the integrity of the mucosal cells increases the epithelial permeability (leak), causing symptoms to flare. Over the next several weeks healing may occur which correlates with the time of clinical remission. Perhaps the epithelium regenerates and for a period of time is 'healthy' and returns to its normal impermeability. Then, whatever events initiated the disease continue and relapse occurs.

Remission may persist for 4–12 months, and hydrodistention may then be repeated as needed. If no remission is obtained, repeat the dilation at least two more times as, in our experience, patients respond to a subsequent dilation.

Sodium oxychlorosene

Sodium oxychlorosene (Clorpactin® WCS-90) is a highly reactive chemical compound that is a modified derivative of hypochlorous acid in a buffered base. Its activity is dependent on the liberation of hypochlorous acid and its resulting oxidizing effects and detergency.

Wishard et al. (1957) treated 20 patients with five weekly instillations of 0.2% sodium oxychlorosene under local anesthesia. Improvement occurred in 14 of the 20 patients, although follow-up was brief. Messing & Stamey (1978), treating 38 patients with 0.4% sodium oxychlorosene, reported significant improvement in 72%.

Ureteral reflux is a contraindication to the use of sodium oxychlorosene. It is recommended that the compound usually be used under anesthesia.

Bladder training

Whatever therapy is successful at alleviating the pain and sensory urgency of IC, the individual afflicted with the disorder will continue to have a small capacity bladder, in part based on sensory urgency and in part because of frequent low volume voiding. In controlled clinical trials, it has been reported that even with good remission of pain and urgency, there is almost no change in urinary frequency over a 12-week period (Parsons & Mulholland, 1987; Mulholland et al., 1990; Parsons et al., 1993). The problem of urinary frequency must be addressed in order to obtain a functional recovery of the bladder.

This is accomplished by training the patients to undergo a program of progressively holding their urine to increase their bladder capacity (Parsons & Koprowski, 1991). This therapy can be directed by a urological nurse. To begin, obtain a three-day voiding profile from the patient (to include time of voiding and a measurement of volume). Determine the average time interval between voids, and gradually increase this interval monthly. For example, if the patient voids every hour, recommend he or she attempt to void every hour and a quarter and at the end of 1 month increase that to an hour and a half. The patient should never progress too quickly because he or she will become discouraged and drop out.

It usually takes three to five months for this bladder training protocol to start to see results. At the end of three to four months, the bladder capacity will increase approximately 2.5 times and there will be a corresponding reduction in urgency and the number of voidings per day.

We also discovered that if patients have minimal or no pain associated with their urinary frequency, bladder training may be the only therapy required and, in fact, the only therapy that is effective. For more details concerning the employment of bladder training, the reader is referred to Parsons & Koprowski (1991).

Antidepressant therapy

Chronic pain and sleep loss cause depression; thus, it is valuable to place most IC patients with moderate or worse symptoms on antidepressant medications. Tricyclic antidepressants have several modes of action that are beneficial. They have side-effects of drowsiness (aids sleep), increase pain thresholds and elevate the mood. If tricyclic antidepressants are used, start with low doses and warn patients they will be tired (for 12–15 hours per day) for the first two to three weeks of therapy. Once they become tolerant to this side-effect, increase slowly, if needed, to a larger dose. Amitriptyline (Hanno et al., 1989) or imipramine can be prescribed in doses beginning at 25 mg (or even 10 mg) one hour before bedtime.

In an uncontrolled trial, amitriptyline was reported by Hanno et al. (1989) to ameliorate the symptoms of IC. Patients were treated with 25 mg of amitriptyline one hour before bedtime for one week; the dose was then increased weekly by 25 mg to 75 mg. Fifty percent of patients responded to this medication.

The exact mechanism of action of amitriptyline is unknown, although it may block H_1 histamine receptors and perhaps mast cell degranulation. More likely the drug raises pain tolerance due to its antidepressant activity.

If fluoxetine (Prozac®) is selected, use 20 mg per day and increase if needed to 40 mg. Sertraline (Zoloft®) is another well-tolerated antidepressant. It can be used at 50 mg per day and increased to 100 mg if needed.

Antidepressant therapy is an important adjunct to treatment. It does not cure IC, but patients function much better with their disabling symptoms if not depressed. In essence, they 'feel better' even if they still void 20 times per day.

Surprisingly, many patients (about 25–30%) improve dramatically with only antidepressant therapy. No matter what other therapy has been initiated, we place all moderately (or worse) symptomatic patients on antidepressants and remove them if they improve and are being successfully managed with some other treatment (e.g. heparin or pentosanpolysulfate).

Conclusion

The exploration of IC, despite its long history, has been fairly recent. Hunner's report of 1914 revealed the ulcerative type of IC, but it was 64 years later that Messing & Stamey (1978) uncovered the non-ulcerative type, increasing diagnosis nine-fold; and it was only nine years ago that work on the first large-scale epidemiological survey of IC began in the USA. The statistics of this study revealed approximately 450 000 existing cases, taking a patient 2–4.5 years to receive a correct diagnosis. The direct medical costs for diagnosis and treatment, as well as the indirect costs due to significant work disability and other limitations of patient functional status, are potentially large. This reality has raised concerns and spurred major findings by NIH and ICA into the search for its etiology and treatment. Nevertheless, there are still no definitive answers to such pertinent issues as etiology, the efficacy of therapeutic options, prevalence, incidence, risk factors, and social and economic costs of IC. Substantive and updated information concerning these issues is much needed if one is to head toward the direction of cure.

References

Bade JJ, Rijcken B & Mensink HJA (1995). Interstitial cystitis in the Netherlands: prevalence, diagnostic criteria and therapeutic preferences. *Journal of Urology*, **154**, 2035–8.

Balagni RK, Hanno PM, Ma M, et al. (1991). Induction of glomerulations in rabbit bladder after exposure to IC urine. *Journal of Urology*, **145**, 258A.

Bohne AW, Hodson JM, Rebuck JW, Reinhard RE (1962). An abnormal leukocyte response in interstitial cystitis. *Jounal of Urology*, **88**, 387.

Brandes LJ & Cheang M (1995). Response to antidepressants and cancer: cause for concern? (Letter to the Editor). *Journal of Clinical Psychopharmacology*, **15**, 84–5.

Brandes LJ, Arron RJ, Bogdanovi RP, Tong J, Zaborniak CLF, Hogg GR, Warrington RC, Fang W & LaBella FS (1992). Stimulation of malignant growth in rodents by antidepressant drugs at clinically relevant doses. *Cancer Research*, **52**, 3796–800.

Brandes LJ, Warrington RC, Arron RJ, Bogdanovi RP, Fang W, Queen GM, Stein DA, Tong J, Zaborniak CL & LaBella FS (1994). Enhanced cancer growth in mice administered daily human-equivalent doses of some H1-antihistamines: Predictive in vitro correlates. *Journal of National Cancer Institute*, **86**, 770–5.

Bumpus HC (1930). Interstitial cystitis. *Medical Clinics of North America*, **13**, 1495–8.

Chelsky MJ, Rosen SI, Knight LC, Maurer AH, Hanno PM & Ruggieri MR (1994). Bladder permeability in interstitial cystitis is similar to that of normal volunteers: direct measurement by transvesical absorption of ^{99m}technetium-diethylenetriaminepentaaccetic acid. *Journal of Urology*, **151**, 346–9.

Close CE, Carr MC, Burns MW, Miller JL, Bavendam TG, Mayo ME & Mitchell ME (1996). Interstitial cystitis in children. *Journal of Urology*, **156**, 860–2.

Dunn M, Pamsden PD, Roberts JBM, Smith JC & Smith PBJ (1977). Interstitial cystitis treated by prolonged bladder distension. *British Journal of Urology*, **49**, 641–5.

Duthie AM (1977). The use of phenothiazines and tricyclic antidepressants in the treatment of intractable pain. *South African Medical Journal*, **51**, 246–7.

Erickson DR, Simon LJ & Belchis DA (1994). Relationships between bladder inflammation and other clinical features in interstitial cystitis. *Urology*, **44**, 655–9.

Fritjofsson A, Fall M, Juhlin R, Persson & Ruutu M (1987). Treatment of ulcer and non-ulcer interstitial cystitis with sodium pentosanpolysulfate: a multicenter trial. *Journal of Urology*, **138**, 508–12.

Hand JR (1949). Interstitial cystitis: report of 223 cases (204 women and 19 men). *Journal of Urology*, **6**, 291–310.

Hanno PM (1994). Diagnosis of interstitial cystitis. *Urology Clinics of North America*, **21**, 63–6.

Hanno PM & Wein AJ (1987*a*). Interstitial cystitis, Part I. *AUA Update Series*, Lesson 9, **9**: 3–7.

Hanno PM & Wein AJ (1987*b*). Interstitial cystitis, Part II. *AUA Update Series*, Lesson 10, **6**: 2–7.

Hanno PM, Buehler J & Wein AJ (1989). Use of amitriptyline in the treatment of interstitial cystitis. *Journal of Urology*, **141**, 846–8.

Hanno PM, Levin RM, Monson FC, Teuscher C, Zhou ZZ, Ruggieri M, Whitmore K & Wein AJ (1990). Diagnosis of interstitial cystitis. *Journal of Urology*, **143**, 278–81.

Held PJ, Hanno PM, Wein AJ, Pauly MV & Cann MA (1990). Epidemiology of interstitial cystitis 2. In *Interstitial Cystitis*, ed. P.M. Hanno, D.R. Staskin, R.J. Krane & A.J. Wein, pp. 29–48. New York: Springer.

Hollander DH (1994). Interstitial cystitis and silk allergy. *Medical Hypotheses*, **43**, 155–6.

Holm-Bentzen M, Jacobsen F, Nerstrom B, Lose G, Kristensen JK, Pedersen RH, Krarup T, Feggetter J, Bates P, Barnard R, Larsen & Hald T (1987). Painful bladder disease: clinical and pathoanatomical differences in 115 patients. *Journal of Urology*, **138**, 500–2.

Holm-Bentzen M, Larsen S, Hainau B & Hald T (1985). Non-obstructive detrusor myopathy in a group of patients with chronic abacterial cystitis. *Scandinavian Journal of Urology and Nephrology*, **19**, 21–6.

Hunner GL (1915). A rare type of bladder ulcer in women: Report of cases. *Boston Medical and Surgical Journal*, **172**, 660–5.

Hunner GL (1918). Elusive ulcer of the bladder. Further notes on a rare type of bladder ulcer with a report of twenty-five cases. *American Journal of Obstetrics*, **78**, 374–95.

Hurst RE, Parsons CL, Roy JB & Young JL (1993). Urinary glycosaminoglycan excretion as a laboratory marker in the diagnosis of interstitial cystitis. *Journal of Urology*, **149**, 31–5.

Iishi H, Tatsuta M, Baba M & Taniguchi H (1993). Enhancement by the tricyclic antidepressant, desipramine, of experimental carcinogenesis in rat colon induced by azoxymethane. *Carcinogenesis*, **14**, 1837–40.

Johansson SL & Fall M (1989). Clinical features, and spectrum of light microscopic changes in interstitial cystitis. *Journal of Urology*, **143**, 1118–24.

Jokinen EJ, Alfthan O & Oravisto KJ (1972). Anti-tissue antibodies in interstitial cystitis. *Clinical and Experimental Immunology*, **11**, 333–9.

Jones CA, Harris M & Nyberg L (1994). Prevalence of interstitial cystitis in the United States. *Journal of Urology*, **151**, 423.

Kalota SJ, Stein PC & Parsons CL (1992). Prevention of acrolein-induced bladder injury by pentosanpolysulfate. *Journal of Urology*, **148**, 163–6.

Koziol JA (1994). Epidemiology of interstitial cystitis. *Urology Clinics of North America*, **21**, 7–20.

Koziol JA, Clark DC, Gittes RF & Tan EM (1993). The natural history of interstitial cystitis: a survey of 374 patients. *Journal of Urology*, **149**, 465–9.

Koziol JA, Adams HP & Frutos A (1995). Discrimination between the ulcerous and the non-ulcerous forms of interstitial cystitis by noninvasive findings. *Journal of Urology*, **155**, 87–90.

Larsen S, Thompson SA, Hald T, Barnard RJ, Gilpin CJ, Dixon JS & Gosling JA (1982). Mast cells in interstitial cystitis. *British Journal of Urology*, **54**, 283–6.

Lilly JD & Parsons CL (1990). Bladder surface glycosaminoglycans is a human epithelial permeability barrier. *Surgery, Gynecology and Obstetrics*, **171**, 143–5.

Long CC, Jessop J, Young M & Holt PJ (1992). Minimizing the risk of post-operative pyoderma gangrenosum. *British Journal of Dermatology*, **127**, 45–8.

Lose G, Frandsen B, Hojensgard JC, et al. (1983). Chronic interstitial cystitis: increased levels of eosinophil cationic protein in serum and urine and an ameliorating effect of subcutaneous heparin. *Scandinavian Journal of Urology and Nephrology*, **17**, 159–61.

Messing EM (1985). Interstitial cystitis and related syndromes. In *Campbell's Urology*, 5th edn, ed. P.C. Walsh, R.F. Gittes, A.D. Perlmutter & T.A. Stamey, pp. 1070–86. Philadelphia: WB Saunders.

Messing EM & Stamey TA (1978). Interstitial cystitis: early diagnosis, pathology and treatment. *Urology*, **12**, 381–92.

Mulholland SG, Hanno P, Parsons CL, Sant GR & Staskin DR (1990). Pentosan polysulfate sodium for therapy of interstitial cystitis. *Urology*, **35**, 552–8.

Nagazawa T & Umegae Y (1990). Sericulturist's lung disease: hypersensitivity pneumonitis related to silk production. *Thorax*, **45**, 233–4.

Nitze M (1907). In *Lehrbuch der Cystoskopie: Ihre Technik ünd Kinsche Bedeutung*, pp. 205–10. Berlin: JE Bergman.

Nordlund JJ & Askenase PW (1983). The effect of histamine, antihistamines and a mast cell stabilizer on the growth of cloudman melanoma cells in DBA/2 Mice. *Journal of Investigative Dermatology*, **81**, 28–31.

Ochs RL, Stein TW, Jr, Peebles CL, Gittes RF & Tan EM (1994). Autoantibodies in interstitial cystitis. *Journal of Urology*, **151**, 587–92.

Oravisto KJ (1975). Epidemiology of interstitial cystitis. *Annals Chirurgiae et Gynaecologicae Fenniae*, **64**, 75–7.

Oravisto KJ (1980). Interstitial cystitis as an autoimmune disease (a review). *European Urology*, **6**, 10–13.

Oravisto KJ, Alfthan OS & Jokinen EJ (1970). Interstitial cystitis. *Scandinavian Journal of Urology and Nephrology*, **4**, 37–42.

Parsons CL & Koprowski P (1991). Interstitial cystitis: successful management by a pattern of increasing urinary voiding interval. *Urology*, **37**, 207–12.

Parsons CL & Mulholland SG (1987). Successful therapy of interstitial cystitis with pentosanpolysulfate. *Journal of Urology*, **138**, 513–15.

Parsons CL & Walker CJ (1996). Cystoscopic changes in IC. *Urology*, **48**, 289–90.

Parsons CL, Boychuk D, Jones S, Hurst R & Callahan H (1990). Bladder surface glycosaminoglycans: an epithelial permeability barrier. *Journal of Urology*, **143**, 139–42.

Parsons CL, Benson G, Childs SJ, Hanno P, Grannum RS & Webster G (1993). A quantitatively controlled method to study prospectively interstitial cystitis and demonstrate the efficacy of pentosanpolysulfate. *Journal of Urology*, **150**, 845–8.

Parsons CL, Housley JD, Schmidt JD & Lebow D (1994). Treatment of interstitial cystitis with intravesical heparin. *British Journal of Urology*, **73**, 504–7.

Parsons CL, Lilly JD & Stein P (1991). Epithelial dysfunction in non-bacterial cystitis (interstitial cystitis). *Journal of Urology*, **145**, 732–5.

Ratner V, Slade D & Greene G (1994). Interstitial cystitis: a patient's perspective. *Urology Clinics of North America*, **21**, 1–5.
Riley JF & West GB (1953). The presence of histamine in tissue mast cells. *Journal of Physiology*, **120**, 528–33.
Sant GR (1990). Interstitial cystitis: pathogenesis, evaluation and treatment. *Urology Annual*, **3**, 171.
Sant GR (1991). Interstitial cystitis. *Monographs in Urology*, **12**, 37–63.
Silk MR (1970). Bladder antibodies in interstitial cystitis. *Journal of Urology*, **103**, 307–9.
Simmons JL (1961). Interstitial cystitis: an explanation for the beneficial effect of an antihistamine. *Journal of Urology*, **86**, 149–55.
Simmons JL & Bunce PL (1958). On the use of an antihistamine in the treatment of interstitial cystitis. *American Surgery*, **24**, 664–7.
Skene AJC (1878). *Diseases of the Bladder and Urethra in Women*. New York: William Wood.
Slade DKA (1989). Interstitial cystitis: a challenge to urology. *Urologic Nursing* January–March.
Smith BH & Dehner LP (1972). Chronic ulcerating interstitial cystitis (Hunner's ulcer). *Archives of Pathology*, **93**, 76–81.
Stewart BH, Persky L & Kiser WS (1968). The use of dimethylsulfoxide (DMSO) in the treatment of interstitial cystitis. *Journal of Urology*, **98**, 671–2.
Theoharides TC (1988). Neuroimmunology of tumor growth: the role of mast cells. *International Journal of Immunopathology and Pharmacology*, **1**, 89.
Theoharides T (1994). Hydroxyzine in the treatment of interstitial cystitis. *Urology Clinics of North America*, **21**, 113–19.
Uragoda CG & Wijekoon PN (1991). Asthma in silk workers. *Journal of Social and Occupational Medicine*, **41**, 140–2.
Wen CM, Ye St, Zhou LX & Yu Y (1990). Silk-induced asthma in children: a report of 54 cases. *Annals of Allergy*, **65**, 375–8.
Wishard WN, Nourse MH & Mertz JHO (1957). Use of Clorpactin® WCS-90 for relief of symptoms due to interstitial cystitis. *Journal of Urology*, **77**, 420.
Wright SC, Zhong J & Larrick JW (1994). Inhibition of apoptosis as a mechanism of tumor promotion. *FASEB Journal*, **8**, 654–60.

7

Temporomandibular Disorders

CAROL M. GRECO, THOMAS E. RUDY AND ANDREW HERLICH

Temporomandibular disorders (TMDs) are a set of clinical conditions characterized by pain in the muscles of the face, head and neck, pain in the temporomandibular joint area, joint sounds, and/or reduced mandibular range of motion. It has been estimated that up to 12% of the population has symptoms consistent with TMDs (Dworkin et al., 1990). Primary care physicians and general dentists are often the first to hear patients complain about this puzzling and persistent pain problem. When primary care physicians are well informed about TMDs, they can educate their patients, as well as provide conservative medical treatments and appropriate referrals.

History

Pain problems associated with the temporomandibular joint (TMJ) and masticatory muscles have been recognized clinically for over 60 years. The first clinical cases were identified by dentists in the 1920s, and the primary responsibility for the diagnosis and treatment of these disorders has remained within the field of dentistry. The evolution of thinking regarding TMDs has included many theories of etiology and pathogenesis, ranging from anatomical features of the TMJ, to occlusal abnormalities, to behavioral origins such as bruxism (grinding the teeth). Many distinct treatments have been applied to TMDs based on presumed pathogenesis or the clinical training of the health care provider. Similarly, several taxonomic systems for classifying orofacial pain problems have been developed over the past two decades (Block, 1980; Eversole & Machado, 1985; Bell, 1986; Fricton et al., 1988; American Academy of Craniomandibular Disorders, 1990). Most of these classification systems lack clear examination guidelines, which makes communication among clinicians and comparison across research studies problematic. With few exceptions (Fricton et al., 1988; Dworkin & LeResche, 1992) these systems fail to acknowledge the complex associations between chronic pain and dysfunction in various aspects of the patients' lives: social, emotional and vocational, as well as masticatory functioning. In recent years the idea that TMDs include several distinct or overlapping clinical conditions is increasingly accepted, as is the notion that multiple causative or exacerbating factors may be present.

Description of temporomandibular disorders

The primary feature of TMDs is orofacial pain. Many patients seeking treatment complain of persistent pain in the muscles of mastication, which may be constant or quite variable in severity and frequency. Pain and tenderness in the area of the TMJ, especially with mandibular movement, also is a common symptom. Often, associated muscles of the head, neck and shoulders become painful as well, and it is not uncommon for TMD sufferers to report frequent headaches. A restricted range of mandibular movement may be present, as well as various joint sounds elicited by jaw movements. Some patients report that their jaw has 'locked' open or closed, and the duration of this sign can range from moments to days.

Diverse combinations of these signs and symptoms can be present in different individuals. For example, a patient may complain of muscle pain but exhibit no joint sounds, another may report popping sounds and joint pain, with limited opening. While joint sounds and limitations in opening may be present, they are not sufficient for a diagnosis; pain must also be present. The pain is often exacerbated by chewing and talking, and patients may avoid favorite foods and social activities due to fear of increased pain. Pain severity and interference with life activities due to pain are thought to be less for many chronic TMD patients compared with patients with chronic headache and chronic back pain (Turk & Rudy, 1990). The severity of the pain and related oral and psychosocial dysfunction is quite variable between individuals as well as in the same person over time (Von Korff, 1995). Although some professions believe that certain TMDs progress through stages of dysfunction, cross-sectional epidemiological studies do not support the idea of progression to further masticatory dysfunction or increased pain with age (Levitt & McKinney, 1994; Carrlson & LeResche, 1995).

Many people with TMDs use over-the-counter medications to reduce their pain. Others seek treatment from dentists and physicians, as well as other health care professionals. Frequently, a patient will not obtain sufficient relief from a particular treatment and will continue to seek further treatments, often becoming more confused and frustrated by the problem as time goes on. The following case studies illustrate some of the variation in symptoms, duration of pain and treatment history typically seen in patients at a TMD clinic.

Case presentations

The following patients were participants in a comprehensive standardized TMD evaluation and treatment program at the University of Pittsburgh's Pain Evaluation and Treatment Institute. The TMD program was funded by a grant from the National Institute of Dental Research. Evaluation procedures included a comprehensive oral/dental examination based on nationally recognized evaluation criteria (Dworkin & LeResche, 1992), a panoramic radiograph, a clinical interview by a psychologist and self-report questionnaires concerning pain and functioning. Most patients received magnetic resonance imaging (MRI) of the TMJ; however, it should be noted that this was a component of the research program. In general, MRI is not recommended in clinical practice due to its expense and evidence that the MRI results may not be significantly associated with treatment outcome (Weissman et al., 1993).

These particular patients were chosen because they illustrate a range of TMD symptoms and psychosocial sequelae of chronic pain. Background information and evaluation results are presented in the following paragraphs. Later in the chapter, following information on epidemiology, pathogenetic hypotheses and guidelines for diagnosis and treatment, the case studies will be revisited to illustrate their response to our standardized conservative treatment.

Case 1

The first patient is a 38-year-old married Caucasian female who came to the University of Pittsburgh's Pain Evaluation and Treatment Institute complaining of constant pain in the muscles of her face and in the TMJ region, frequent headaches and occasional pain in the muscles of her neck and shoulders. Her pain varied in severity, with flare-ups each morning and most weekday afternoons. She reported that her symptoms had started abruptly 10 months earlier, with no identifiable precipitating event. She had not previously sought treatment for her pain symptoms; instead she had been taking three acetaminophen tablets to reduce her pain.

Oral/dental evaluation

On clinical examination, the patient showed no limitations in mandibular opening. Unassisted opening without pain was 48 mm, and maximum opening regardless of pain was 50 mm. No joint sounds were detected on opening, either with or without stethoscope assistance. Her TMJ was painful to palpation, as were several muscles sites on the head and neck. Occlusal wear on the lower incisors was observed. No abnormalities were observed on the panoramic radiograph or on the TMJ MR images.

Psychosocial interview and questionnaires

The patient reported a strong tendency to clench her teeth together, during both daylight hours and during sleep. In addition, she reported biting her nails, chewing on pens and pencils, and a habit of jutting or thrusting her jaw forward. She reported that her pain interfered substantially with her ability to work; however, she never missed work due to her symptoms. Instead, she suffered and tried to perform to the best of her ability. Although she loved her job as a hospice organization administrator, she considered it very stressful. By her own report, she was felling distressed and overwhelmed, both by her persistent, puzzling pain and also by her stressful job. She indicated that her pain problem interfered with her ability to perform household chores, and sometimes she reduced her social activities due to her persistent pain.

Case 2

The second patient is a 56-year-old married African-American woman who came to the TMD pain treatment project at the University of Pittsburgh seeking treatment for jaw pain, which had been ongoing for the previous 14 years. Her primary complaints were pain in the TMJ area, primarily on the left side, headaches and soreness in the upper back. She reported that there was always some pain present, and that approximately once per week she had an excruciating pain flare lasting for up to two days. The patient was not able to identify any specific precipitants, and she stated that the symptoms gradually increased over time. Her treatment history included three previous intraoral appliances (splints) which she no longer possessed, and physical therapy in the form of transcutaneous electrical nerve stimulation (TENS) and heat treatment. At the time of her evaluation she was taking acetaminophen with codeine several times per week and extra-strength buffered aspirin on a daily basis to manage her pain. In addition to her jaw pain, the patient had been diagnosed with osteoarthritis in the right knee.

Oral/dental evaluation

The patient's mandibular opening ability was within normal limits, at 36 mm unassisted opening without pain, and 42 mm maximum opening regardless of pain. Crepitus was detected from the left TMJ upon opening, and pain in both the left and right TMJ area was elicited by palpation. Several intra- and extraoral muscle sites were also painful to palpation, including the muscles of the neck and shoulders. No abnormalities were apparent on panoramic radiograph. MRI of the TMJ revealed degenerative changes in the left mandibular condyle including flattening of the condyle and some spur formation. The left intra-articular meniscus or disc appeared to be anteriorly displaced and irregular in shape. The right TMJ was seen as normal.

Psychosocial interview and questionnaires

The patient revealed that chewing, talking, cold damp weather and time pressures or rushing were associated with increases in her jaw pain. She acknowledged several oral parafunctional behaviors that had the potential for increasing pain, such as grinding her teeth at night, clenching her teeth during the day, biting her lips, and holding the telephone between her ear and shoulder. She reported that her pain symptoms caused a great deal of interference with her social, recreational and household activities. As a retired court reporter, she was no longer working, but she had many community and family activities and interests. In addition to decreasing her enjoyment and performance of these activities, her pain symptoms made her feel quite distressed and out of control of her life. She reported depressed mood, sleep problems, fatigue and irritability. Despite her reports of affective distress and high pain severity and interference, the patient appeared energetic in the interview, and highly motivated for treatment.

Epidemiology

Epidemiological research in the area of TMDs has focused primarily on estimates of prevalence rates for signs and symptoms, and descriptions of characteristics of TMD cases versus controls (Von Korff, 1995). Signs and symptoms of TMDs are not uncommon in the general population. Clicking sounds have been found in 8–29% of children aged 7–18 years and 8–41% of adults; crepitation occurs in up to 16% of asymptomatic people (Fricton & Schiffman, 1995). Recent population-based questionnaire data in the USA indicate a prevalence rate of 12% for TMD-related pain, which includes complaints of persistent pain in the TMJ area and the muscles of the face (Dworkin et al., 1990). Another extensive survey of over 42 000 USA households estimated the prevalence rate of jaw joint or facial muscle pain in adults to be 6% (Lipton et al., 1993). In Scandinavia, estimates of prevalences rates ranged from 16% to 59% for reported symptoms, and from 33% to 86% for clinical signs (Carlsson, 1984).

The discrepancy between US studies and northern European studies may not reflect the true differences between these populations, but instead may be due to the fact that the definitions used for TMD problems and the methods of investigation varied extensively. The lack of an agreed set of criteria for diagnosing and classifying TMDs has certainly hampered previous epidemiological studies. Depending on which diagnostic criteria are used, studies may classify individuals as TMD cases or not, resulting in wide variability in prevalence rates across studies. For example, some studies rely on self-report of pain and dysfunction, whereas others may include diverse clinical assessment procedures (Carlsson & LeResche, 1995).

Temporomandibular disorder prevalence across sex and age groups

Early epidemiological studies did not find great differences in prevalence of signs and symptoms of TMDs between men and women in the general population (Carlsson & LeResche, 1995). The patients who present for treatment at TMD clinics, however, are predominantly female. Possible explanations for the sex difference in treatment seeking include a difference in tolerance to pain and other physical symptoms (Lipton et al., 1993), and a sex role or psychosocial differences in the acceptability of seeking help for a pain problem. There is also some question as to whether there is a difference between men and women in the presence of estrogen receptors in the TMJ (Abubaker et al., 1993; Campbell et al., 1993), and whether men and women differ in susceptibility to joint and musculoskeletal problems (Dworkin et al., 1990). The reasons why females are more likely to predominate in groups of TMD patients in treatment are probably multiple, and may be a result of the interactions of various social and biological factors.

While signs and symptoms of TMD such as pain to palpation of the masticatory muscles and TMJ clicking are not uncommon among children and adolescents, they are less common than in adults, and the severity of symptoms is generally mild (De Boever & van den Berghe, 1987). A longitudinal investigation of children and adolescents indicated a slight increase in prevalence in signs and symptoms as children grow older, but also a great fluctuation in signs and symptoms over time, with many who initially had TMJ clicking at age 15 years showing no clicking at age 20 years, and vice versa (Magnusson et al., 1986).

Findings from both longitudinal and cross-sectional studies suggest that TMD problems may decrease rather than increase over time. A longitudinal epidemiological study of older adults indicated that joint sounds fluctuate over time in this age group, and that symptoms of TMD tend to decrease with increasing age (Osterberg et al., 1992). Using a sample over 10 000 TMD patients from the USA, Levitt & McKinney (1994) found that severity and prevalence of joint dysfunction were lower among older age groups than younger age groups.

Economic costs

Temporomandibular disorders are common in the general population; however, there is great deal of variability in the extent to which individuals continue to seek treatments for the problem. In a large-scale epidemiological study of persons belonging to a health maintenance organization in the Northwestern United States (Group Health Cooperative of Puget Sound), the prevalence rate of temporomandibular disorders was 21.1% (Von Korff, 1995). Only one-quarter of those with TMDs (23%) had been treated for the disorder. As with other intermittent pain conditions such as headache, many people simply tolerate their symptoms or learn to minimize them through self-care such as eating soft foods, taking nonprescription pain medications, and avoiding wide mandibular opening. However, an alternative explanation for the relatively low rate of treatment-seeking is that the treatments may be quite costly. Many patients report that their insurance companies do not cover costs of TMD treatment. This can lead to a large financial burden for patients whose pain is severe. In the Puget Sound study, of the TMD patients who sought treatment, 29% had seen at least three different providers previously, and 12% had been to five or more providers. Of participants in a jaw pain research study at the University or Pittsburgh, 58% had been treated at least one time previously. Sixty one percent indicated that they relied on pain medications at least three times per week, adding to the financial costs of this disorder. Although there have been no research studies to date on the actual economic costs of TMDs to patients or to society, many patients report no previous treatments due to the costs involved. Others, overwhelmed by pain, report spending thousands of dollars for treatments prior to seeking treatment at the University of Pittsburgh's TMD treatment project.

Confirmations

Psychosocial and behavioral classification of patients with temporomandibular disorders

Turk & Rudy (1987, 1988) have proposed a classification system for chronic pain based on the empirical integration of psychosocial and behavioral data in assessing the psychological features of chronic pain patients. The primary hypothesis was that certain modal patterns in psychological assessment data recur in chronic pain patients and that these patterns represent a homogeneous subgroup of patients that are relatively independent of medical or dental diagnoses. To assess the psychosocial and behavioral factors, Turk & Rudy (1988) used the West Haven–Yale Multidimensional Pain Inventory (WHY MPI: Kerns et al., 1985). The MPI consists of a set of empirically derived scales designed to assess pain patients' appraisals of pain severity, interference with social and familial activities, impact on their lives, current mood state, responses from significant others and the performance of common daily activities.

Rudy et al. (1989) have demonstrated that TMD patients could be classified reliably into one of three subgroups based on the perceived impact of pain and associated symptoms on their lives, psychological distress, activity levels and responses by significant others to symptoms. These investigators used a multivariate statistical approach to classification. A cluster analysis was performed on the MPI scales to derive homogeneous subgroups of TMD patients according to similarities among their pattern of responses to the various MPI scales. This approach identifies mutually occurring groups of patients and can be compared with alternative a priori methods such as used in the Research Diagnostic Criteria for Temporomandibular Disorders (RDC/TMD).

The empirically derived classification developed by Rudy et al. (1989) for TMD patients identified one subset of patients (46%) who were characterized by high levels of pain and psychological distress, low levels of perceived control over their life, and low levels of common daily activities: 'dysfunctional' patients (DYS). A second group (22%)

were characterized by feelings of low social support and a high frequency of negative responses by significant others and thus were labeled as 'interpersonally distressed'. Approximately 32% of the patients comprised a group labeled 'adaptive copers', as they reported lower levels of emotional distress and higher levels of perceived control while remaining quite active. These three subgroups did not differ from each other on the basis of duration of pain, sex and age, or in terms of RDC Axis I examination findings, including radiographic studies.

In another study, Turk & Rudy (1990) compared TMD patients with chronic back pain or headache and found that regardless of diagnosis, the majority of patients could be classified reliably into one of these three groups. All three syndrome groups, however, were represented in each of the subgroups identified. Thus, it is possible that TMD, headache or chronic back pain patients who are classified within the same subgroup may be more similar to each other than patients with the same physical diagnosis but who were classified within different psychosocial subgroups.

Recently Rudy et al. (1995) completed a study designed to evaluate the differential response of 133 TMD patients classified within the three psychosocial behaviorally based subgroups described above to a conservative, standardized treatment. The treatment consisted of the combination of an intraoral appliance, biofeedback and stress management. Follow-up assessments were conducted 6 months after treatment termination. The results demonstrated that as a group, patients significantly improved and maintained improvements on physical, psychosocial and behavioral measures ($p < 0.0001$) external to the measures used in the classification system. Comparisons across patient subgroups, however, revealed differential patterns of improvement on the outcome measures. Most notably, reliable change indices demonstrated that the patients classified into a subgroup characterized by the greatest degree of psychological distress (DYS) showed significantly greater improvements on measures of pain intensity ($p < 0.001$), perceived impact of TMD symptoms on their lives ($p < 0.001$), depression ($p < 0.01$) and negative thoughts ($p < 0.001$), compared with 'interpersonally distressed' and 'adaptive copers' patient groups. 'Interpersonally distressed' patients also displayed treatment changes that were uniquely different from those found for 'adaptive coper' patients (e.g., changes in pain intensity). These findings support the clinical utility of the psychosocial-behavioral classification system and suggest that individualizing treatments based on patient characteristics may improve treatment efficacy. Additionally, these findings have important methodological implications for TMD treatment outcome studies, i.e., combining heterogeneous samples in treatment outcome studies without statistically controlling for subgroup differences (e.g., by blocking) may result in nonsignificant findings. The treatment provided may have been very effective, but only for a subset of patients.

Dysfunctional TMD patients, i.e., those patients who are found to have high levels of psychological disruption, pain severity, depression and disability, provide a unique therapeutic challenge. We completed a study (Turk et al., 1996) designed to evaluate whether a tailored treatment intervention for patients classified as DYS was more effective than a generic therapeutic approach. Fifty TMD patients classified as DYS were randomly assigned to one of two treatment conditions: (1) a flat plane interocclusal appliance and biofeedback-assisted relaxation training (IA/BF), and (2) IA/BF treatment plus cognitive therapy (CT) for depression (IA/BF+CT). Both groups received six weekly treatment sessions, followed by post-treatment and six-month follow-up evaluations. Multivariate analyses of nine indices that measured physical, psychosocial and behavior changes indicated both groups displayed significant improvements at six months (all $p < 0.001$). Compared with IA/BF patients, IA/BF + CT patients displayed significantly larger changes ($p < 0.001$), particularly on measures of pain severity and depression. These results suggest that DYS TMD patients in general demonstrate and maintain significant improvements on physical as well as psychological and behavioral measures following treatments that targets each of these three components. Thus, including a specific component tailored to the DYS patient characteristics, namely depression and disability, added incrementally to the outcome.

Role of injury/macrotrauma

Facial pain and disability may develop gradually or abruptly following a direct injury to the face, head or neck, or an indirect injury such as whiplash sustained during a motor vehicle accident. Trauma could result in direst damage to the structures of the TMJ, arthritic processes, or damage to the masticatory muscles or related soft tissues. Retrospective studies indicate that many TMD patients report a history of overt or indirect trauma. In a sample of 661 patients seeking treatment for TMD, 284 (43%) reported extrinsic trauma to their head or neck as the precipitating factor in the onset of symptoms (Harkins & Martenay, 1985). Between 44% and 79% of TMD clinic patients report a history of either MVA or other direct trauma, whereas only 13% of dental patients without pain report such history (Pullinger & Seligman, 1991). Although many TMD patients report past trauma, chronic facial pain may not be a common outcome of injury. In a recent study of 20 672 compensation claims following MVAs, only 28 people (0.14% of claims) sought compensation for TMDs (Probert et al., 1994). In a prospective study of 155 post-MVA trauma cases, 15% had facial pain immediately following the accident, but symptoms had diminished after one month and had resolved in all patients by 12 months (Heise et al., 1992). Although complaints of symptoms consistent with TMDs are not common following MVAs, past trauma may be an important causative factor for a subset of TMD patients.

Contradictions

Occlusal factors

During the 1930s to 1960s, the idea that poor occlusion was associated with TMJ problems prevailed (McNamara et al., 1995). Malocclusion, or a 'bad bite' is still thought by many clinicians to be an important causative factor in jaw pain and joint problems. Occlusal factors that have been considered important are skeletal anterior open bite (in which the front teeth do not touch when the mouth is closed), overjet or horizontal overlap of the teeth, crossbite and lack of posterior occlusal support. Most research, however, has shown little or no relationship between these isolated occlusal factors and TMD diagnostic groups. Recent research by Pullinger et al (1993) used combinations of occlusal features in asymptomatic controls and strictly defined subgroups of TMD patients. These authors found that some occlusal features, such as skeletal anterior open bite and several missing posterior teeth, occurred mainly in patients and rarely in healthy subjects; however, these features were rare in patients as well as in normals, which limits their diagnostic usefulness. The authors concluded that many of the occlusal features that were traditionally believed to be influential contribute only minor amounts to risk for TMD, and that occlusion cannot be considered the most important factor in the development of TMDs.

Pathogenetic hypotheses

Despite the prevalence of signs and symptoms of TMDs, the etiology of TMDs is poorly understood. There is virtually no definitive information available concerning the etiology of TMDs. Although some patients readily identify a specific onset event (such as an injury to the face, head or neck) related to the development of their pain symptoms, most report that their symptoms developed without warning and with no particular onset event. Just as the signs and symptoms associated with TMDs are complex and multiple, so are the potential causative factors. Table 7.1 lists potential causative or exacerbating factors that should be considered in the evaluation of TMDs. Reviewed below is one of the more common etiological models that encompasses both structural, environmental and behavioral factors.

Table 7.1. *Potential causative, predisposing or exacerbating factors for temporomandibular disorders*

(1) Traumatic onset events
  (a) Direct blow to the jaw or face
  (b) Indirect injury, such as whiplash injury from a motor vehicle accident
  (c) Prolonged wide mouth opening
(2) Cumulative strain or microtrauma, not associated with a particular onset event
  (a) Bruxism
  (b) Oral parafunctional habits
  (c) Habitual poor jaw posture and head posture
(3) Physical factors
  (a) Malocclusion
  (b) Arthritis
  (c) Skeletal abnormalities
  (d) Previous trauma
(4) Psychosocial factors that can exacerbate perceived pain
  (a) High level of perceived stressors
  (b) Depressive symptoms
  (c) Anxiety

Psychophysiological models of temporomandibular disorders

Over the past two decades, psychological factors increasingly have been recognized by many theorists dealing with the etiology and treatment of TMDs. Although other psychological factors have received some attention (e.g., personality, emotional characteristics), to date, psychophysiological models of TMD appear to be the most popular psychologically based explanations for the development and/or maintenance of TMD.

The basic assumption of this model of TMD is that this persistent pain condition results from the interaction of potentially stressful environmental events, inadequate coping abilities, and a predisposing organic or psychological condition, or diathesis. If the adversive stimulation to the individual is very intense or recurrent and the individual lacks adequate coping skills, a stereotyped response may develop in an unfavorably disposed body system. In TMD problems, this unfavorable disposition may be due to overutilization of masticatory muscles (e.g. nocturnal bruxism), a structural problem (e.g., internal derangement of the TMJ), observational learning (e.g., learned oral behaviors from a parent, such as chewing on a pencil to find the answer to a problem), and so forth.

In TMD, the individual response stereotype is believed to manifest itself as a localized hyper-reaction in the muscles of mastication. As the response becomes prolonged, the sympathetic nervous system becomes dysregulated and the sustained hyper-reactivity of these muscles may lead to local ischemia and reflex muscle spasm. Muscle hyperactivity may be mediated by the extrapyramidal gamma-motoric system, which is closely linked to the limbic system and thus very susceptible to emotional influences. With sustained muscular hyperactivity, pain develops as a consequence of local ischemic hypoxia and pain-eliciting irritants from hypoxic cells (e.g., lactic acid). These irritants may cause nociceptive receptors to become increasingly sensitized. The resulting muscle pain then may act as a new stressor and thus perpetuate a vicious pain–tension cycle. The cycle, once started, tends to perpetuate itself. Additionally, once a muscle has been subjected to a myospastic episode it tends, for reasons not yet understood, to become more susceptible to future episodes (Buxbaum et al., 1989).

Although the relationship between psychophysiological and structural factors in TMD remains unclear, several authors (Laskin, 1980; Buxbaum et al., 1989) have suggested that just as articulating structural pathologies can adversely affect the neuromusculature, so too can long-standing neuromuscular problems produce organic changes in the articulating elements of the TMJ. Moreover, secondary organic changes may become self-perpetuating because they result in altered oral patterns with attendant reinforcement of the initial spasm and pain. Thus, TMDs may be conceptualized as a continuum, in that what initially may have been primarily a functional, psychophysiological disorder may in time lead to structural changes in the TMJ. The reverse etiological order also may occur (Buxbaum et al., 1989).

Diagnostic and treatment approaches

Although interest in TMDs has spanned many decades and at least two continents (North America and Europe) much confusion remains about etiological factors. In addition, the plethora of distinct diagnostic systems developed over the years by various clinicians and investigators has added to this confusion. Without a universally accepted classification system, it is difficult for practitioners and investigators to compare observations and communicate about epidemiological and treatment outcome research results. To remedy this situation research diagnostic criteria (RDC/TMD) (Dworkin & LeResche, 1992) were developed by an international group. The RDC project sought to develop a measurable and reproducible set of clinical criteria for the most common forms of TMD, using both physical examination and evaluation of psychosocial functioning. The RDC/TMDs include a clear and detailed set of examination and classification procedures for physical TMD conditions, and also provide guidelines for evaluating psychosocial disability associated with temporomandibular disorders. Much work remains on establishing the validity and reliability of the examination and classification procedures, as well as determining the clinical utility of the diagnostic system. The RDC/TMDs holds promise for improving the research on TMDs.

Classification of temporomandibular disorder subgroups using the research diagnostic criteria Axis I

Axis I of the RDC includes the clinical TMD diagnoses and is divided into three groups. Table 7.2 outlines the three groups and various subdivisions within these groups. Group I includes the most common painful muscle disorders: (Ia) myofascial pain and (Ib) myofascial pain with limited opening. To classify a patient into group Ia, there must be self-reported ongoing pain in the muscles of mastication and related muscles of the neck and shoulders, as well as pain reported upon the dentist's palpation of at least three out of 20 intraoral and extraoral muscle sites. For classification into group Ib, limited mandibular opening (less than 40 mm pain-free unassisted opening, and passive stretch of 5 or more millimeters beyond the pain-free opening) is required in addition to the criteria for Ia.

The second group of disorders is the disc displacement group. The assignment of a group II classification is made on the basis of clinical signs and does not require a report of pain. There are three possible group II disorders, and each joint may receive one or no group II diagnoses. These represent variation from the normal intra-articular placement of the cartilage disc that cushions the surfaces of the condyle and articular eminence during jaw movements and rest. The most common displacement is an anteriorly displaced disc. During the translation phase of mandibular opening and closing, in which the rotated condyle moves parallel to the surface of the articular eminence, the disc may be restored to its normal position, creating a popping sound as it moves into place. This is called disc displacement with reduction and this phenomenon would warrant a group IIa diagnosis. A group IIb diagnosis, disc displacement without reduction with limited opening, is given if the displaced disc does not click or pop back into place and interferes with the range of motion such that opening is less than 35 mm. A group IIc classification, disc displacement without reduction without limited opening, is made if the displaced disc does not interfere with normal opening. These disc displacements can sometimes be inferred by the presence of clicking or popping sounds in the joint, although nonreducing displacements without limited opening may require imaging techniques for detection.

Table 7.2. *Diagnostic subgroups of temporomandibular disorders according to Research Diagnostic Criteria Axis I*

Group I: Muscle diagnoses
  (a) Myofascial pain
  (b) Myofascial pain with limited opening (< 40 mm)
Group II: Disc displacements
  (a) Disc displacement with reduction
  (b) Disc displacement without reduction, with limited opening ($\leqslant 35$ mm)
  (c) Disc displacement without reduction, without limited opening
Group III: Arthralgia, arthritis, arthrosis
  (a) Arthralgia
  (b) Osteoarthritis of the TMJ
  (c) Osteoarthrosis of the TMJ

Note: TMJ, temporomandibular joint.

Group III disorders include arthralgia (IIIa), osteoarthritis of the TMJ (IIIb), and osteoarthrosis of the TMJ (IIIc). The criteria for arthralgia (IIIc) requires a report of ongoing pain in the joint, such as during maximum opening, and TMJ pain on palpation. A joint would be classified as IIIb, osteoarthritis, if coarse crepitus is present in addition to arthralgia or if imaging reveals a degenerative condition of the joint structures. A group IIIc classification would be assigned if coarse crepitus is present or a degenerative condition is determined on imaging, but there is no pain on palpation or during movement. As with group II, each joint may receive only one diagnosis from group III.

Differential diagnosis

When considering a diagnosis of TMD, it is important to rule out certain other problems whose symptoms may at first seem to mimic those of TMDs. These include trigeminal neuralgia, impacted molars and other dental problems that can cause facial pain. Certain rare muscle disorders, such as muscle spasm, myositis and contracture, must be ruled out before the patient can receive a group I diagnosis. Before assigning a group III diagnosis, polyarthritides, acute traumatic injury and infection in the joint must be ruled out.

Research diagnostic criteria Axis II: pain-related disability and psychological status

Recognizing that the extent of disability and distress associated with a chronic TMD condition may not have a direct correspondence to abnormalities in the structure and function of the masticatory muscles and TMJ (Rudy et al., 1989), the developers of the RDC/TMDs proposed a separate system for classifying the global severity of the pain condition. The proposed classification system, which has not yet been validated, includes questions on pain intensity, pain related jaw disability, depression and nonspecific physical symptoms. More information on RDC Axis II can be found in Dworkin & Le Resche (1992). An alternative method for understanding the TMD patient's extent of pain severity and disability is through the West Haren–Yale Multimensional Pain Inventory (Kerns et al., 1985), which is described in the Confirmations section of this chapter.

Widespread acceptance of the RDC/TMDs, and the growing recognition of the multidimensional nature of the chronic pain experience are factors that should continue to improve the treatment outcome research on TMDs. Now more than ever, experts agree that the physical, psychosocial and behavioral components of the pain problem all should be addressed through various treatment components.

Treatments for TMDs vary widely, from education and reassurance to surgical intervention. When a patient complains of facial pain symptoms to the family doctor or primary care physician and TMD is suspected, a referral should be made to a qualified dentist to diagnose TMD. Ideally, the referral should be to a dentist who specializes in TMDs and who works with other health professionals to provide comprehensive multifaceted treatment. Summarized below are several conservative interventions that can be provided by a primary care physician, with assistance from other professionals as needed.

Conservative treatment strategies for primary care

Education and reassurance

TMD symptoms can be confusing and distressing as well as painful to patients. Patients' fears may make the problem worse. Reassuring the patient that TMD problems sometimes end as spontaneously as they began may help to dispel fears. Many patients fear that symptoms such as clicking and popping will progress to greater disturbances in functioning. Providing them with the information that 20–30% of the population experiences joint sounds without pain may reassure patients that joint sounds are normal.

Jaw rest

Although referral to a qualified dental professional for appliance therapy may be indicated, especially if the patient reports bruxism, there are several other simple methods for promoting jaw rest which can help to reduce muscle and joint pain. Optimizing jaw and head posture can be important for many TMD patients. Many patients habitually adopt a 'teeth together' mouth posture, and do not realize that this causes extraneous muscle tension. Developing a 'teeth apart' posture reduces muscle tension and over time can help to reduce pain. Asking patients to be aware of general posture also is recommended. A slumped posture or head forward posture can put undue strain on the muscles of the neck, head and shoulders, and may contribute to TMD pain. Patients who work on computers should be aware that improper height of the keyboard or monitor also can contribute to muscle problems. Reducing parafunctional oral habits, such as daytime clenching, gum chewing and biting on fingernails, pens and pencils can also promote jaw rest. Table 7.3 presents a list of patient self-help strategies, including oral habit reduction, dietary suggestions and general stress management.

Flare management

There are several simple strategies that a patient may use to manage acute pain flares, including cold therapy, moist heat therapy and over-the-counter anti-inflammatory medication. During the first 24–48 hours of a flare, using ice or a cold pack until numbness occurs (no more than 10 minutes), can help to reduce pain and swelling. For an ice massage, freeze some water in a paper or Styrofoam cup and then tear off the bottom to expose the ice and massage the painful area gently until if feels numb. Another easy method for cold treatment is to wrap a bag of frozen peas or corn in a dishtowel, and apply it to the painful area. Moist heat may be alternated with cold to manage a flare. The easiest method is to wet a washcloth with hot water (but not hot enough to burn the skin) and apply to the painful area for 10–20 minutes. Some patients will discover that alternating heat and cold is helpful for reducing discomfort, others will prefer only one or the other.

Pharmacological treatment options that may require pain specialist consultation

Rational treatment of TMDs can include pharmacological adjuncts to optimize other treatment modalities such as splint therapy, physical therapy or biofeedback. Analgesic medications are a first line consideration for pharmacological therapy. They include common over-the-counter medications such as acetaminophen, aspirin or ibuprofen. Unfortunately, the latter two medications are limited in their usefulness by the potential side-affects of gastric irritation. Additionally, the over-the-counter dosing of ibuprofen is limited to the recommended 200 mg every 4–6 hours. In many instances, the dosing is too low to bring about any real analgesic or anti-inflammatory results. Most practitioners utilize ibuprofen in the 400 mg range and at least three times per day (Gray et al., 1994; Haas, 1995). Ibuprofen may be utilized as high as 800 mg every 6 hours during the acute phase of the

Table 7.3. *Reducing temporomandibular joint pain symptoms*

Temporomandibular joint pain symptoms are frequently associated with increased levels of jaw muscle activity. Following the suggestions listed below can significantly decrease the amount of pain many people experience

(1) Activities you can control:
  Sleep on your back, not on your side or stomach
  Do not open your mouth overly wide (e.g. yawning, shouting, biting into a large food item)

(2) Pay attention to your diet:
  Avoid extra chewy or large food items that require wide mouth opening
  Avoid harder foods that require greater muscle activity (e.g., raw carrots)
  Prepare foods so they can be eaten without requiring overly wide opening of mouth (e.g., slice an apple instead of biting into the whole fruit)

(3) Behavior to avoid:
  Clenching your teeth
  Biting your lips or tongue
  Chewing on pens or pencils
  Biting the side of your mouth
  Cupping your chin in your hand
  Resting your head with your hand on the side of your face
  Biting your nails
  Thrusting or jutting your jaw forward
  Holding the telephone between your chin and shoulder
  Chewing gum
  Bracing your jaw by holding your front teeth together
  Smoking cigarettes, cigars or pipes

(4) Develop relaxation strategies:

Stressful situations, such as when you are anxious, angry or under pressure, often lead to increased muscle tension. Become more aware of these situations and be extra careful to avoid tensing your jaw muscles at such times. *The following strategies can help you to relax* your muscles before and during stressful situations
  Take deeper and slower breaths
  Repeat the word 'relax' as a reminder to keep calm
  Focus on positive thoughts: look for the possibilities, not just the problems in a situation

process. Other useful nonsteroidal anti-inflammatory medications include diflunisal (500 mg every 12 hours), naproxen (250 mg every 6 hours), ketorolac (10 mg every 6 hours) and flurbiprofen (50 mg every 6 hours).

If nonsteroidal anti-inflammatory medications have insufficient responses, then the addition of an opiate such as codeine (60 mg every 4–6 hours) or oxycodone (5 mg every 4 hours) may be useful. Opiates plus nonsteroidal anti-inflammatory drugs are a powerful and effective combination in treating acute TMD pain. Opiates are limited by the side-effects of gastrointestinal upset, constipation, sedation, respiratory depression (in the sensitive or frail patient) and, in the long term, they present the potential for chemical dependency and tolerance (Haas, 1995). Oral preparations of meperidine pentazocine have little increased benefit over codeine or oxycodone in the treatment of TMD pain.

Chronic, debilitating TMD pain that persists despite comprehensive multidisiplinary treatment may necessitate the long-term use of opiates. These may include sustained release oral preparations of morphine, oxycodone or methadone. Fentanyl patches should be reserved only as a last resort. Before embarking on the use of these opiate preparations, consultation with a pain specialist would be prudent to prevent over- or underdosing. Cessation of the use of these compounds requires a gentle taper schedule that may be simplified when a pain specialist assists the primary care practitioner in their use.

Skeletal muscle relaxants have been used to break muscle spasms in acute TMD pain flares. Drugs such as cyclobenzaprine (Flexeril®), methocarbamol (Robaxin®), orphenadrine (Norflex®) or carisoprodol (Soma®) have all been used successfully to help to reduce painful spasms particularly in patients who have myofascial type pain; however, there has been little research to support the efficacy of their use. Additionally, their usefulness has been limited by the side-effects of sedation and dizziness (Haas, 1995).

Tricyclic antidepressant compounds are useful in the treatment of chronic TMD pain. Their dosing for analgesia and improved sleep tends to be significantly less than the dosing for depression (Haas, 1995). Successful use in terms of reduced pain and improved sleep with amitriptyline, desipramine or nortriptyline, has occurred within one week of initiation of therapy. Side-effects such as xerostomia, weight gain, sedation, dysrhythmias and other drug interactions may limit or preclude their use in certain patients.

Short-term use of benzodiazepines may be helpful in anxious patients with severe muscle spasms. Diazepam, alprazolam, nitrazepam and temazepam have been used to create anxiolysis and induce sleep. As a result, muscle spasms may diminish or disappear. The usefulness of benzodiazepines is limited by the side-effects of sedation, paradoxical anxiety and significant chemical dependency (Gray et al., 1994; Haas, 1995).

Finally, there is a place for intraarticular injections of long-acting steroids such as dexamethasone, methyl prednisolone, and possibly trimcinolone. These injections should be performed only by a practitioner who is quite familiar with the anatomy of the TMJ (Gray et al., 1994; Haas, 1995).

Treatments provided by other professionals

Some of the more common treatments for TMDs provided by dentists, psychologists and physical therapists are described below. Although the various treatments are described separately, based on the roles of the treatment providers, it is important to remember that treatment efforts can and should be coordinated. Due to the multifactorial nature of TMDs, with their potentially interacting structural, behavioral and psychological features, multidisciplinary treatment is recommended, particularly for more chronic cases.

Dental professionals can provide intraocclusal appliance (splint) therapy

Probably the most frequent treatment provided to patients with TMDs is splint therapy. A splint is a clear acrylic appliance that is custom made to fit over the upper or lower teeth. Generally, the occlusal surface is flat to allow for the normal sliding motions of the mandible. The splint also should cover the full arch of the mandible or maxilla to provide contact for all of the teeth. One goal of splint therapy is to reduce strain on the muscles and joint by providing an increased distance between the upper and lower teeth. The splint also is thought to promote reduction in parafunctional oral habits such as nocturnal and diurnal grinding and clenching, which also reduces excess strain on the masticatory system. Several studies support the effectiveness of splint therapy in reducing bruxism (Solberg et al., 1975) and myalgia (Greene & Laskin, 1972; Agerberg & Carlsson, 1974; Clark et al., 1981). In some studies, appliances have been shown to reduce clicking as well as pain in many patients (Anderson et al., 1985; Moloney & Howard, 1986; Clark et al., 1988); however, in one study clicking sounds returned after discontinuation of the splint (Lundh et al., 1985). In a randomized controlled trial, Turk et al. (1993) found splint therapy to be as effective as biofeedback/stress management training for pain reduction. When combined, the treatments were more effective than either one alone.

Some clinicians recommended full-time splint use (except for eating and oral hygiene) and others may prescribe it only for night-time use. It is not uncommon for patients to use a night splint indefinitely to control the effects of bruxing. Full-time (day and night) splint therapy should not be continued indefinitely because there is reason to suspect that very long-term use irreversibly changes the natural occlusal relationships of the upper and lower teeth.

Psychologists can provide behavioral interventions, biofeedback and stress/pain management training

It is increasingly recognized among professionals who treat pain patients that chronic pain is a multidimensional experience, comprising physical or structural components, affective or emotional factors and psychosocial and cognitive components. Psychosocial factors such as anxiety and depressive symptoms are very important to assess among TMD patients, particularly because they have been found to be predictive of treatment outcome (Fricton & Olsen, 1996).

Behavior change

During discussions with the patients, many oral-parafunctional behaviors may be identified that can exacerbate the pain problem. These may include clenching the teeth during the daytime, chewing gum, chewing on fingernails, pens or pencils, smoking and jutting the mandible forward. These behaviors add unnecessary activity to the muscles and excess loading to the joint. Education on parafunctional oral habits is a common component of TMD treatment, and many patients report significant reductions in pain as a result of eliminating such behaviors; however, habits can be difficult to change. Ideally, a clinician and patient will together develop a strategy on when the behaviors occur, how to become more aware of the behaviors and how to replace them with more adaptive behaviors, such as a relaxed jaw posture. In ongoing treatment, the patient has repeated chances to report on success and the problems around modifying these behaviors, and the clinician can be a partner who helps the patient maintain motivation for change. In a recent study, change in oral habits during a comprehensive treatment program was significantly associated with reductions in pain and disability, accounting for 16% of the variance in TMJ pain, perceived pain severity, and interference with life activities after treatment (Greco et al., 1996).

Biofeedback

Several randomized studies provide support for the effectiveness of biofeedback-assisted relaxation training on TMD pain and dysfunction (Dahlstrom & Carlsson, 1984; Hijzin et al., 1986; Turk et al., 1993). Biofeedback has been compared with splint therapy and found to have comparable beneficial effects and, in one case, continued improvement was noted in the biofeedback group six months after treatment had ended (Turk et al., 1993). Electromyographic (EMG) biofeedback is used to train patients to relax the muscles of the face, develop a relaxed facial posture and maintain facial muscle relaxation while imagining personally relevant stressful events. Surface electrodes are attached to the masseter muscles and patients receive visual or auditory feedback on their muscle tension. In addition to the skills mentioned above, biofeedback can serve to reinforce to the patient the value of reducing oral habits and can give patients who have been coping with chronic pain a sense of self-control over their muscle tension and associated pain. It is very important for patients to practice the skills learned in the biofeedback session at home and at work. The patient and clinician can work together to assign times for practicing this 'homework', such as after each meal and while driving to and from work.

Stress management/pain management training

Many patients report that TMD pain is worse during stressful times. This may be due to increased jaw clenching in response to stress, or excess muscle tension in general; therefore, stress management and pain management can be important components of a TMD treatment program. Through ongoing collaboration with the clinician, the patient can learn relaxation skills, cognitive techniques for reducing stress reactions to events and methods for distracting attention away from pain. When these skills are solidified through ongoing practice, they can be very helpful in reducing mild to moderate pain and preventing pain flare-ups. For patients who are in greater emotional distress, stress management techniques such as cognitive therapy aimed at decreasing distorted or dysfunctional thoughts can provide added benefits in terms of reduction of depressive symptoms (Turk et al., 1996).

Researchers in chronic pain have long recognized an association between chronic pain and depression. Clinicians who work with chronic pain patients tend to agree that many, but certainly not all, of these patients show depressive symptoms such as sleep and appetite problems, depressed mood and a lack of interest in activities. One study of TMD patients found that 13.5% endorsed clinically elevated scores on a depression inventory (Wright et al., 1991). Another study reported that 30% of TMD patients showed evidence of major depression during a clinical interview (Kinney et al., 1992). When signs and symptoms of depression are encountered during comprehensive evaluation for TMDs, it is important for the psychologist to address these issues during treatment, as treatment outcome may be affected (Turk et al., 1996).

Physical therapists can provide therapeutic exercises and apply modalities

Most research on physical therapy interventions for TMDs consist of clinical reports rather than randomized controlled trials (Decker et al., 1995). Many authors emphasize the beneficial effects of physical therapy exercises on a mandibular range of motion and pain and on the tenderness associated with TMDs. In addition, one controlled study (Au & Klineberg, 1993) found an exercise regimen to be associated with significant reductions in joint sounds among pain-free young adults with clicking and popping. Some of the frequently used exercises for increasing jaw function and reducing pain include: (1) postural exercises to reduce strain on the masticatory and cervical muscles and on the joint, (2) isometric exercises to improve muscle and joint coordination and strengthen the muscles, (3) gentle stretching exercises to improve joint and muscle range of motion, and (4) quick repetition of small opening motions to improve the biomechanical functioning of the joint and jaw muscles (Rocabado & Iglarsh, 1991). Such exercises can be taught to the patient for home use; however, ongoing appointments with the physical therapist are necessary to ensure the proper use of exercises and to monitor success.

Various modalities are frequently applied by physical therapists to promote relaxation and pain reduction; however, there is a lack of controlled trials for determining their efficacy for TMDs (Mohl et al., 1990). Some of the common modalities include the application of heat and cold, ultrasound, electrical stimulation, soft tissue mobilization and joint mobilization.

Heat, particularly moist hot packs, are thought to promote muscle relaxation, increase blood flow and reduce pain. Cold therapy may be provided in the form of a vapocoolant spray or cold packs. Cold can provide counter-stimulation to painful areas and allow the patient to stretch the muscles. In a well-designed and controlled study, the combination of vapocoolant spray and stretching exercises was more effective than exercise alone and no intervention for patients with myofascial pain (Burgess et al., 1988). Cold pack application also is intended to reduce the acute inflammation of the muscles and joint through a decreased circulation.

Ultrasound is high frequency inaudible acoustic vibrations that are thought to produce both thermal and nonthermal physiological effects. The thermal effects are similar to those expected by surface application of moist heat. Ultrasound is also thought to decrease the viscosity of collagen and allow increased mobility of the muscles and joint. Higher frequencies provide stimulation to areas within 2 cm of the surface, while deeper structures are treated by lower frequency vibrations (Gunn, 1991). TENS and other devices are thought to provide counter-stimulation and promote relaxation of the muscles, and thereby reduce pain; however, the research results on their effectiveness for TMDs is mixed (Clark et al., 1990).

The treatments available for TMDs are multiple, and there are many reports of their success. Many of the treatments have not been tested thoroughly in well-designed randomized, controlled trials with sufficient follow-up periods. It is common in clinical practice to encounter a TMD patient who has tried several treatments that were each effective for a limited period. It is necessary, therefore, to continue to assess symptoms and progress over time, and it is highly recommended that various health care professionals remain involved in the treatment program.

Case studies revisited

Summary of the standardized treatment program

Both patients were enrolled in a standardized conservative, comprehensive treatment program at the Pain Evaluation and Treatment Institute, University of Pittsburgh. The program, which was part of a research study funded by the National Institute of Dental Research, consisted of a mandibular flat-plane intraoral appliance to be worn full time initially and worn not at all by the end of the program, and six $1\frac{1}{2}$ hour weekly biofeedback/stress management sessions. The sessions were focused on skill development in several areas. For biofeedback training, surface EMG electrodes were applied to the masseter muscles. Computer-controlled auditory feedback directly corresponding to the patient's muscle tension was used to help the patient to learn to reduce jaw muscle tension and develop appropriate jaw posture. The stress management consisted of: (1) education about the association of stress, muscle tension and pain; (2) cognitive coping skills training to control reactions to pain and stress; (3) progressive muscle relaxation training; and (4) homework assignments to practice relaxation skills without biofeedback instrumentation. A more detailed description of the treatment program and methodology can be found in Rudy et al (1995) and Turk et al. (1996).

Response to treatment

Case 1

The patient was dismayed about the idea of wearing the intraoral appliance full-time, except for eating and brushing her teeth. She was sure that it would interfere with her speaking ability at work. She was told that most patients adjust their speech automatically, and she was instructed to read aloud at home for a few minutes per day with the splint in her mouth in order to facilitate comfort with speaking. By the second session, she had adjusted well to wearing the splint, and had told her staff about the treatment program so that they would not be surprised by seeing her wearing the splint.

In the biofeedback session, the patient was surprised by her high level of facial muscle tension. Over the first two biofeedback sessions, she was able to reduce her muscle tension substantially. This reduction was associated with a decrease in jaw pain during the session. The EMG feedback and pain decrease convinced her that lowering muscle tension was a good idea for her. She began to feel that she was developing some control over a problem that had seemed inexplicable previously. She was asked to practice relaxing her face several times per day for a few minutes at a time, using a posture that she had learned during her biofeedback session. She chose to perform most of her practice sessions at work. As she built this practice into her day, she began to realize just how tense and stressed she felt while at work. She felt as if she repeatedly responded to each new problem as though it were a crisis. She realized that holding her muscles tight was not helping her to solve problems, but instead was causing her to have more pain. She resolved to change the way she responded to stressors at work, both emotionally and physically. She knew that a change of behavior and attitude might have many positive consequences; pain could be reduced and she could be a good role model for problem solving for her staff.

During the sessions, the patient was taught progressive muscle relaxation (PMR), a whole body relaxation exercise that helps people to achieve a deep state of relaxation through tensing and then letting go of tension in various muscle groups. The exercise ends with visualization of a favorite place, chosen by the patient, which is associated with feelings of well-being and safety. She was instructed to practice this exercise, which takes approximately 15–20 minutes, at least once each day. She practiced most evenings just before getting ready for bed. One of the benefits of repeated practice of PMRs is that patients become skilled at relaxing their body quickly and easily. The patient began to practice a brief version of the PMR during her workday. She focused on the muscles of the back, neck and head, and used visualization of her family's cabin in the woods as her special place.

By the fourth treatment session, the patient reported that she rarely used her intraoral appliance. By the final session, she was not using it at all. She had adopted a relaxed jaw posture as her normal, automatic posture, and she rarely caught herself clenching her teeth in response to problems at work or other stressors. In addition, she built a brief relaxation break into her workday, in which she relaxed her whole body and thought of her special place. She felt that this kept her pain to a minimum, and also helped her to maintain a positive and productive attitude at work. No longer in constant pain, she was usually completely pain free, with weekly or biweekly pain flares lasting only 1–2 hours. She also had eliminated her use of pain medications.

When the patient was seen for a six-month follow-up, her TMD symptoms had continued to improve. She continued to use facial and general relaxation techniques, and rarely used her splint, which she saw as a 'last line of defense' against a pain flare. She did not use medications. She continued to report 'major improvement' in her TMD symptoms compared with her initial presentation.

On the basis of her pretreatment oral/dental evaluation, the patient had been given a group Ia diagnosis of Myofascial Pain and a group IIIa diagnosis of Arthralgia. At her posttreatment evaluation, none of the TMJ and muscle sites was painful to palpation. In addition, her test scores on the Multidimensional Pain Inventory (MPI) indicated that her level of activity had increased and that depressed mood had significantly decreased. This conservative treatment program, aimed at providing jaw rest and teaching skills for pain reduction and prevention, was highly effective for this individual who initially was quite distressed by the constant muscle and joint symptoms she had been experiencing.

Case 2

This patient had no difficulty adjusting to wearing her splint on a full-time basis. She was not sure how helpful it would be, as she had tried splints before with limited success. When the rationale of the splint as a 'short-term helper' during the skills training phase of treatment, with gradual reduction of splint use and replacement with self-management strategies was explained to her, she was motivated to continue.

In the initial biofeedback session the patient was able to reduce the tension in her masseter muscles substantially. In the second session, however, she felt what she called a 'muscle spasm' during the feedback session. She focused on her breathing and on the words 'get out from under the pain' and was soon free of this extra discomfort. She reported being pleased at her ability to control her reaction to the 'spasm' and avoid tensing up further in response to it.

The patient was taught the PMR exercise in session two. She reported that the feeling of deep relaxation was so pleasant that she would definitely build it into her daily routine. During a subsequent session, however, she reported that the tensing of the muscles aggravated her knee pain. As a result of this, and because the patient was easily able to achieve a relaxed state due to her diligent practice of PMR, we decided to discontinue the tensing of muscles and focus only on cognitive imagery for relaxing the muscles. She developed her own particular images to facilitate relaxation: she would breathe and visualize water flowing over her painful knee, over the painful muscles and joints of her face, and she would envision the water washing the pain away. The patient noticed that as she continued to practice her relaxation techniques, she was able to reduce the duration and intensity of her pain flares.

By the end of treatment, she was using her splint only occasionally, when she was performing physically demanding work. She routinely used relaxation techniques to manage her knee pain and the occasional flare-ups of TMD pain. She reported major improvement in her TMD symptoms as a result of treatment. When the patient came back to the clinic for a six month follow-up visit, she reported that she had undergone knee surgery, and that the relaxation techniques had helped her immensely during her rehabilitation process.

According to the RDC/TMDs, the initial diagnosis at the patient's oral/dental evaluation included group Ib Myofascial Pain with limited opening, group IIc Disc Displacement without reduction without limited opening, and a group IIIb osteoarthritis of the left TMJ. At the post treatment evaluation, pain on palpation of the TMJs was absent, and no muscle pain was present. It is unlikely that our treatment halted the degenerative changes shown on MRI. The patient's symptoms, however, were significantly reduced during the treatment program. She was able to generalize the skills she was taught and used them successfully to cope with other ongoing pain problems. In addition, the MPI testing results indicated that she reported a greater sense of control over her life and less emotional distress after the treatment. Additionally, the MPI scores showed that her perceived pain, which had decreased in severity, was no long causing a great deal of interference with her life's activities.

These case studies illustrate the benefits of a brief and conservative but comprehensive treatment program that focuses not only on physical examination parameters, but also the contributions of new skills and the reduction of parafunctional oral behaviors.

Conclusion

Temporomandibular disorders are a widespread problem that can present in diverse ways across individuals and within individuals over time. There may be masticatory muscle pain, as well as pain in the related muscles of the head and neck. Pain in the TMJ and joint sound upon opening also are frequently observed. A limitation in mandibular opening also may be present. TMDs are actually a collection of clinical conditions that may overlap and are not considered a single disorder. Subgroups of TMDs include: (1) muscle disorders, (2) TMJ disc displacements, and (3) arthralgia, arthritis or arthrosis.

When evaluating the patient who presents with orofacial pain, it is important to consider not only the physical signs and symptoms, but also the patient's perceptions of the pain, its interference with his or her life activities, and the effects of oral parafunctional behaviors on pain. Although some patients with persistent TMD pain also show depressive symptoms and/or problems managing anxiety, these are not the cause of their TMD. Rather, the cognitive patterns and behavioral manifestations (e.g., excess muscle tension) associated with these features may exacerbate the pain problem, and therefore should be addressed in a manner that makes their presumed contribution clear to the patient.

There are a number of noninvasive treatments that are effective for reduction of the pain associated with TMDs, including medications, intraoral appliances, biofeedback and stress management, and physical therapy exercises and modalities. TMD problems, especially those of short duration, can be managed effectively by primary care physicians. For more persistent, chronic problems, a multidisciplinary comprehensive approach is recommended. In our experience, few TMD patients are in need of invasive approaches such as TMJ injections or surgery.

Acknowledgment

The preparation of this paper was supported in part by USPHS Research Grant R01 DE07514 from the National Institute of Dental Research, National Institutes of Health, Bethesda, MD 20892.

References

American Academy of Craniomandibular Disorders: Craniomandibular Disorders: Guidelines for Evaluation, Diagnosis and Management. (1990). Chicago: Quintessence Publishing Company.

Abubaker AO, Raslan WF & Sotereanos GC (1993). Estrogen and progesterone receptors in temporomandibular joint discs of symptomatic and asymptomatic persons: a preliminary study. *Journal of Oral and Maxillofacial Surgery*, **51**, 1096–100.

Agerberg G & Carlsson GE (1974). Late results of treatment of functional disorders of the masticatory system: a follow-up questionnaire. *Journal of Oral Rehabilitation*, **1**, 309–16.

Anderson G, Schulte JK & Goodkind RJ (1985). Comparative study of two treatment methods for internal derangement of the temporomandibular joint. *Journal of Prosthetic Dentistry*, **53**, 392–7.

Au AR & Klineberg IJ (1993). Isokinetic exercise management of temporomandibular joint clicking in young adults. *Journal of Prosthetic Dentistry*, **70**, 33–9.

Bell WE (1986). *Temporomandibular Disorders: Classification, Diagnosis, Management*. Chicago: Year Book Medical Publishers.

Block SL (1980). Differential diagnosis of craniofacial–cervical pain. In *The Temporomandibular Joint*, 3 edn, ed. B. G. Sarnat & D. M. Laskin, pp. 348–421. Springfield, IL: Charles C. Thomas.

Burgess J, Sommers E, Truelove EE & Dworkin, SF (1988). Short-term effects of two therapeutic methods on myofascial pain and dysfunction of the masticatory system. *Journal of Prosthetic Dentistry*, **60**, 606–10.

Buxbaum JD, Myslinski NR & Myers DE (1989). Dental management of orofacial pain. In *Handbook of Chronic Pain Management*, ed. C. D. Tollison, pp. 297–316. Baltimore: Williams and Wilkins.

Campbell JH, Courey MS, Bourne P & Odziemiec C (1993). Estrogen receptor analysis of human temporomandibular disc. *Journal of Oral and Maxillofacial Surgery*, **51**, 1101–5.

Carlsson GE (1984). Epidemiological studies of signs and symptoms of temporomandibular joint pain dysfunction: a literature review. *Austalian Prosthodontic Society Bulletin*, **14**, 7–12.

Carlsson GE & LeResche L (1995). Epidemiology of temporomandibular disorders. In *Temporomandibular Disorders and Related Pain Conditions*, ed. B. J. Sessle, P. S. Bryant & R. A. Dionne, pp. 211–26. Seattle: IASP Press.

Clark GT, Beemsterboer PL & Rugh JD (1981). Nocturnal masseter muscle activity and the symptoms of masticatory dysfunction. *Journal of Oral Rehabilitation*, **8**, 279–86.

Clark GT, Lanham F & Flack, VF (1988). Treatment outcome for consecutive TMJ clinic patients. *Journal of Craniomandibular Disorders*, **2**, 87–95.

Clark GT, Adachi NY & Doman MR (1990). Physical medicine procedures affect temporomandibular disorders: a review. *Journal of the American Dental Association*, **121**, 151–62.

Dahlstrom L & Carlsson S (1984). Treatment of mandibular dysfunction: the clinical usefulness of biofeedback in relation to splint therapy. *Journal of Oral Rehabilitation*, **11**, 277–84.

De Boever JA & van den Berghe L (1987). Longitudinal study of functional conditions in the masticatory system in Flemish children. *Community Dentistry and Oral Epidemiology*, **15**, 100–3.

Decker KL, Bromaghim CA & Fricton JR (1995). Physical therapy for temporomandibular disorders and orofacial pain. In *Orofacial Pain and Temporomandibular Disorders*, ed. J. R. Fricton & R. B. Dubner. New York: Raven Press.

Dworkin SF, Huggins KH, LeResche L, Von Korff M, Howard J, Truelove E &

Sommers E (1990). Epidemiology of signs and symptoms in temporomandibular disorders: clinical signs in cases and controls. *Journal of the American Dental Association*, **120**, 273–81.

Dworkin SF & LeResche L (eds) (1992). Research diagnostic criteria for temporomandibular disorders. *Journal of Craniomandibular Disorders: Facial and Oral Pain*, **6**, 301–55.

Eversole LR & Machado L (1985). Temporomandibular joint internal derangements and associated neuromuscular disorders. *Journal of the American Dental Association*, **110**, 69–79.

Fricton JR & Olsen T (1996). Predictors of outcome for treatment of temporomandibular disorders. *Journal of Orofacial Pain*, **10**, 54–65.

Fricton JR & Schiffman EL (1995). Epidemiology of temporomandibular disorders. In *Orofacial Pain and Temporomandibular Disorders*, ed. J. R. Fricton & R. Dubner. pp. 1–14. New York: Raven Press.

Fricton JR, Kroening RJ & Hathaway KM (1988). *TMJ and Craniofacial Pain: Diagnosis and Management*, St Louis, MO: Ishiyaku Euroamerica.

Gunn N (1991). Ultrasound: current concepts. *Clinical Management*, **11**, 64–9.

Gray R, Davies SJ & Quayle AA (1994). A clinical approach to temporomandibular disorders. *British Dental Journal*, **177**, 101–6.

Greco CM, Rudy TE & Turk DC (1996). Oral habit change and reduction of pain and disability among TMD patients. *American Pain Society 15th Annual Scientific Meeting*.

Greene CS & Laskin DM (1972). Splint therapy for the myofascial pain-dysfunction (MPD) syndrome: a comparative study. *Journal of the American Dental Association*, **84**, 624–8.

Haas DA (1995). Pharmacologic considerations in the management of temporomandibular disorders. *Journal of the Canadian Dental Association*, **61**, 105–14.

Harkins SJ & Martenay JL (1985). Extrinsic trauma: a significant precipitating factor in temporomandibular dysfunction. *Journal of Prosthetic Dentistry*, **54**, 271–2.

Heise AP, Laskin DM & Gervin AS (1922). Incidence of temporomandibular joint symptoms following whiplash injury. *Journal of Oral and Maxillofacial Surgery*, **50**, 825–8.

Hijzen T, Slangen J & Van Houweligen H (1986). Subjective, clinical and EMG effects of biofeedback and splint treatment. *Journal of Oral Rehabilitation*, **13**, 529–39.

Kerns RD, Turk DC & Rudy TE (1985). The West Haven–Yale Multidimensional Pain Inventory (WHYMPI). *Pain*, **23**, 345–56.

Kinney RK, Gatchel RJ, Ellis E & Holt C (1992). Major psychological disorders in chronic TMD patients: implications for successful management. *Journal of the American Dental Association*, **123**, 49–54.

Laskin DM (1980). Myofascial pain-dysfunction syndrome: etiology. In *The Temporomandibular Joint: A Biological Basis for Clinical Practice*, ed. B. Sarnat & D. Laskin, pp. 289–99. Springfield, IL: Charles C. Thomas.

Levitt SR & McKinney MW (1994). Validating the TMJ scale in a national sample of 10 000 patients: demographic and epidemiological characteristics. *Journal of Orofacial Pain*, **8**, 25–35.

Lipton JA, Ship JA & Larach-Robinson D (1993). Estimated prevalence and distribution of reported orofacial pain in the United States. *Journal of the American Dental Association*, **124**, 115–21.

Lundh H, Westesson P, Kopp, S & Tillstrom B (1985). Anterior repositioning splint in the treatment of temporomandibular joints with reciprocal clicking: comparison with a flat occlusal splint and an untreated control group. *Oral Surgery, Oral Medicine, Oral Pathology*, **60**, 131–6.

Magnusson T, Egermark-Eriksson I & Carlsson GE (1986). Five year longitudinal study of signs and symptoms of mandibular dysfunction in adolescents. *Journal of Craniomandibular Practice*, **4**, 338–44.

McNamara JA, Seligman DA & Okeson JP (1995). The relationship of occlusal factors and orthodontic treatment to temporomandibular disorders. In *Temporomandibular Disorders and Related Pain Conditions*, vol. 4, ed. B. J. Sessle, P. S. Bryant & R. A. Dionne, pp. 399–427. Seattle, Washington: IASP Press.

Mohl ND, Ohrbach RK, Crow HC & Gross AJ (1990). Devices for diagnosis and treatment of temporomandibular disorders. Part III, Thermography, ultrasound, electrical stimulation and EMG biofeedback. *Journal of Prosthetic Dentistry*, **63**, 472–7.

Moloney F & Howard JA (1986). Internal derangements of the temporomandibular joint: anterior repositioning splint therapy. *Australian Dental Journal*, **31**, 30–9.

Osterberg T, Carlsson GE, Wedel A & Johansson U (1992). A cross-sectional and longitudinal study of craniomandibular dysfunction in an elderly population. *Journal of Craniomandibular Disorders–Facial and Oral Pain*, **6**, 237–46.

Probert TCS, Wiesenfeld D & Reade PC (1994). Temporomandibular pain dysfunction disorder resulting from road traffic accidents: an Australian study. *International Journal of Oral and Maxillofacial Surgery*, **23**, 338–41.

Pullinger AG & Seligman DA (1991). Trauma history in diagnostic subgroups of temporomandibular disorders. *Oral Surgery, Oral Medicine, Oral Pathology*, **71**, 529–34.

Pullinger AG, Seligman DA & Gornbein JA (1993). A multiple regression analysis of the risk and relative odds of temporomandibular disorders as a function of common occlusal features. *Journal of Dental Research*, **72**, 968–79.

Rocabado M & Iglarsh ZA (1991). *Musculoskeletal Approach to Maxillofacial Pain*. Philadelphia: Lippincott.

Rudy TE, Turk DC, Zaki HS & Curtin HD (1989). An empirical taxometric alternative to traditional classification and temporomandibular disorders. *Pain*, **36**, 311–20.

Rudy TE, Turk DC, Kubinski JA & Zaki HS (1995). Differential treatment responses of TMD patients as a function of psychological characteristics. *Pain*, **61**, 103–12.

Solberg WK, Clark GT & Rugh JD (1975). Nocturnal electromyographic evaluation of bruxing patients undergoing short-term splint therapy. *Journal of Oral Rehabilitation*, **2**, 215–23.

Turk DC & Rudy TE (1987). Toward a comprehensive assessment of chronic pain patients: a multiaxial approach. *Behavior Research Therapy*, **25**, 237–49.

Turk DC & Rudy TE (1988). Toward an empirically-derived taxonomy of chronic pain patients: integration of psychological assessment data. *Journal of Consulting Clinical Psychology*, **56**, 233–8.

Turk DC & Rudy TE (1990). The robustness of an empirically derived taxonomy of chronic pain patients. *Pain*, **43**, 27–35.

Turk DC, Zaki HS & Rudy TE (1993). Effects of intraoral appliance and biofeedback/stress management alone and in combination in treating pain and depression in patients with temporomandibular disorders. *Journal of Prosthetic Dentistry*, **70**, 158–64.

Turk DC, Rudy TE, Kubinski JA, Zaki HS & Greco CM (1996). Dysfunctional patients with temporomandibular disorders. Evaluating the efficacy of a tailored treatment protocol. *Journal of Consulting and Clinical Psychology*, **64**, 139–46.

Von Korff M (1995). Health services research and temporomandibular pain. In *Temporomandibular Disorders and Related Pain Conditions*, ed. B. J. Sessle, P. S. Bryant & R. A. Dionne, pp. 227–36. Seattle: IASP Press.

Weissman JL, Rudy TE, Curtin HD & Zaki HS (1993). MR findings and treatment outcome in TMD patients. *Journal of Dental Research*, **72**, 193.

Wright J, Deary IJ & Geissler PR (1991). Depression, hassles and somatic symptoms in mandibular dysfunction syndrome patients. *Journal of Dentistry*, **19**, 352–6.

8

Chest Pain Syndromes

LAWSON R. WULSIN

The modern history of functional chest pain syndromes begins with 'soldiers heart', first described in 1860 by British physicians during the Crimean War, when previously healthy soldiers developed debilitating chest pains (Castell, 1992). At the same time on the American side of the Atlantic, DaCosta described 'irritable heart' in Civil War soldiers (Jarcho, 1959). In 1883 Kronecker & Meltzer reported that mental distress was associated with esophageal contractions, and by the end of the century Osler's *Principles and Practice of Medicine* had made the terms 'oesophagismus' and 'pseudoangina' familiar to physicians, linking both conditions to hysterical women and neurasthenic men (Osler, 1892).

All of these early descriptions of chest pain syndromes note an association with anxiety, but Jones & Lewis (1941) published the first large study of the psychological aspects of patients with recurrent chest pain and found unusually high frequencies of acute anxiety (17%), chronic anxiety state (14%), psychopathic personality (18%), depression (12%) and hysteria (11%).

Sophisticated studies of the pathophysiology of chest pain in patients without serious heart disease began with Likoff's report of 15 women with recurrent chest pain, abnormal electrocardiograms (ECGs), and normal coronary angiograms (Likoff et al., 1967). That same year Kemp et al. (1967) reported evidence for cardiac ischemia by ECG and stress testing in 27% of a sample of 50 patients with recurrent chest pain and normal coronary angiograms. More recently Cannon (1988, 1991) has described the hemodynamics and associated features of the syndrome of 'microvascular angina' in patients with normal coronary arteries and recurrent chest pain. And during the 1970s and 1980s the relationship between chest pain and the various esophageal motility disorders and esophageal reflux were well described (Langevin & Castell, 1991; Richter, 1991*b*). Finally, the advent of more precise criteria for psychiatric diagnoses in the early 1980s has led to more precise descriptions of the associations between psychiatric disorders and recurrent chest pain (Beitman et al., 1991; Katon et al., 1988).

Definition

The term 'syndrome' implies a lower level of classification than a discrete disease, such as coronary artery disease. The frequent need for this lower level of classification comes from the fact that good primary care physicians find a discrete medical etiology for chest pain in fewer than 20% of patients who present with undiagnosed recurrent chest pain (Kroenke & Mangelsdorrf, 1989).

'Functional' chest pain syndromes are not easily traced to the diseased heart, or any other single organ system. These syndromes consist of: (1) recurrent chest pain, which is usually maintained by (2) multiple contributing factors, and which occurs in patterns of quality, duration and severity that are (3) not typical of common medical disorders, such as coronary artery disease or costochondritis.

Case presentation

Ms A is a 40-year-old white women with a history of asthma, diabetes, high blood pressure and depression, who had episodic bouts of chest pain over several years that eventually led to two evaluations by cardiologists, the most recent being in June 1995, resulting in her second normal coronary angiogram. Her medications included triamcinolone inhaler, albuterol, insulin and paroxetine.

In March of 1996 she began a series of seven visits to emergency rooms over the next six months, for a combination of chest pain and shortness of breath. Eventually she was admitted to the hospital in September 1996 for atypical chest pain, a myocardial infarction was ruled out, and the psychiatrist was called to evaluate the psychiatric contributions to her chest pain. She met all the criteria for severe panic disorder, often with several moderate attacks a day, and in fact she acknowledged having been given the diagnosis of panic disorder several years before, a diagnosis that she and her doctor had lost sight of in the flurry of medical evaluations. Furthermore, she reported progressive depressive symptoms since the death of her mother four years previously, a topic she could only discuss through a rush of tears.

Ms A was the oldest of four children raised by a chronically ill mother, so she had become a caregiver early in her life. She married a man almost 40 years older than herself and had nine children by him, the oldest of whom is mentally ill and living at home. Ms A has a family history of heart disease and asthma and her 78-year-old husband has congestive heart failure and emphysema. Chest pain speaks with a loud voice in this family.

Ms A responded dramatically to identification of the diagnoses of panic disorder and depression, patient education, initiation of a trial of clonazepam and increasing her dose of paroxetine. Her chest pain initially reduced in frequency and severity, followed by several relapses with exacerbations of her chest pain behaviors, but overall her functioning has improved consistently since clarification of the psychiatric diagnoses and increasing her psychotropic medications. Rehabilitation will require persistent treatment of the biological (asthma), psychological (panic and depression) and social (caregiver in a demanding family system) contributions to her chest pain syndrome.

Prevalence

The prevalence of chest pain syndromes varies with the clinical setting. Richter et al. (1989) estimated that each year in the USA, of the identified 180 000 new cases of chest pain with normal coronary arteries, as many as 50% have esophageal abnormalities. As this estimate is based only on those who have coronary angiograms, Richter considered 90 000 new cases per year of chest pain associated with esophageal abnormalities to be 'grossly underestimated'.

Nationally, two-thirds of those who present to the emergency department with chest pain are sent home, and over 80% of those sent home have noncardiac diagnoses. The distribution of these noncardiac diagnoses in one study of our large urban academic emergency department in Cincinnati (Rouan et al., 1987) was 45% 'atypical' chest pain, 23% musculoskeletal chest pain, 10% unknown, 9% gastrointestinal and 1% anxiety. In this study, conducted in 1984–85, 1045 chest pain patients were released from the emergency department (67% of all chest pain patients seen), and of these 922 (88%) had noncardiac initial diagnoses. The large proportion of patients diagnosed with 'atypical' chest pain (45%) is common and these patients often get little or no effective treatment.

Doubting the accuracy in this study of the frequency of 1% anxiety (a number which reflected the tendency for emergency physicians to generate a spontaneous psychiatric diagnosis to explain chest pain), we assessed 334 consecutive patients presenting to the same emergency room with chest pain (Yingling et al., 1993). Using self-report measures for panic disorder (Zung Self-Rating Anxiety Scale and the Panic Disorder Self-Rating Scale) and depression (Beck Depression Inventory) administered within two days after the emergency department visit, we found that 35% of those presenting with chest pain screened positive for either psychiatric disorder (23% for depression, 18% for panic disorder). Emergency department physicians, however, only documented a psychosocial contribution to the chest pain in 5.7% of this sample. We concluded that symptoms of depression and panic disorder are common among emergency department chest pain patients, are likely to contribute to the chest pain syndrome, and are unlikely to be recognized and treated.

Some 10–30% of patients with recurrent chest pain who undergo coronary angiography have normal coronary arteries (Kemp et al., 1986; Papanicolaou et al., 1986). Although these people may have functional evidence of ischemia by ECG or stress testing, their mortality is similar to that of age- and sex-matched normal cohorts (Pamelia et al., 1985; Miller et al., 1988). One follow-up study found a morbidity rate of 0.2% and a mortality rate of 0.3% (Wielgosz et al., 1984; Kemp et al., 1986).

Of those with recurrent chest pain and normal coronary angiograms 30–40% may have panic disorder (Katon et al., 1988; Beitman et al., 1989*b*). As many as 50% have esophageal abnormalities (Richter et al., 1989) and primarily motility disorders, such as nutcracker esophagus or esophageal sphincter spasm, or esophageal reflux. Nutcracker esophagus may be the most common esophageal motility disorder in the chest pain population; 27–48% of patients with chest pain and abnormal esophageal motility have nutcracker esophagus (Richter et al., 1989).

Economic costs

Studies of the functioning of patients with recurrent chest pain and normal coronary arteries suggest that half of these patients have poor return-to-work rates and high levels of health service utilization during the year following the normal angiogram (Levy & Winkle, 1979; Ockene et al., 1980). Richter et al. (1987) have found that the chest pain patients with normal coronary arteries and esophageal disorders receive an average of 1.2 prescriptions per month, visit the emergency department 2.2 times a year and are hospitalized 0.8 times a year for further evaluation of chest pain, resulting in approximately $3500 spent per year for medical expenses related to chest pain. Richter (1991*b*) has estimated that in the USA about $400 million per year is spent on the direct medical costs of noncardiac chest pain. Much of the impetus for recent research on patients with chest pain syndromes has been driven by these observations of low functioning and high utilization. Chest pain has become an expensive problem for our society.

Confirmations

The most promising current hypothesis on the mechanism of chest pain syndromes postulates that the essential common feature in these patients is abnormal visceral pain perception. This hypothesis arose from observations of abnormally low pain thresholds in esophageal balloon distention studies (Richter et al., 1986; Bradley et al., 1991), somatic preoccupations in panic disorder (Katon, 1989) and acute sensitivity in some chest pain patients to the catheter tip during heart catheterizations, compared with patients with coronary artery disease who could not feel the catheter at all (Cannon, 1995).

Shapiro et al. (1988) first reported abnormal visceral pain perception during cardiac procedures among patients with recurrent chest pain and normal coronary arteries. He found that in some of these patients their characteristic chest pains could be provoked by: (1) catheter movement in the right atrium, and (2) intra-atrial boluses of normal saline in 10 of 11 chest pain subjects with normal angiograms and exercise-induced ECG changes suggestive of ischemia. Paradoxically, most subjects with coronary artery disease could feel neither stimulus.

Cannon et al. (1990) then provoked characteristic chest pain in 86% of 36 subjects with normal angiograms by pacing their heart rates of five beats per minute higher than resting heart rate. Studies of flow dynamics showed no difference in pain thresholds between those with microvascular dysfunction and those without, which suggests that abnormal pain perception is more important than abnormal flow in the provocation of the characteristic pain. Again, like normal controls, patients with coronary artery disease or valvular heart disease who had reported angina could rarely feel any of these stimuli.

Cannon & Benjamin (1993) have proposed that rather than viewing chest pain as the stimulus we should consider the possibility that often chest pain may be the normal response to abnormal sensory perceptions of common physiological processes, such as right ventricular filling pressures or cardiac pacing. These patients with abnormal visceral pain perception may represent 'the opposite end of the spectrum from "silent ischemia" in patients with coronary artery disease, in which even severe myocardial ischemia may go unrecognized because of defective nociceptor activation or afferent sensory transmission or processing in the brainstem'.

Similar observations of heightened visceral sensitivity to pain have been reported in patients with irritable bowel syndrome (Ritchie, 1973; Lynn & Friedman, 1993). Whether the lower pain threshold in patients with chest pain syndromes applies to somatic pain perception in all areas of the body or is limited to particular viscera has not been well studied. Nor do we know what percentage of patients with chest pain syndromes have measurably lower pain thresholds in the target organ systems.

The strongest confirmation of the abnormal visceral nociception hypothesis comes from the one controlled treatment study of chest pain in 60 patients with normal coronary angiograms (Cannon et al., 1994). Compared with placebo and clonidine, imipramine treatment over three weeks was associated with a significant reduction in chest pain, regardless of baseline abnormalities in cardiac, esophageal or psychiatric measures. The imipramine effect was independent of improvement in psychiatric symptoms, which suggests that the mechanism for the effect was through a reduction in visceral pain perception. This finding calls for further confirmation through replication.

Contradictions

Research into the factors which contribute to chest pain syndromes has led to the development of at least four other major hypotheses: (1) esophageal spasm, (2) esophageal irritation, (3) smooth muscle dysfunction, and (4) microvascular angina. The shortcomings of each of these hypotheses has led to the elaboration over the past five years of the fifth hypothesis: abnormal visceral pain perception, which incorporates much of the thinking of the earlier hypotheses (Cannon & Benjamin, 1993; Cannon, 1995) and attempts to resolve the contradictions. A closer look at these alternative mechanisms shows the current status of the competing hypotheses and the contradictions which require resolution.

Pathogenetic hypotheses

Esophageal spasm – in the forms of nutcracker esophagus, hypertensive lower esophageal sphincter, and diffuse esophageal spasm – offers an intuitively appealing explanation for noncardiac chest pain, invoking images of ischemia in esophageal smooth muscle as the source of the pain. In support of this possibility over 40% of those with esophageal abnormalities and normal coronary arteries have abnormal high-amplitude peristaltic contractions (Brand et al., 1977). Measures of intraesophageal pressures have repeatedly correlated only weakly with pain reports. Contractions often occur without pain, and pain may resolve without relaxation of the contractions. Furthermore, because of the rich blood supply to the esophagus, even severe spasm rarely induces ischemia in the esophageal smooth muscle (Richter et al., 1989).

Esophageal reflux induces chest pain by stimulation of esophageal chemoreceptors, in contrast to mechanoreceptor stimulation in esophageal spasm. Gastroesophageal reflux disease is the most common esophageal cause of noncardiac chest pain, occurring in over 40% of chest pain patients with normal coronary arteries (DeMeester et al., 1982; Hewson et al., 1991; Richter 1991*b*). Twenty-four-hour monitoring studies have shown that over half of the chest pain episodes cannot be explained by abnormal pH readings or abnormal esophageal pressure readings (Richter, 1991*b*). Reflux and spasm may contribute, but they do not explain most chest pain episodes. The mechanism for esophageal chest pain remains unknown (Richter et al., 1989; Clouse, 1992).

The search for more subtle mechanisms of chest pain than could be explained by esophageal studies or coronary angiograms led to the description initially of 'syndrome X' by Kemp (1973) in his analysis of a study by Arbogast & Bourassa (1973), who showed that patients with chest pain and normal coronary arteries had evidence of ischemia by ECG, but metabolic and hemodynamic flow data showed no sign of ischemia during stress. Cannon (1991) then demonstrated, in a series of studies, abnormally limited vascular responses at the arteriolar level of the coronary circulation in response to various challenges such as electrical pacing, exercise and pharmacological challenge with ergonovine and dipyridamole. This evidence for limited coronary flow reserve led to the hypothesis that 'microvascular angina' might explain some portion of the chest pain syndromes. The evidence points to intramyocardial prearteriolar arteries and abnormal arteriolar endothelial cell functioning as possible sites for the 'lesions' (Cannon, 1993); however, many studies have failed to find metabolic or hemodynamic evidence of ischemia in samples selected for the presence of limited coronary flow reserve (Cannon et al., 1992), so for now the microvascular angina hypothesis remains an intriguing but unproven explanation for a minority of chest pain syndromes.

Observations that patients with chest pain syndromes often had disorders at several sites of smooth muscle function (such as hypertension, esophageal motility disorders, asthma and other respiratory conditions, headaches) led to the hypothesis that chest pain reflected a generalized autonomic dysregulation of smooth muscle function (Cannon, 1991). To examine this possibility, Cannon studied 87 patients with chest pain and normal coronary angiograms, looking for abnormalities of the coronary microcirculation and esophageal motility (Cannon et al., 1990). They found that patients with dysfunction in one organ were highly likely to also have dysfunction in the other.

This smooth muscle dysfunction hypothesis seeks to incorporate the data on the high prevalence of panic disorder and depression by postulating that these psychiatric disorders are associated with centrally mediated dysregulation of the autonomic nervous system that innervates smooth muscle. Data describing such dysregulation have been sketchy.

Diagnostic approaches and treatment

Diagnosis

As cardiac disease is the one common cause of chest pain that is also immediately lethal, the evaluation of new chest pain (first episode) must begin with a focus on cardiac and respiratory causes. Esophageal disorders and psychiatric disorders are unlikely until the chest pain becomes recurrent. In the context of a good history and physical examination the evaluation of first episode chest pain can usually rule out life-threatening cardiac and respiratory causes with cardiac enzymes and other common blood tests, ECG and chest radiographs. Life-threatening causes of chest pain usually require hospitalization for initial management.

Other causes of first episode chest pain can be managed in the outpatient setting, and here the challenge is how to evaluate and treat the patient in the most cost-effective manner (Figure 8.1) (Richter, 1991*a*). It is useful to provisionally classify these less urgent conditions as primarily: (1) gastrointestinal, (2) chest wall, (3) psychiatric, or (4) other cardiac causes, although multiple factors may contribute to the chest pain. Provisional hypotheses about the factors contributing to the chest pain will guide the priorities of the evaluation.

The two essential components of the initial management of first episode chest pain are: (1) patient education, and (2) establishing a sound relationship with a primary care doctor. A well-informed patient is less likely to go searching for expensive answers than one who is frightened because of ignorance, and the relationship with a primary care doctor becomes the key to efficient evaluation when chest pains recur. The pattern of emergency room visits and consultations can be guided efficiently only by a primary care doctor who remains responsible for the patient across settings and disciplines.

For patients with recurrent chest pain a broad careful history, including family history, focusing on cardiac, gastrointestinal and psychiatric histories, lays the foundation for further investigations (Figure 8.2)

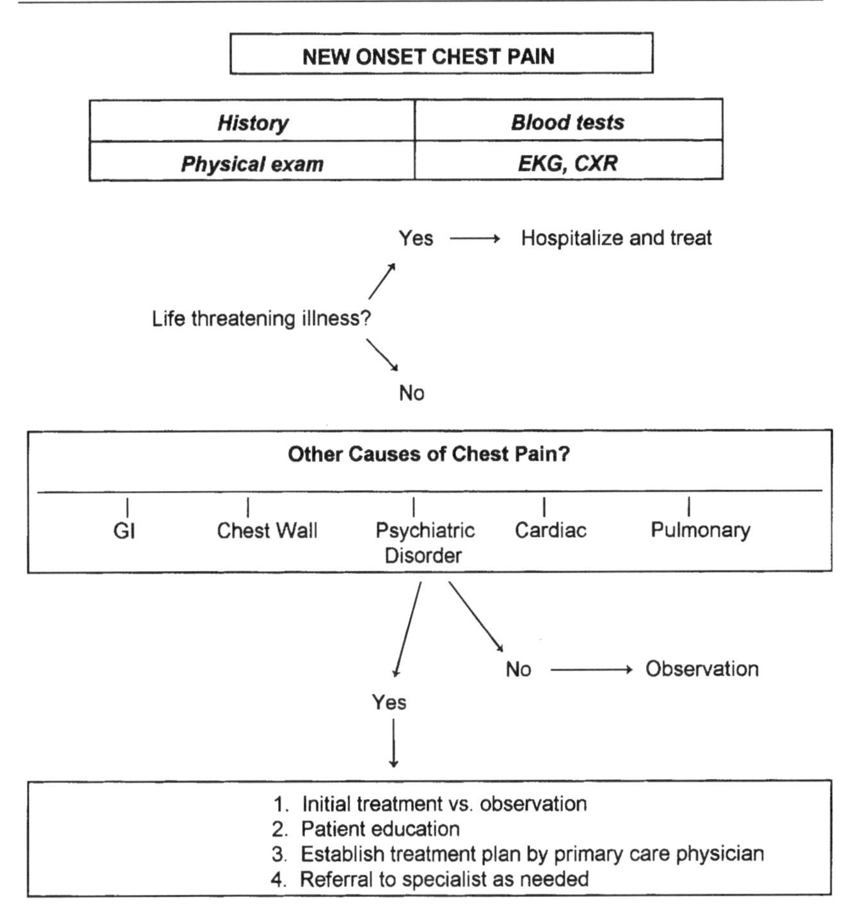

Figure 8.1. Algorithm for evaluating patients with new onset of chest pain. CXR, chest radiograph; EKG, electrocardiogram; GI, gastrointestinal. (From Richter, 1991*a*.)

(Richter, 1991*a*). Screening for depression and anxiety disorders (see below) is easy, inexpensive and often productive. The evaluator must keep in mind the multiple factors that possibly contribute to a single chest pain syndrome; finding one explanation does not eliminate the need to search for others. People with coronary artery disease do sometimes develop panic disorder and the combination can be particularly troublesome (Zaubler & Katon, 1996).

For patients with prominent gastrointestinal symptoms and/or history, the most productive next step is an evaluation for acid reflux, including the Bernstein acid perfusion test in the primary care office. For patients with positive or equivocal findings an aggressive trial of H_2 antagonists or omeprazole may be the most cost-effective approach

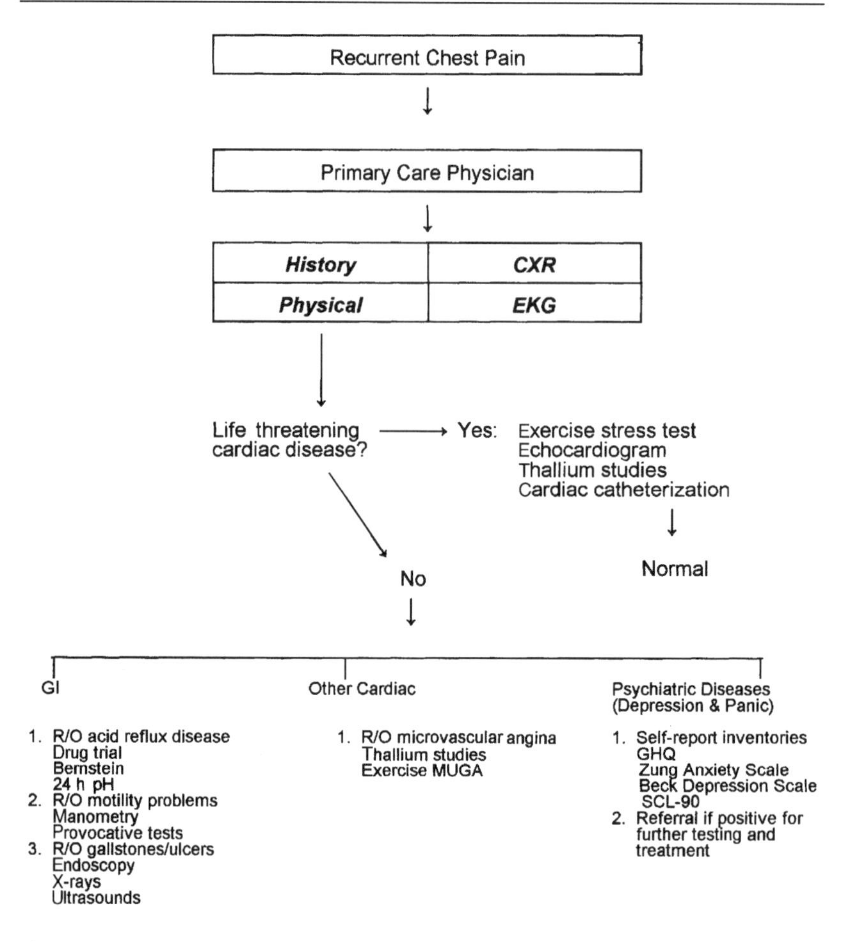

Figure 8.2. Algorithm for evaluating patients with recurrent chest pain. CXR, chest radiograph; EKG, electrocardiogram; GI, gastrointestinal; R/O, rule out; GHQ, general health questionnaire; SCL-90, Hopkins Symptom Check List-90. (From Richter, 1991*b*.)

(Richter, 1991*a*). Patients with a negative Bernstein test and persistent pain may be referred to a gastroenterologist for 24-hour pH monitoring. The next step, which also requires a gastroenterology consultation, is to search for esophageal motility problems through esophageal manometry and provocative tests, such as edrophonium and balloon distention.

For patients with recurrent chest pain a cardiology consultation is often useful, particularly for evaluating whether a thallium stress test or a coronary angiogram is necessary to rule out coronary artery disease. For a substantial minority of patients a negative evaluation for coronary artery disease will be reassuring and sufficient. Microvascular angina can usually be diagnosed by reversible thallium perfusion defects or abnormal left ventricular ejection fraction response to exercise by radionuclide angiograph (Richter, 1991*a*).

Psychiatric disorders are best identified by a careful psychiatric history, including a family history combined with screening measures. Prime-MD (Spitzer et al., 1994) provides a combination of a screening questionnaire and a structured interview for the five most common psychiatric disorders in primary care (mood disorders, anxiety disorders, substance abuse, somatoform disorders and eating disorders). Other screening measures that have been used in primary care settings include the Beck Depression Inventory (Beck et al., 1961), the General Health Questionnaire (Goldberg & Hillier, 1979) and the Zung Anxiety Scale (Zung, 1971). Positive responses on these screening measures or evidence in the psychiatric history of current or past psychiatric disorders warrants a psychiatric consultation.

Treatment

Several principles guide the treatment of chest pain syndromes. First, multiple causes may require multiple treatments, which must be coordinated by a single clinician. Second, outcomes are judged by doctors and patients; it is not sufficient for a good outcome to rule out coronary artery disease and nutcracker esophagus if the patient's chest pain persists and functioning at home and work do not improve. On the other hand, if the doctor and patient agree, a good outcome may include improved functioning despite persistent chest pain at a tolerable level, once the contributing factors have been satisfactorily identified. Third, comorbid disorders should be optimally treated to reduce the interaction effect of one disorder on the other, such as coronary artery disease and panic disorder. Fourth, as with other chronic pain syndromes, clear graded treatment goals and careful symptom monitoring are the best protection against dissatisfied patients and frustrated doctors.

The best treatment study of chest pain patients with normal coronary angiograms (Cannon et al., 1994) showed that imipramine 50 mg/day significantly improved chest pain in a double-blind, placebo-controlled three week trial of imipramine compared with clonidine in 60 patients. This study, conducted at the National Heart, Lung and Blood Institute, in the USA, began with a five-week single-blind placebo washout phase. The double-blind treatment phase compared imipramine 50 mg/day with clonidine 0.1 mg/day with placebo for five weeks. Evaluations at baseline and during treatment included exercise treadmill testing of cardiac function, radionuclide angiography, cardiac catheterization with pacing, esophageal motility testing, esophageal sensitivity testing and a structured diagnostic interview for psychiatric disorders.

The response to imipramine did not depend on the presence at baseline of cardiac, esophageal or psychiatric abnormalities, nor did it depend on the improvement of psychiatric symptoms. The authors postulate that imipramine reduced chest pain through a visceral analgesic effect. Until further studies elaborate on this finding, both clinical wisdom and the results of this one controlled trial suggest that imipramine (or possibly other tricyclic antidepressants) is a good first choice drug for the management of recurrent chest pain (except in the postmyocardial infarction period). Subtherapeutic antidepressant doses may be sufficient for the chest pain effect alone; however, in patients with clinical depression or panic disorder higher doses may be necessary to resolve the chest pain syndrome as well as the comorbid psychiatric disorder.

Clouse (1992) conducted a six-week placebo-controlled trial of trazodone (150 mg/day) in 29 patients referred to the esophageal manometry laboratory for evaluation of esophageal motor dysfunction. Less than half of the sample met the criteria for current psychiatric disorder (generalized anxiety disorder 46%, major depression 31%). The trazodone group showed significant improvement in esophageal symptom distress relative to placebo at six weeks but not at three weeks. The reduction in distress was not accompanied by parallel changes in esophageal pressures and the study did not assess visceral pain sensitivity. The findings of Clouse's study are similar to those of Cannon's later study, both of which find that low doses of these antidepressants reduce distress without altering key measures of visceral functioning. The effect appears to be independent of improvement in psychiatric symptoms.

Another pharmacological option implied by these studies of imipramine and trazodone is to try serotonin reuptake inhibitors (fluoxetine, paroxetine, sertraline, fluvoxamine), which are effective adjuncts in other chronic pain syndromes. These newer antidepressants are better tolerated than the tricyclics and are commonly used in the primary care setting, in spite of their current high costs.

Conclusions

An understanding of the history and the current pathogenetic mechanisms of chest pain syndromes provides a roadmap for efficiently evaluating chest pain patients. A systematic approach to each of the factors contributing to the patient's recurrent chest pain is best coordinated by a primary care physician over the course of the syndrome.

Effective treatments exist for many of the contributing conditions, including the condition of abnormal visceral nociception.

References

Arbogast R & Bourassa MG (1973). Myocardial function during atrial pacing in patients with angina pectoris and normal coronary arteriograms: comparison with patients having significant coronary artery disease. *American Journal of Cardiology*, **32**, 257–63.
Beck AT, Ward CH, Mendelson M, Mock J & Erbaugh J (1961). An inventory for measuring depression. *Archives of General Psychiatry*, **4**, 561–71.
Beitman BD, Basha IM, Trombka LH, Jayaratna MA, Russell B, Flaker G & Anderson S (1989*a*). Pharmacotherapeutic treatment of panic disorder in patients presenting with chest pain. *Journal of Family Practice*, **28**, 177–80.
Beitman BD, Mukerji V, Kushner M, Thomas AM, Russell J & Logue MB (1991). Validating studies for panic disorder in patients with angiographically normal coronary arteries. *Medical Clinics of North America*, **75**, 1143–55.
Beitman BD, Mukerji V, Lamberti JW, Schmid L, DeRosear L, Kushner M, Flaker G & Basha I (1989*b*). Panic disorder in patients with chest pain and angiographically normal coronary arteries. *American Journal of Cardiology*, **63**, 1399–403.
Bradley AL, Scarinci IC & Richter JE (1991). Pain threshold levels and coping strategies among patients who have chest pain and normal coronary arteries. *Medical Clinics of North America*, **75**, 1189–202.
Brand DL, Martin D, Pope CE II (1977). Esophageal manometrics in patients with angina-like chest pain. *American Journal of Digestive Diseases*, **22**, 300–5.
Cannon RO III (1991). Cardiovascular investigations regarding pathophysiology and management. *Medical Clinics of North America*, **75**, 1097–118.
Cannon RO III (1993). Chest pain with normal coronary angiograms. *New England Journal of Medicine*, **328**, 1706–7.
Cannon RO III (1995). The sensitive heart: a syndrome of abnormal cardiac pain perception. *Journal of the American Medical Association*, **273**, 883–7.
Cannon RO III & Benjamin SB (1993). Chest pain as a consequence of abnormal visceral nociception. *Digestive Diseases and Sciences*, **38**, 193–6.
Cannon RO & Epstein SE (1988). 'Microvascular angina' as a cause of chest pain with angiographically normal coronary arteries. *American Journal of Cardiology*, **61**, 1338–43.
Cannon RO III, Cattau EL Jr, Yakshe PN et al. (1990). Coronary flow reserve, esophageal motility and chest pain in patients with angiographically normal coronary arteries. *American Journal of Medicine*, **88**, 217–22.
Cannon RO III, Camici PC & Epstein SE (1992). Pathophysiological dilemma of syndrome X. *Circulation*, **85**, 883–92.
Cannon RO III, Arshed AQ, Mincemoyer R, Stine AM, Gracely RH, Smith WB & Benjamin SB (1994). Imipramine in patients with chest pain despite normal coronary angiograms. *New England Journal of Medicine*, **330**, 1411–17.

Castell DO (1992). Chest pain of undetermined origin: overview of pathophysiology. *American Journal of Medicine*, **92** (Suppl. 5A), 5A-2S–5A-4S.
Clouse RE (1992). Psychopharmacologic approaches to therapy for chest pain of presumed esophageal origin. *American Journal of Medicine*, **92** (Suppl. 5A), 5A-106S–113S.
DeMeester TR, O'Sullivan CC, Bermudez G, Midell AI, Cimochowski GE & O'Drobinak J (1982). Esophageal function in patients with angina-type chest pain and normal coronary angiogram. *Annals of Surgery*, **196**, 488–98.
Goldberg DP & Hillier VF (1979). A scaled version of the General Health Questionnaire. *Psychological Medicine*, **9**, 139–450.
Hewson EG, Sinclair JW, Dalton CB & Richter JE (1991). Twenty-four hour esophageal pH monitoring. The most useful test for evaluating non-cardiac chest pain. *American Journal of Medicine*, **90**, 576–583.
Jarcho S (1959). Functional heart disease in the civil war (daCosta, 1871). *American Journal of Cardiology*, **29**, 809–17.
Jones M & Lewis A (1941). Effort syndrome. *Lancet*, **ii**, 813–18.
Katon W (1989). *Panic Disorder in the Medical Setting*. National Institute of Mental Health. DHHS Pub. No. (ADM) 89–1629. Washington, DC: Supt. Of Docs., US Government Print Office.
Katon W, Hall ML, Russo J. et al. (1988). The relationship of psychiatric illness to coronary arteriographic results. *American Journal of Medicine*, **84**, 1–9.
Kemp HG (1973). Left ventricular function in patients with the anginal syndrome and normal coronary arteriograms. *American Journal of Cardiology*, **32**, 375–6.
Kemp HG, Elliott WC & Gorlin R (1967). The anginal syndrome with normal coronary ateriolography. *Transections of the Association of American Physicians*, **80**, 59.
Kemp HG, Kronmal RA, Vliestra RE & Frye RL (1986). Seven year survival of patients with normal or near normal coronary arteriograms: a CASS registry study. *American Journal of Cardiology*, **7**, 479–83.
Kroenke K & Mangelsdorrf AD (1989). Common symptoms in ambulatory care: incidence, evaluation, therapy and outcome. *American Journal of Medicine*, **86**, 262–6.
Kronecker H & Meltzer S (1883). Der schluckmechanismus, seine erregung und seine hemmung. *Archives of Anatomy and Physiology*, 7 (Suppl.), 328–62.
Langevin S & Castell O (1991). Esophageal motility disorders and chest pain. *Medical Clinics of North America*, **75**, 1045–63.
Legrand V, Hodgson JM, Bates ER, Averon FM, Manaris GB & Vogel RA (1985). Abnormal coronary flow reserve and abnormal radionuclide exercise test results in patients with normal coronary angiograms. *American Journal of Cardiology*, **6**, 1234–53.
Levy EB & Winkle RA (1979). Continuing disability of patients with chest pain and abnormal angiograms. *Journal of Chronic Diseases*, **32**, 191–6.
Likoff W, Segal BL & Kasparian H (1967). Paradox of normal selective coronary arteriograms in patients considered to have unmistakable coronary heart disease. *New England Journal of Medicine*, **276**, 1063–6.

Lynn RB & Friedman LS (1993). Irritable bowel syndrome. *American Journal of Medicine*, **88**, 217–22.

Miller TD, Taliercio CP, Zinsmeister AR & Gibbons RJ (1988). Prognosis in patients with an abnormal exercise radionuclide angiogram in the absence of significant coronary artery disease. *Journal of the American College of Cardiologists*, **12**, 637–41.

Ockene IS, Shay MJ, Alpert JS, Weiner BH & Dalen J (1980). Unexplained chest pain in patients with normal coronary arteriograms. *New England Journal of Medicine*, **303**, 1249–52.

Osler W (1892). *Principles and Practice of Medicine*. New York: D. Appleton.

Pamelia FX, Gibson RS, Watson DD, Craddock GB, Sorowatka J & Beller GA (1985). Prognosis with chest pain and normal thallium-201 exercise scintigrams. *American Journal of Cardiology*, **55**, 920–6.

Papanicolaou MN, Califf RM, Hlatky MA, McKinnis RA, Lee KL & Pryor DB (1986). Prognostic implication of angiographically normal and insignificantly narrowed coronary arteries. *American Journal of Cardiology*, **58**, 1181–7.

Richie J (1973). Pain from distention of the pelvic colon by inflating a balloon in the irritable colon syndrome. *Gut*, **14**, 125–32.

Richter JE (1991*a*). Practical approach to the diagnosis of unexplained chest pain. *Medical Clinics of North America*, **75**, 1203–8.

Richter JE (1991*b*). Gastroesophageal reflux disease as a cause of chest pain. *Medical Clinics of North America*, **75**, 1065–80.

Richter JE, Barish CF & Castell DO (1986). Abnormal sensory perception in patients with esophageal chest pain. *Gastroenterology*, **91**, 1141–6.

Richter JE, Dalton CB, Bradley LA & Castell DO (1987). Oral nifedipine in the treatment of non-cardiac chest pain in patients with the nutcracker esophagus. *Gastroenterology*, **93**, 21–2.

Richter JE, Bradley LA & Castell DO (1989). Esophageal chest pain: current controversies in pathogenesis, diagnosis and therapy. *Annals of Internal Medicine*, **110**, 66–78.

Rouan GW, Hedges JR, Toltzis E, Goldstein-Wayne B, Brand D & Goldman L (1987). A chest pain clinic to improve the follow-up of patients released from an urban university teaching hospital emergency department. *Annals of Emergency Medicine*, **16**, 1145–50.

Shapiro LM, Crake T & Poole-Wilson PA (1988). Is altered cardiac sensation responsible for chest pain in patients with normal coronary arteries? Clinical observations during cardiac catheterization. *British Medical Journal*, **296**, 170–1.

Spitzer RL, Williams JBW, Kroenke K, Linzer M, deGray FV, Hahr SR, Brody D & Jonson JD (1994). Utility of a new procedure for diagnosing mental disorders in primary care. *Journal of the American Medical Association*, **272**, 1749–56.

Wielgosz AT, Fletcher RH, McCants CB, McKinnis RA, Harey TL & Williams RB (1984). Unimproved chest pain in patients with minimal or no coronary disease: a behavioral phenomenon. *American Heart Journal*, **108**, 67–72.

Yingling KW, Wulsin LR, Arnold LM & Rouan GW (1993). Estimated prevalences of panic disorder and depression among consecutive patients seen in

an emergency department with acute chest pain. *Journal of General Internal Medicine*, **8**, 231–5.
Zaubler TS & Katon W (1996). Panic disorder and medical comorbidity: a review of the medical and psychiatric literature. In *Panic Disorder: Critical Issues in Treatment*. Bulletin of the Menninger Clinic, **60** (2, Suppl. A), A12–A38.
Zung WWK (1971). A rating instrument for anxiety disorders. *Psychosomatics*, **XII**, 371–9.

9

Repetitive Strain Injury

STEPHEN P. TYRER

The term, repetitive (or repetition) strain injury (now often abbreviated to RSI), was first used in 1982 in a report from the Australian National Health and Medical Research Council and was widely reported in the Australian subcontinent. In the USA the term used for the same 'disease' is cumulative trauma disorder and the favored description in the UK is work-related upper limb disorder. The essential features of the disorder, injury caused by repetitive movements leading to strain of the musculo-ligamentous structures, is encapsulated in the words repetitive strain injury. The status of this disorder continues to arouse controversy because of the lack of objective findings in the sufferers from this condition and uncertainty about how far the disorder is work related (Tyrer, 1994*a*).

History

Work-related upper arm symptoms are not new. In 1713 Ramazzini described pain in the arms in scribes and notaries which he believed was due to the constant use of quill pens for writing, poor seating and excessive mental labor. The scribes were said to be worked hard by their masters, with few breaks so that they would not cause their master any financial loss. The features of repetitive activity, faulty posture during work and stress associated with the activity have been described by numerous authors subsequently.

Symptoms of pain and fatigue in the arms in writers in the British Civil Service were reported by Sir Charles Bell in 1833 and were thought to be due to the availability of steel-nibbed pens, which had been introduced in place of the quill variety (Bell, 1833). Thirty years later, Samuel Solly, senior surgeon of St Thomas' Hospital, London, described severe and persistent arm pain accompanied by pins and needles, numbness in the fingers, cold feelings and fatigue in the affected arm (Solly, 1864). These symptoms were found in men whose occupation required them to write excessively and the syndrome from which they suffered was therefore called scriveners' palsy.

The association of nervous problems with these symptoms was raised by the neurologist, Sir William Gowers, at the end of the last century. From his experience, he found that 'those of distinctly nervous temperament, irritable, sensitive, bearing overwork and anxiety badly' were most frequently affected (Gowers, 1892). Gowers further stated that any condition that 'lowers the tone of the nervous system, may doubtless act as a predisposing cause' and he found it 'remarkable how many patients were enduring anxiety from family trouble, business worry or weighty responsibilities'. It is of relevance that at the time that Gowers wrote there was a recession in England and employers had no problem in filling vacant positions. Gowers described this condition as an 'occupation neurosis'.

Although writers' cramp was reported in the first years after Gowers' original observations it was then only described sporadically until the early years of the next century. At this time the Morse code was introduced and telegraphists had to learn a new technique which involved frequent repetitive movements of the fingers. In 1908, a doctor examining telegraphists who were complaining of pain in the arms claimed that symptoms of cramp, pain and weakness were due to muscle failure owing to the rapid repetitive movements involved in operating Morse code. Within a three-year period almost 60% of the work force were reporting symptoms of muscle weakness, cramp or pain that they attributed to the new technology. As a result, a committee was commissioned and reported that the cause of the symptoms was due to 'a nervous instability on the part of the operator and to repeated fatigue due to the complicated movements required for sending messages' (Great Britain and Ireland Post Office, 1911). The committee explained that this condition was not simply due to muscular fatigue but was a result of a 'nervous breakdown', the first time this concept was introduced into the English language but now used more widely to describe stress-related acute psychiatric illness.

Further outbreaks of occupationally related muscle weakness and pain were reported sporadically from Japan and Scandinavia in the mid-twentieth century and seem to have been associated with the increased emphasis on occupational medicine that was being developed at this time. In the early 1980s what was termed a major epidemic of arm and neck pain occurred in Australia. The symptoms were thought by occupational physicians to be due to new work practices and the description of tenosynovitis was used to describe the new disease. The workers' unions were alarmed, publicized the condition and gave lists of symptoms that informed workers whether or not they had RSI. Many self-help groups were set up to support the workers. Many more women were affected than men and groups such as WRIST (Women's Repetitive Injury Support Team) were formed. Surprisingly, the first report postulating that fast, repetitive movements were responsible for the pain and fatigue was over a decade before large numbers of the workforce began to suffer from RSI (Ferguson, 1971). This original report described that 14% of keyboard telegraphists had RSI but it was only later that it was found that 25% of telegraphists in Sydney were affected but only 4% in Melbourne, despite similar practices in both cities. Although patients were thoroughly investigated with radiographs, imaging techniques, scans, electromyography, tissue biopsy and blood tests, no consistent organic lesion could be found.

Almost 4000 reports of RSI were made between 1981 and 1985 and then the incidence quickly declined. Although in part this was because a number of litigants claiming that their injuries were directly attributed to their work failed to persuade courts that this was the case, the publicity that was given to the whole area helped to change ergonomic practices at work as well as recognizing that workers under stress were more prone to develop these symptoms.

In the USA, the condition of what was described as cumulative trauma disorder, which effectively is identical with RSI, increased later than in Australia but rose from fewer than 7 cases per 100 000 workers in 1986 to over 21 cases per 100 000 by 1989 (Bureau of Labor Statistics, 1990).

The common characteristics of each of the 'outbreaks' of muscle pain and fatigue were the introduction of new technology, a belief by the workers that the employers were driving them too hard and the recognition that not all individuals developed these symptoms but only those who were under stress. It is because of the association of these symptoms to social and psychological factors that RSI has been described as a psychosocial disease. The rapid rise in the incidence of RSI cases in Australia in the mid-1980s has been attributed to a number of social and demographic factors. At this time the trade union movement was powerful in Australia and was genuinely concerned about permanent injuries to workers. They asked for work health and safety officers to be stationed in workplaces for early recognition of RSI and each worker was issued with 'the sufferers' handbook'. This focus on symptoms made the workers much more concerned about their physical welfare and encouraged sickness and absence. Lawyers took an acquisitive interest in the condition and saw the potential for employer negligence litigation and set themselves up as 'RSI negligence claim specialists'. It has been said that the so-called industrial rehabilitation experts who first labelled workers as having RSI were in part responsible for the 'epidemic' reaching such large proportions.

Despite the furore over the Australian epidemic of RSI, there has always been a steady stream of sufferers from upper limb pain syndromes which the complainants believe are due to their work practices. Although the early writers claimed that the majority of people who had RSI were in boring, understimulating, low-paid jobs (Ireland, 1988) it is important to note that at least two groups of people who enjoy their work have a higher frequency of arm pain, fatigue and stiffness than would be expected by chance. These groups are musicians and those who interpret conversation by sign language for deaf people. The majority of musicians are self-employed and are not covered by insurance policies that enable them to live comfortably if they have to give up their profession. The incidence of persistent pain occurring in musicians, which is sufficiently severe to prevent them from carrying out their activities, is estimated at almost 0.5% (Fry, 1986). This suggests that factors other than boring occupation or financial gain are responsible for this condition. It behoves us to determine what comprises this syndrome, what factors lead to its exhibition and what pathological changes can be found with are unique to this disease entity.

Definition

Definitions of RSI emphasize the putative etiology of the condition rather than listing characteristic symptoms and signs. This is not satisfactory and it is more sensible to divide those disorders that are thought to result from repetitive movements into two main groups:

Clinical conditions with demonstrable pathology.
Those ill-defined symptom complexes with diffuse aching, weakness and muscle tenderness.

Clinical conditions with demonstrable pathology

There are well-described conditions that may be related to repetitive movements, particularly of the upper limbs. These include:

De Quervain's stenosing tenosynovitis.
Supraspinatus tendinitis
Peritendinitis crepitans
Carpal tunnel syndrome
Cubital tunnel syndrome (entrapment of the ulnar nerve at the elbow)
Lateral epicondylitis (tennis elbow)
Medial epicondylitis (golfer's elbow)

Rotator cuff syndrome
Dupuytren's contracture

The conditions indicated above have been reported to be related to work practices and the extent to which occupationally related activities cause these conditions is indicated in approximate order of decreasing frequency. Each of these illnesses is associated with clearly identifiable disease processes that can be ascertained by nerve conduction studies, radiographs, ultrasound or magnetic resonance imaging (MRI) scans, or at operation. Although some are related to repetitive movements, e.g., carpal tunnel syndrome from the use of vibrating tools, these diseases are separate from what is normally termed RSI.

Repetitive strain injury and other symptom complexes

RSI is defined both by its symptoms and relationship to work practices.

Pain is invariably present and in the majority of cases diffuse tenderness can be elicited in the muscle bellies that have been involved in the action that has been reported to cause the problem. Skin rolling tenderness can also often be detected, particularly over the upper trapezius. The muscle groups most frequently involved include the neck and shoulder muscles, in particular the trapezius, both the flexor and extensor muscles of the forearm and the small muscles of the hand. Weakness is nearly always present but is difficult to assess reliably because the patient finds that contraction of the affected muscle causes pain and so tests to assess muscle power are poorly performed. In those who have had symptoms for some time there is often evidence of reduced muscle bulk, which is usually due to underuse of the affected muscles. Persistent tingling has been reported associated with numbness but deep tendon reflexes are preserved and there is no objective evidence of afferent nerve abnormalities on standard testing. Symptoms normally affect the upper limbs but similar symptoms have been reported in the lower limbs, particularly in athletes.

The Occupational Repetition Strain Injuries Advisory Committee of the New South Wales Government Department of Industrial Relations in Australia have proposed a three-stage system indicating the progress of symptoms in individuals who suffer from RSI.

Stage 1 Aching and tiredness of the affected limb occurring during the work shift but settling overnight and on days off work. There is no significant reduction in work performance and no physical signs. This condition can persists for months and is reversible.

Stage 2 Symptoms failing to settle overnight, causing sleep

disturbance and associated with a reduced capacity for repetitive work. Physical signs may be present. The condition usually persists for months.
Stage 3 Symptoms persisting at rest, with disturbed sleep and pain occurring with non-repetitive movement. The person is unable to perform light duties and experiences difficulty with nonoccupational tasks. Physical signs are present. The condition may persist for months or years.

Consistent signs of injury, elicited either on physical examination or by objective physical measures are meager. Standard nerve conduction studies reveal no abnormality and, indeed, if these are present the diagnosis needs to be revised. Much attention has been paid to temperature changes occurring during the course of RSI. In an elegant study Cooke et al. (1993) showed that patients with RSI had increased vasodilatation of the hands compared with controls and also decreased vasomotor activity, although the vasomotor response to cold stress was similar to normal subjects.

How far the symptoms that occur in RSI are related to work-related practices is a debate that is still not settled. In an extensive literature review to determine how far work factors were responsible for the symptoms of RSI it was shown that the studies carried out were flawed by poor medical diagnostic criteria and none of the studies reviewed established a causal relationship between work activities and distinct medical conditions (Vender et al., 1995). It has been shown that workers carrying out identical movements every day are more likely to complain of symptoms that those who rotate activities on a regular basis (Higgs et al., 1992). In the majority of individuals with symptoms arising from work practices symptoms were not persistent and were normally relieved after weekend rest. The factors that cause such symptoms to become persistent are difficult to identify. Abnormal postures, leading to muscle imbalance and associated pressures on nerves have been reputed to cause the typical symptoms (Higgs & Mackinnon, 1995).

In summary, RSI consists in a soft tissue disorder, manifest by pain, tenderness and muscle weakness. There are no standard diagnostic tests that are consistently abnormal in this condition. Although there is some evidence of increased temperature of the painful muscles, thermal dysregulation is not found. The condition, by definition, is presumed to result from repetitive practices usually sustained at work. Concrete evidence of such an association is lacking but there may be a relationship between abnormal posture and unvarying work practices (Tyrer, 1994*b*).

Case presentation

Mrs D, a married woman aged 37 years, was employed as a typist and secretary to a senior management executive in the city of London. She originally worked as a shorthand typist and reported no major work problems until shortly after a word processing machine was introduced into the office. Five months after being trained on the word processor Mrs D started to complain of weakness in both hands and tingling in the finger tips, particularly on the right side. She found that her symptoms improved with rest. These symptoms occurred at a period that Mrs D was spending more time at her word processor because of an increased volume of work. Mrs D was working for up to 8.5 hours a day with only 45 minutes break for lunch.

An improvement occurred in Mrs D's symptoms when the amount of work reduced in the winter months but returned again the following spring when more typing was required. In addition to symptoms of weakness and tingling she also developed a burning feeling in her palms and pouring cold water on her hands was associated with a feeling of heat from the liquid. She later developed weakness in her forearms. Shortly after this Mrs D started to drop items because she was not able to pinch her thumb and fingers together sufficiently strongly. This was associated with a gradual feeling of pain in the arm, ascending up to the elbow. Her sleep became worse, she continued to have pain over the weekends even though she was not working, and after a number of periods off work she was placed on long-term sick leave.

On examination at this time Mrs D was found to have altered sensation in both index fingers over both the proximal and distal part of the fingers, with reduced sensation over the distal part of the middle and ring fingers. The right hand was very slightly warmer than the left. Administration of a cold liquid was associated with a feeling of heat on this hand but not on the left hand. There was no evidence of muscle weakness in the elbows, forearms or shoulders, although it was noted that movements of the forearm and shoulder were carried out with some difficulty.

Radiographs to both hands reported no bone abnormality or tissue swelling. Thermography showed minimally increased uptake over the palmar surface of the hands. A radioisotope bone scan showed very slightly increased uptake in both wrists but elsewhere this was of normal distribution.

Mrs D commenced legal proceedings against her employer on the grounds of her RSI being caused by the new word processor and the excessive demands that were made for her to complete work at the time of increased industrial activity. She has now been discharged from her post and is receiving Invalidity Benefit.

Prevalence

The prevalence of RSI is related to the decade in which this is reported, country, type of occupation, season and age of the sufferer. Considerable variations in prevalence have been reported, reflecting the largely subjective nature of complaints in this syndrome and the relationship between the onset of these and new work practices. At times, the term 'epidemic' to refer to the considerable increase in reports of this condition is a term that is justifiably warranted (Lucire, 1986). It is instructive to consider details of the prevalence of this condition in a historical context.

In 1908, telegraphists' cramp, a disorder with a low sporadic incidence, was added to the list of diseases to be compensated under the UK Workmen's Compensation Act of 1906 on the evidence of the union's doctor that cramp was muscular failure caused by the rapid repetitive movements of the new Morse telegraphy (Great Britain and Ireland Post Office, 1911). Within four years 30% of the workforce were reporting symptoms of cramp, fatigue and pain and in some offices almost two-thirds of the workforce complained of these. The incidence of similar symptoms in the USA at this time was between 4% and 10%, despite more intensive work practices than were carried out by the British workers (Great Britain and Ireland Post Office, 1911). When changes were made in the work situation the prevalence reduced considerably.

Other countries had similar rapid rises in the reported cases of work-related upper arm syndromes. Almost 40 years ago in Japan between 10% and 28% of punch card perforators, typists, telephone operators, keyboard operators and process workers described such symptoms and the Japanese Ministry of Labor introduced ergonomic measures in 1964 to reduce the length of hours at work (Nakaseko et al., 1982). At this time the prevalence of such symptoms in Australia was estimated as being between 1% and 5%. In 1982 the Australian National Health and Medical Research Council produced a document called Approved Occupational Health Guide – Repetition Strain Injuries, and suggested that such injuries might be avoided by extensive alteration of work practices.

Following this paper there was a rapid increase in claims for compensation for RSI. Employers in occupations which included repetitive practices received claims from over 5% of the payroll and up to 30% in some places (Hadler, 1986). The prevalence of RSI has reduced considerably in Australia over the past eight years because of the combination of tighter diagnostic precision and more stringent interpretation of the evidence for work being a causative factor. In attempting to relate the prevalence of the symptoms of RSI with working conditions it is relevant to note that at any one time a tenth of the population has pain in the arm or neck, or both (Hadler, 1986) and a third of the population has a morbidity risk of suffering such symptoms (Lawrence, 1969). The equivalent of the RSI in the USA, cumulative trauma disorder, has been reported to lead to more than 50% of all illnesses that are due to occupational factors (Sommerich et al., 1993). One survey reported that 78% of a population at risk because of vigorous repetitive arm movements had some symptoms of the disease (Taylor & Pitcher, 1984), although the definitions of RSI given in this article were not clearly stated.

Economic costs

The economic dimensions of repetitive strain injuries of upper extremities have been recently analyzed for the US population (Webster & Snook, 1994). The database explored comprised the computerized claims records of Liberty Mutual Insurance Company for 1989. The search identified 6607 cases, representing 0.83% of all disability claims. Claims that required no medical or indemnity payments were not included in this sample. Costs were assessed in 1992, allowing at least two years for each claim to settle; a settlement was in fact obtained for 92% of all claims. The mean cost per case was $8070, which was substantially greater than the company's average payment ($4075) for a worker's compensation claim. Medical costs constituted one-third of the payments, the rest being disbursed as indemnity payments for lost wages. The total payments amounted to 1.64% of all compensable costs of this commercial insurer; using this ratio to extrapolate to the entire insurance industry, the authors estimated that the annual cost of this syndrome in the USA in 1989 was approximately $563 million.

Confirmations

As RSI does not fulfil at present the definition of a disease it is difficult to provide relevant information to indicate definitely whether individuals have or have not got this condition. There are nevertheless a number of features that occur in people who complain of painful hands or wrists, associated with numbness or tingling, with concomitant loss of strength or poor coordination in the affected joints, and who carry out frequent movements of the hands and/or arms.

In the first instance, it is vital to exclude known pathological entities, including De Quervain's stenosing tenosynovitis, peritendinitis crepitans, carpal tunnel and cubital tunnel syndromes, lateral and medial epicondylitis, rotator cuff syndrome and Dupuytren's contracture. The physician is normally able to determine by physical examination whether there is a likelihood of these conditions being present.

Conditions involving tenosynovitis always include signs of crepitus and tenderness along the line of a tendon sheath, or in some occasions immediately proximal to this. De Quervain's syndrome affects the extensor tendons of the thumb and the flexor tendons to the thumb and middle and ring fingers. Peritendinitis crepitans also affects the thumb in the 'crossover' zone of the thumb extensor tendons. This is a prescribed disease in the UK Department of Health Schedule of Industrial Diseases. It has been found that there are five main factors leading to this disease: (1) occupational change giving rise to unaccustomed movement, (2) resumption of work after absence, (3) repetitive movements, (4) direct local trauma, and (5) local strain (Thompson et al., 1951).

The essential clinical features of carpal and cubital tunnel syndrome are due to compression of the median and ulnar nerve, respectively, and these can be confirmed by electromyogram (EMG) studies. Although many have assumed that carpal tunnel syndrome is associated with repetitive movements at work, Nathan et al. (1988), in a study of 471 industrial employees from 27 occupations in four industries, found no consistent association between the type and level of occupational hand activity and the prevalence or the severity of nerve conduction defects.

Lateral and medial epicondylitis (commonly termed tennis and golfer's elbow, respectively), are painful conditions affecting the outer and inner parts of the elbow. In tennis elbow, pain occurs over the elbow and may spread along the forearm as far as the wrist and is aggravated by extending the wrist and fingers against resistance. This condition is common, affecting 1–3% of the population, occurs most frequently between the ages of 40 and 60 years, a precipitating factor is absent in most cases and the majority of sufferers are not manual workers.

The pathology of these epicondylitides is uncertain but it is thought that there is a tear or some other traumatic change in the muscles or tendons adjoining the epicondyle of the humerus. This condition has similarities to RSI in that the disease is diagnosed from symptoms rather than signs on physical examination and there is little objective confirmatory evidence of a disease process.

Rotator cuff syndrome, otherwise known as impingement or painful arc syndrome, is a condition in which rotation of the shoulder is usually full but is painful through a certain arc of the movement. It is due to a tendon or tendons (rotator cuff) around the shoulder joint becoming partly trapped. Hawkins & Abrams (1987) have stated that 'individuals who excessively use their arms above the horizontal are especially at risk for developing (this syndrome)'. It is known that these symptoms are common among swimmers and field athletics sports, particularly among those with overhead actions (Hawkins & Kennedy, 1980). It is presumed that the syndrome is due to reduced blood supply to the tendon of the supraspinatus muscle which increases with age and is affected by the position of the shoulder. Again, there are no simple objective tests that can be employed to determine the definite presence or absence of rotator cuff syndrome.

The syndrome should be distinguished from rotator cuff tear due to traumatic rupture of the supraspinctus tendon, which normally occurs following a fall on the outstretched arm. In this condition abduction is extremely painful or impossible.

Thoracic outlet syndrome is a condition in which an identifiable anatomical abnormality such as a cervical band or un-united fracture of the clavicle compresses the brachial plexus, giving rise to pain in the root of the neck or shoulder and radiating down the arm, usually the ulnar aspect. By definition it is not due to occupational practice.

Dupuytren's disease and later contracture is a disfiguring condition, at first shown by no more than a nodular thickening of the palmar fascia, associated with tethering of the skin. Early (1962) examined the hands of 5000 workers at Crewe Locomotive works in Cheshire, UK, and found that the incidence of Dupuytren's contracture in heavy manual workers was similar to that observed amongst clerical workers. Similar observations were shown by Fisk in 1985. Genetic factors are important in the genesis of this disease (Ling, 1963) and it is noteworthy that those of Chinese, Indian or African-Caribbean stock rarely develop this condition.

Pathological findings in patients with repetitive strain injury

Objective measure of pathological dysfunction in patients with RSI have been carried out in only a few centers. The areas that have been investigated include temperature and blood flow changes, vibration threshold and response to topical application of capsaicin.

The normal response to the vasoconstrictive stimulus of cold is a fall in temperature and blood flow that occurs both at the site of the cold stimulus and elsewhere in the body. Investigations carried out at St Bartholomew's Hospital in London in patients with RSI have shown vasodilation of vessels in the affected hand which was decreased following exposure to contralateral cold challenge to the other arm. This pattern is similar to that found in control subjects but different from patients with complex regional pain syndromes (Cooke et al., 1993). Although this study was carried out on only a small number of subjects the different response of RSI patients compared with those with sympathetically mediated pain in complex regional pain syndromes suggested to the authors that patients with RSI were unlikely to develop sympathetic pain syndromes.

Greening & Lynn (1998) have shown that patients with RSI have evidence of both A_β fiber and C fiber abnormalities. They demonstrated that patients with RSI and office keyboard workers have a higher threshold to vibration in the median nerve compared with control subjects. This was increased further in the RSI patients after use of the keyboard but only on the right side, whereas there was a fall in threshold in the control group. In addition, the RSI patients had a significantly raised threshold to vibration on stimulation of the ulnar nerve, which was not shown by either the office workers or controls. At suprathreshold stimulation 82% of the RSI group experienced a painful response to vibration whereas none of the other office workers or control subjects had this changed sensory response. There was a close correlation between the degree of pain experienced and this raised threshold.

These findings, coupled with the evidence that those working on office machinery have a higher threshold to vibration than control subjects, suggest that there is a relationship between frequent arm movements and these objective neurological findings. Nevertheless, interpretation of these results is still open to debate. It is known that aching of the limbs following frequent work usually subsides with 24–48 hours with rest and it is not known whether there is a concomitant change in the vibration threshold in such patients. The changes observed may be reversible. Furthermore, RSI sufferers, because of the very nature of their symptoms, carry out fewer arm movements following the onset of pain and the changes observed may be due to lack of use.

These results indicating changes in peripheral afferent input are supported by workers in Australia who demonstrated an elevation in threshold and a reduction in the amplitude of the cerebral event related potential (ERP) in response to carbon dioxide laser stimulation of the pain affected limb in sufferers from RSI (Gibson et al., 1991). The assumption is that the central nervous system processing of incoming noxious information is altered by increased peripheral nociceptive input.

It is known that primary afferent C and A_Δ signs with polymodal nociceptors are the major fibers involved in the transmission of nociceptive stimuli to the central nervous system. Activation of these fibers also induces a neurogenic flare response which is thought to occur through axon reflex mechanisms (Holzer, 1988; Maggi & Meli, 1988). Capsaicin, an extract of red peppers, releases substance P from sensory neurons (Gamse et al., 1979). When capsaicin is applied to denervated skin no flare response occurs and further studies have shown that, in general, patients with evidence of neurogenic pain have a decreased flare response (LeVasseur et al., 1990). If indeed patients with RSI have altered peripheral afferent conduction this should be detected by the administration of capsaicin.

In a study examining capsaicin-induced neurogenic vasodilatation and flare responses in a large series of patients with RSI and age-matched control volunteers, a reduction in capsaicin-induced vasodilation in the painful limb was observed, with a strong association between the severity of clinical pain and the degree of reduction in neurogenic vasodilatation (Helme et al., 1992). Furthermore, the latent period to onset of the response was increased in the affected painful limb. A surprising finding in this study was an increase in capsaicin-induced vasodilation in the unaffected limb.

There are a number of hypotheses to explain these findings. It is known that a pain stimulus can elicit a sympathetic vasoconstrictor response and it may be that capsaicin administration leads to greater sympathetic vasoconstriction in subjects with RSI. It is possible that there is a generalized alteration in sympathetic vasoconstrictor tone in subjects with RSI but there was no evidence of abnormal sympathetic functioning on clinical testing in these patients. It is more likely that there is a change in the responsivity of thc primary afferent neurons because of the pain experienced. Repeated stimulation of polymodal nociceptors has been shown to reduce the size of the axon reflex flare to subsequent stimuli (Carpenter & Lynn, 1981). This may be due to a depletion of the vasoactive neuropeptides from the local axon terminals following a period of chronic activation.

It is difficult to explain the increased flare response in the unaffected limb of patients with RSI. It could be that these patients have a reduced pain threshold to mechanical stimuli and it is of interest that a lower dose of capsaicin is required for the activation of vasodilation in patients with fibromyalgia (Littlejohn et al., 1987).

Notwithstanding, these results indicate that there are definite pathological abnormalities in subjects with RSI that are directly related to the degree of pain experienced. These findings lend weight to the contention by a number of authors that RSI is a form of chronic pain syndrome (Brooks, 1993) and that the abnormalities described above are simply a reflection of the degree of pain experienced.

Psychological and psychiatric findings

Virtually all investigations examining the psychological and psychiatric status of patients with RSI show that affected subjects have higher levels of depression on both self-report and observer rating scales for depression, have a somewhat greater number of previous psychiatric conditions prior to the onset of RSI, reduced activity and a greater propensity to somatize psychological problems (Helme et al., 1992).

Virtually all of the well-controlled studies that have been carried out on RSI patients demonstrate that there is a higher reported frequency of depression and anxiety (Bammer & Bignault, 1988; Spence, 1990). Furthermore, symptoms of depression have been shown to predict both chronicity and the development of more severe musculoskeletal problems and pain (Westgaard and Jansen, 1992; Lenio & Magni, 1993). The degree of depression and anxiety on the self-rating scales are not greatly different from similar findings in patients with chronic pain (Bammer & Bignault, 1988; Tyrer et al., 1989). It is difficult to determine cause and effect, but some authors have stated that RSI is indeed a chronic pain syndrome and sufferers are similar to those with chronic painful states arising from other causes (Brooks, 1993). This same author has stated that the degree of pain expressed by RSI patients far exceeds that which would normally be expected from a pain group with physical detectable injuries.

One study has shown that symptoms of depression predict subsequent development of musculoskeletal problems and incapacity (Lenio & Magni, 1993) but it is important to note that most investigators involving RSI workers find that the majority of sufferers have not had previous psychiatric illnesses. It has been proposed that somatization of psychological problems serves an adaptive function by attributing such difficulties to an external physical cause (Goldberg & Bridges, 1988), and in a number of sufferers from RSI this link has been suggested (Lucire, 1986). In this regard, it has been shown that sufferers from RSI have greater denial of nonorganic problems and a tendency to focus on somatic rather than psychological interpretations of problems (Helme et al., 1992).

Sufferers from RSI can reduce their activity considerably and the reduction in capsaicin-induced vasodilation reported in the Australian studies was closely correlated with the decrease in activity reported (Helme et al., 1992). It is possible that this increase is a consequence of disuse.

Contradictions

The major controversy concerning the diagnosis of RSI is concerned with how far this entity is a disease in its own right and to what degree it is a psychosocial condition that has been encouraged by employees' organizations and doctors' beliefs of work-related injury. Secondary debates are concerned with how far RSI is a chronic pain syndrome and whether there is sympathetic nerve dysfunction in this condition.

To fulfill the criteria for a condition to be delineated as a disease entity, causative factors need to be clearly known, the majority of those people exposed to these factors should develop the disease and there needs to be a clearly defined constellation of symptoms and signs with objective evidence of pathology that is different from other illnesses. On these criteria RSI does not fulfill the standards required to indicate that it is a clearly separate disease; however, there have been developments in the past few years that suggest a clearer idea of what organic causative factors are present in this condition.

The history of the development of 'epidemics' of work-related upper arm conditions strongly suggest that beliefs about the condition being related to work-related injury, contributed to massive increases in reporting. Lucire (1986) has explained how this can arise. A constellation of symptoms that is described as a disease receives sympathetic attention with widespread publicity and there is no challenge at first to an incorrect attribution of cause. A powerful agent or force is considered to be responsible for the disease in question. Early reporting of these currently alarming symptoms influences others to claim the same gains as those who have already been affected and who have received compensation. The instruments causing the problems, keyboard and computer terminals, become symbols of physical danger to which those who are vulnerable, dissatisfied or bored react in an exaggerated way. It was only when it is demonstrated that most individuals do not develop such symptoms and that correct ergonomic practices reduce the incidence of the condition that the incidence of new cases is reduced.

There seems little doubt that the rapid increase of reported RSI in the early 1980s in Australia was due to a combination of these factors. A similar 'epidemic' of a different illness occurred 40 years ago in the Royal Free Hospital in London. Nurses living in the hospital nursing home developed symptoms of pyrexia, muscle weakness, vertigo and pain that was described so succinctly that the term 'Royal Free disease' was used to describe it (McEvedy & Beard, 1970). It is now recognized that the symptoms described are very similar to what is now termed 'chronic fatigue syndrome'. Cooper (1993) has proposed that such 'socially transmitted psychopathology' arises in a group of closely connected individuals in whom there is strong emotional tension. Spread of the 'disease' in this emotionally charged climate occurs when a 'carrier', somebody who manifests major symptoms of the disorder, provides a model that others follow by imitation. It is only when there is publicity from such a 'carrier' that the epidemic takes hold. Thus, in the Australian National University in Canberra in 1986 the cost of RSI was over Aus$1 million whereas in Flinders University in South Australia only one employee was found that had this condition, despite identical work practices in both centers (Y. Lucire, personal communication).

The massive increase in the incidence of RSI in Australia in the mid-1980s and the considerable decrease in numbers of patients suffering from this condition when compensation rules were changed and workers' organizations were encouraged not to press for financial redress strongly suggests that these factors played a part in the outbreak of RSI in Australia. Although there have also been changes in ergonomic practices it is unlikely that these changes have been responsible for the considerably reduced lack of reports of this condition. The studies that have been carried out among the sufferers from RSI have shown a greater incidence of previous psychiatric illnesses and mental health problems in those suffering from RSI at this time and it seems likely that those vulnerable to stresses because of previous adverse experiences were prone to develop these symptoms.

If this hypothesis is correct, the assumption is that keyboard operators develop some muscle aching and strain with continuous repetitive work but the majority do not attribute their problems to injury and as their symptoms go away with rest they pay no more attention to them. The vulnerable individual is worried that he or she has caused irreversible muscle or joint damage, takes time off work, does not use the affected limb in case further damage results and a combination of disuse and a chronic painful state result. The hope of compensation may further affect return to full function. Furthermore, workers who adopt abnormal postures when using keyboards and computer terminals render themselves more prone to musculoskeletal strains when they are carrying out repetitive movements. It has also been proposed that those individuals who are anxious tend to adopt more hunched and unsatisfactory positions when carrying out their work and it is for this reason that these individuals develop the symptoms of RSI.

An alternative view of the etiology of RSI has been proposed by the American authors, Phillip Higgs & Susan Mackinnon (1995). These authors believe that the fact that the incidence of RSI has reduced considerably in Australia is not indicative of resolution of the problem because of politico-economic measures but that the problem has been driven underground. The establishment of large numbers of Web sites on the Internet all concerned with RSI certainly indicates that many people believe they have symptoms attributable to repetitive work. Examination of the information in the articles provided by these self-help groups reveals a level of sophistication and knowledge about injuries affecting the arms and hands that is certainly convincing to the unbiased observer (see Computer-related Repetitive Strain Injury and Harvard RSI Action Home Page).

Higgs and Mackinnon believe that maintenance of abnormal or prolonged posture, positions or movements associated with many work activities lead to muscle imbalance and consequent pressure and stretching of affected nerves. If muscles affecting a certain activity are underused, opposing muscle groups are usually employed more frequently and intensely. Muscles in either a shortened or lengthened position will be at a mechanical disadvantage and therefore less effective. Pain results from short and tight muscles, particularly when these are stretched. There will consequently be hypertrophy of the overused group of muscles and the underused group will be weak. This combination contributes to maintenance of the abnormal posture and muscle imbalance. The authors stress that certain positions make the worker more likely to develop such muscle imbalance. In particular, forward flexion of the neck and extension of the head with a slouched position of the shoulders leads to overuse of the sternomastoid, scalene pectoralis minor, trapezius, rhomboid and levator scapulae muscles and underuse of the middle and lower trapezius and serratus anterior muscles.

These abnormal positions directly increase the pressure around the nerve or stretch the nerve, resulting in chronic nerve compression. This leads to decreased blood flow to the nerve causing fibrosis in and around the nerve. This process tethers the nerve, which is rendered less mobile and leads to pain on normal movements. The authors claim that chronic nerve compression is slowly progressive unless there is a major change in posture and movement. As the nerves involved are only compressed during certain movements, standard electrophysiological investigations of nerve function are normal when the affected muscles are at rest as they are during normal electromyogram studies. Percussion over a site of entrapment leads to tingling down the affected nerve (Tinel's sign). Where the muscles of the wrist are involved, flexion or extension of this joint produces paresthesia in the median nerve distribution (Phalen's sign). A positive Tinel and Phalen's sign is frequently found in sufferers from RSI.

Although the authors carefully note that this explanation of the symptoms of RSI is not yet established by pathological findings, they have proposed further trials (Mackinnon & Novak, 1994). Although this hypothesis brings together previous knowledge in this area and is attractive to those who suffer from this condition, this explanation does not indicate why the vast majority of people involved in repetitive tasks do not develop these complaints. Is this simply the result of abnormal posture or is it that those individuals who maintain these postures outside the work environment or continue to use their upper limbs away from work develop the condition? It is also difficult to explain why vast numbers of the work force in Australia in the 1980s and in Japan in the 1960s developed such symptoms unless it is postulated that the postural abnormalities resulted from anxiety and worry about possible work-related injury.

Pathogenetic hypotheses

The three main hypotheses to explain RSI concern the medical, psychological and sociological models of illness.

The medical model hypothesis attributes the origin of RSI to the adoption of abnormal postures when carrying out an activity for long periods of time, the extent of the problem depending upon the degree of heavy work, direct load bearing and lack of rest. The abnormal strains to which muscles and nerves are exposed lead to muscle overuse, and nerve entrapment. Those subjects who are overweight and have short limb length are particularly at risk from developing the condition.

The sociological hypothesis is that on the development of new technology there is a change in the perception of endemic symptoms of upper limb pain which are considered to represent injury. A liberal compensation system contributes to enhanced reporting of the condition.

The psychological/psychiatric hypothesis is that people who are vulnerable to stresses because of early environmental trauma or previous psychiatric illness are prone to misinterpret work-related upper arm symptoms, reduce activity and become disabled as a result of the fear of injury and muscle disuse.

Diagnostic and treatment approaches

Diagnosis

The aims of clinical evaluation of patients with suspected RSI are to determine the diagnosis as far as possible and to decide on how far the disorder identified is related to work.

A full history should be taken of the sufferer's present symptoms, when they arose and their development over time. It is usual for patients with RSI to have had previous episodes of wrist or upper arm pain and often these have developed in the work environment. Associated nonpainful symptoms should be sought, including questions concerned with sleep, mood and activity. All of these are likely to be considerably affected adversely. The sufferer from RSI can usually identify a particular circumstance which has led to an acute exacerbation of their problem and which has caused them to stop work. The circumstances of this event should be inquired about in particular detail, with careful description of the particular work practices in which the person was involved at the time of the acute onset of symptoms. Inquiry should be made from the occupational physician at the patient's place of work and it is often valuable to seek the advice of the foreman or supervisor at the workplace to obtain information on work practices and on the individual's attitude to work (Tyrer, 1987). In patients who seek compensation for work-related injuries there is frequently resentment between the worker and his or her immediate superior and this is a factor which increases subsequent illness behavior.

Inquiry should be made about past surgical and medical conditions, particularly those involving the musculoskeletal system. Any previous history of psychiatric illness should be sought, paying attention to stress-related factors. Details of past and current domestic, social and occupational problems should be obtained and during this exercise it can usually be determined whether there are particular events to which the patient is particularly vulnerable. The personality attributes of the sufferer should be determined; some who have RSI have a long-standing resentful and paranoid attitude and are inclined to blame others for problems that have arisen in their life.

Examination of the patient includes assessment of posture, range of motion and movement patterns, full neurological examination to exclude nerve entrapment and nerve injury and examination of their mental state.

Observation of the patient's standing posture frequently demonstrates a poked forward position of the chin, head and neck with sloping of the shoulders (Figure 9.1). The arms tend to be held by the side with the palms facing backwards. Passive stretching of the shoulder and arm muscles frequently elicits tenderness. Grip is usually considerably reduced in the affected limb and on abduction of the shoulder the scapula may move in an uncoordinated fashion because of underuse of the lower trapezius muscle and overuse of the upper trapezius and rhomboid muscles. Slight winging of the scapulae may also be noted on lowering the arms.

During examination of the muscle groups sensory symptoms may be elicited. Wrist flexion or extension produces paresthesia in the thumb, index and middle fingers and over the thenar eminence (Phalen's sign). Pronation of the forearm when associated with flexion of the wrist and ulnar deviation produces paresthesia in the radial sensory nerve distribution in patients with compression of this nerve. Elbow flexion produces paresthesia in the ring and little fingers in individuals with cubital tunnel syndrome. Sensory testing should include two-point

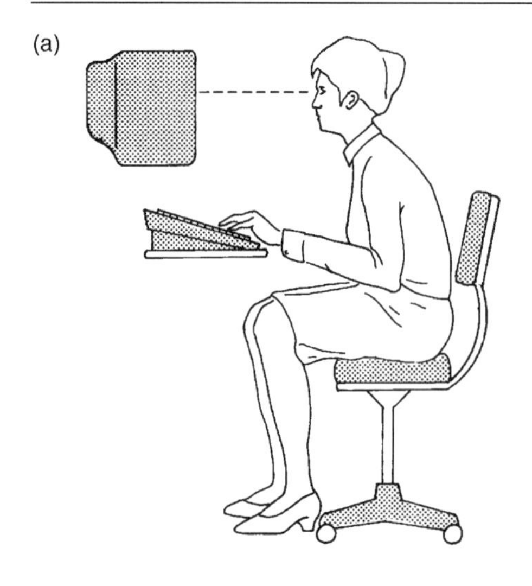

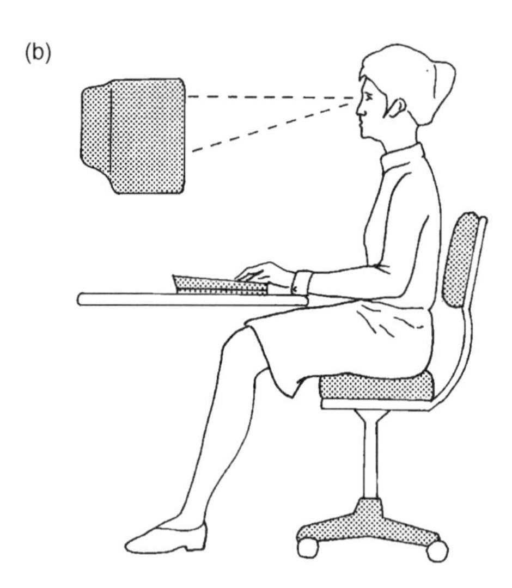

Figure 9.1. (a) Incorrect position for keyboard work. Note flexed posture of neck, head and shoulders with flexion of elbows because of raised keyboard. (b) Correct position for keyboard work. Note that the spine is straight, the neck is neither flexed nor extended, the elbows are extended and the keyboard is lowered. (Drawn by Joseph Rankin.)

discrimination and threshold testing of vibration and pressure (Mackinnon, 1992). Although not part of the standard clinical examination, topical administration of capsaicin over the affected site has been found to produce a reduced flare response compared with application over the same site on the contralateral limb (Helme et al., 1992).

Mental state examination should include assessment of possible depression, including facial expression, evidence of tearfulness and pessimistic attitudes as well as both somatic and psychic evidence of anxiety. It is often valuable to ask the patient to complete a self-rating mood scale such as the Hospital Anxiety and Depression Scale (HAD) (Zigmond & Snaith, 1983) or the Beck Depression Inventory (Beck et al., 1961).

Following the history and physical examination, pathological conditions such as nerve entrapment syndromes, tendon-related disorders (including tennis and golfers' elbow), complex regional pain syndromes and hand-arm vibration syndrome should be identified. These conditions are separate from RSI and should be treated appropriately. Investigations to confirm the presence or absence of such disorders will include electroneurophysiological studies of nerve conduction in the affected parts, an examination of threshold to vibration (which can be carried out with a fair degree of accuracy during the clinical examination by applying the base of a vibrating C tuning fork over a bony point in the distribution of the supposed affected nerve), thermographic techniques and MRI (Patten, 1995). Apart from an increased threshold to vibration that has been noticed in sufferers from RSI, these tests will not reveal conclusive abnormalities in patients with RSI alone.

Management

The management of a patient with RSI involves both treatment of the patient's condition and prevention of work-related risk factors that may have caused or aggravated the condition.

The affected body part should be rested for a time following diagnosis of the condition. In practice the patient will have usually ensured that the affected limb has not been used. Although some authors say that rest should be prescribed for at least two weeks (Rempel et al., 1992) most would consider that this period is too long and there should be a gradual increase in active movement after five to eight days of rest. The use of ice over the affected area may provide symptomatic relief. Immobilization of the appropriate joint, coupled with administration of anti-inflammatory drugs, may be of benefit but splinting the affected joint or immobilization for long periods is counter-therapeutic. Although local corticosteroid injections have been recommended, the evidence for their value is meager.

The most important point to get across to the sufferer from RSI is that the individual concerned has the greatest potential to treat his or her condition. The abnormal postures that have been adopted by the patient should be demonstrated to the individual concerned and education about the positions to adopt to decrease nerve compression should be given. In symptoms involving the wrist, the wrist joint should be kept in a neutral position, neither extended or flexed. Excessive forearm pronation should be avoided and it may be advisable to recommend to the patient that they carry out regular supination activities of the forearm and wrist at regular intervals during the day (see Figure 9.2). Elbow flexion should be avoided.

If there is evidence of muscle imbalance this should be managed by specific physiotherapy exercises, supervised by an experienced physiotherapist, with regular practice by the patient. The aim of physiotherapy initially should be to stretch short and tight muscles (Travell & Simons, 1983) and once the patient has achieved a full and pain-free range of motions of the neck, shoulder and wrist, strengthening exercises are begun. There may be advantages in adding light weights after the patient has remained free from pain for some time and the muscles have shown an increase in muscle bulk. Many patients are overweight and dietary advice may be needed as well as a specific exercise program.

It is vital to examine work practices in detail. If sufferers from RSI are identified early, at stage 1 or stage 2, the individual should be able to return to work. If the person is aware that changes have been made at his or her work station to improve matters, this is going to have a positive psychological effect and encourage rehabilitation.

It is not known what percentage of sufferers from RSI return to work after assessment of their condition. Most who seek compensation do not return to similar work and most of those who develop the symptoms described in stage 3 are not likely to return to work if their symptoms have been present for longer than a few weeks. The beliefs of the patients are very important in this regard. If the sufferer believes that a particular movement or problem has caused their symptoms and it has been shown that this problem has been overcome by a new technique the individual concerned may be more likely to return to productive occupation. Alteration of the work station should be made so that the worker does not have to lean forward and the arms should be kept in a low position with the elbows extended (see Figure 9.1). Breaks should be taken during the day at least once every 2 hours and it may be advisable to supinate the forearm and stretch the neck muscles at these times (Sundelin & Hagsberg, 1989). A lumbar roll to support a normal lumbar curve in the lower back also encourages better posture. As far as possible raising of the hands above the head should be avoided and it may be necessary to lower the work station.

The results of abnormal posture take years to develop and several

(a)

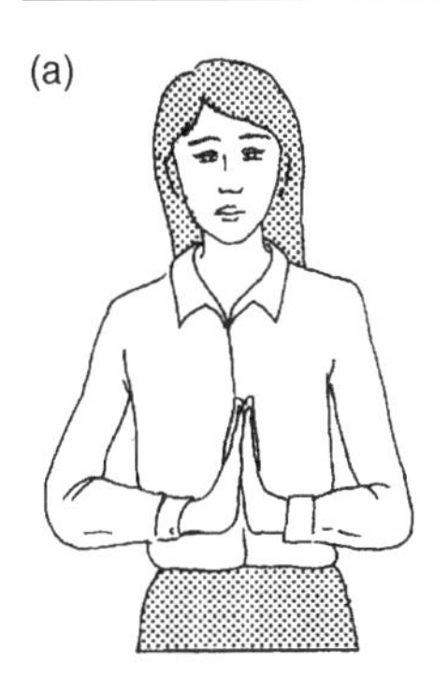

(b)

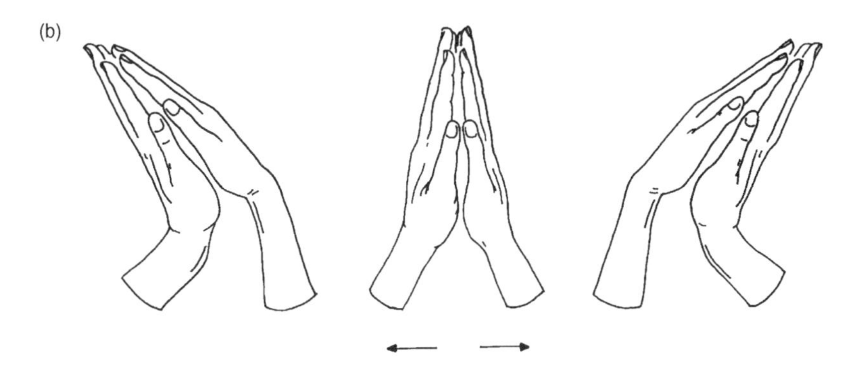

Figure 9.2. Exercises to stretch and relax the extensor muscles of the wrist. The 'prayer position' is adopted first and then the wrists are alternately stretched and relaxed. (Drawn by Joseph Rankin.)

months of physiotherapy and exercise are required to bring about symptomatic improvement. The individual with RSI should be forewarned about the long time it takes to improve matters but slow and regular exercises should be encouraged, with a gradual increase in activity throughout the treatment period.

Conclusion

RSI is a misleading term that includes symptoms of pain, muscle weakness and tingling associated with tenderness of the affected muscles. Although the term implies that repetitive movement is responsible for the condition, abnormal postures and prolonged periods of work are more important in causing the syndrome than repetitive movements. There are few objective tests that can be used to identify abnormalities in this condition, although a reduced flare response to the application of capsaicin and an increased threshold to vibration have been reported. Although sudden increases in the incidence of this condition have been associated with changes in work practice and attribution of these to injuries processes, the majority of sufferers from this condition do not have a primary psychiatric illness and are not seeking sickness benefit or compensation. Treatment involves correction of abnormal postures, a graded program of exercises and alterations in work practice if abnormalities can be identified in ergonomic design.

References

Australian National Health and Medical Research Council (1982). *Approved Guide to Occupational Health.* Camberra: The National Health and Medical Research Council.

Bammer G & Bignault L (1988). More than a pain in the arms: a review of the consequences of developing overuse syndromes. *Journal of Occupational Health of Australia and New Zealand*, **4**, 389–97.

Beck AT, Ward CH, Mendelson M, Mock JE & Erbaugh JK (1961). An inventory for measuring depression. *Archives of General Psychiatry*, **4**, 561–71.

Bell C (1833). Partial paralysis of the muscles of the extremities. In *The Nervous System of the Human Body*. Washington, DC: Duff Green.

Brooks, P. (1993). Repetitive strain injury. *British Medical Journal*, **307**, 1298.

Bureau of Labor Statistics (1990). *Reports on Survey of Occupational Injuries and Disease in 1977–1989*. Washington, DC: Bureau of Labor Statistics, US Department of Labor.

Carpenter SE & Lynn B (1981). Abolition of axon reflex flare in human skin by capsaicin. *Journal of Physiology*, **310**, 69–70.

Cooke ED, Steinberg MD, Pearson RM, Fleming CE, Toms SL & Elusasade JA (1993). Reflex sympathetic dystrophy and repetitive strain injury: temperature and microcirculatory changes following mild cold stress. *Journal of the Royal Society of Medicine*, **86**, 690–3.

Cooper B (1993). Single spies and battalions: the clinical epidemiology of mental disorders. *Psychological Medicine*, **23**, 891–907.

Early PS (1962). Population studies in Dupuytren's contracture. *Journal of Bone and Joint Surgery*, **44B**, 602–13.

Ferguson D (1971). An Australian study of telegraphist's cramp. *British Journal of Industrial Medicine*, **28**, 280–5.

Fisk G (1985). The relationship of manual labour and specific injury to Dupuytren's disease. In *Dupuytren's Disease* (G.E.M. Monograph), 2nd English edn, ed. J. T. Hueston & R. T. Tubiana, pp. 104–105. Edinburgh: Churchill Livingstone.

Fry HJH (1986). Overuse syndrome in musicians: prevention and management. *Lancet*, **ii**, 728–31.

Gamse R, Molnar A & Lembeck F (1979). Substance P release from spinal cord slices of capsaicin. *Life Sciences*, **25**, 629–36.

Gibson SJ, Le Vasseur SA & Helme RD (1991). Cerebral event-related responses induced by CO_2 laser stimulation in subjects suffering from cervico-brachial syndrome. *Pain*, **47**, 173–82.

Goldberg DP & Bridges KW (1988). Somatic presentations of psychiatric illness in primary care settings. *Journal of Psychosomatic Research*, **32**, 137–44.

Gowers WR (1892). *A Manual of Diseases of the Nervous System*, 2nd edn, pp. 710–30. London: J & A Churchill.

Great Britain and Ireland Post Office (1911). *Department Committee on Telegraphists' Cramp Report*. London: His Majesty's Stationery Office.

Greening J & Lynn B (1998). Vibration sense in the upper limb in patients with repetitive strain injury and a group of at risk office workers. *International Archives of Occupational Medicine*, **71**, 29–34.

Hadler NM (1986). The Australian and New Zealand experiences with arm pain and backache in the workplace. *Medical Journal of Australia*, **144**, 191–5.

Hawkins RJ & Abrams JC (1987). Impingement syndrome in the absence of rotator cuff tear. *Orthopedics Clinics of North America*, **18**, 373–82.

Hawkins RJ & Kennedy JS (1980). The impingement syndrome in athletes. *American Journal of Sports Medicine*, **8**, 57–62.

Helme RD, Le Vasseur SA & Gibson SJ (1992). RSI revisited: evidence for psychological and physiological differences from an age, sex and occupation matched control group. *Australia and New Zealand Journal of Medicine*, **22**, 23–9.

Higgs PE & Mackinnon SE (1995). Repetitive motion injuries. *Annual Review of Medicine*, **46**, 1–16.

Higgs P, Young, VL, Seaton M, Edwards B & Freely C (1992). Upper extremity impairment in workers performing repetitive tasks. *Plastic and Reconstructive Surgery*, **90**, 614–20.

Holzer P (1988). Local effector functions of capsaicin-sensitive sensory nerve endings: involvement of tachykinins, CGRP and other neuropeptides. *Neuroscience*, **24**, 739–68.

Ireland DCR (1988). Psychological and physical aspects of occupational arm pain. *Journal of Hand Surgery*, **13B**, 5–9.

Lawrence JS (1969). Disc degeneration. Its frequency and relationship to symptoms. *Annals of Rheumatic Diseases*, **28**, 121–37.

Lenio P & Magni G (1993). Depressive and distress symptoms as predictors of low back pain, neck-shoulder pain and other musculo-skeletal morbidity: a 10 year follow-up of metal industry employees. *Pain*, **53**, 89–94.

LeVasseur SA, Gibson SJ & Helme RD (1990). The measurement of capsaicin-sensitive sensory nerve fiber function in elderly patients with pain. *Pain*, **41**, 19–25.

Ling RSM (1963). The genetic factor in Dupuytren's disease. *Journal of Bone and Joint Surgery (Br)*, **45B**, 709–12.

Littlejohn GO, Weinstein G & Helme RD (1987). Increased neurogenic inflammation in fibrositis syndrome. *Journal of Rheumatology*, **14**, 1022–5.

Lucire Y (1986). Neurosis in the work place. *Medical Journal of Australia*, **145**, 323–7.

Mackinnon SE (1992). Double and multiple 'crush' syndromes: double and multiple entrapment neuropathies. *Hand Clinics of North America*, **8**, 369–90.

Mackinnon SE & Novak CB (1994). Clinical commentary: pathogenesis of cumulative trauma disorder. *Journal of Hand Surgery (Am)*, **19A**, 873–83.

Maggi CA & Meli A (1988). The sensory-efferent function of capsaicin-sensitive sensory neurons. *General Pharmacology*, **19**, 1–43.

McEvedy CP & Beard AW (1970). Concept of benign myalgic encephalomyelitis. *British Medical Journal*, **1**, 11–15.

Nakaseko M, Tokunaga R & Hosokawa M (1982). Occupational cervicobrachial disorder in Japan. *Journal of Human Ergonomics (Tokyo)*, **11**, 7–16.

Nathan PA, Meadows KD & Doyle L (1988). Occupation as a risk factor for impaired sensory conduction of the median nerve in the carpal tunnel syndrome. *Journal of Hand Surgery (Br)*, **13B**, 167–70.

Patten RM (1995). Overuse syndromes and injuries involved in the elbow: MR imaging findings. *American Journal of Roentgenology*, **164**, 1205–11.

Ramazzini B (1713). *De Morbis Artificum*. Diatriba. Padua. (translated by W. C. Wright). Chicago: University of Chicago Press, 1940.

Rempel DM, Harrison RJ & Barnhart S (1992). Work-related cumulative trauma disorders of the upper extremity. *Journal of the American Medical Association*, **267**, 838–42.

Solly S (1864). Scrivener's palsy, or the paralysis of writers. *Lancet*, **ii**, 709–11.

Sommerich CM, McGlothlin JD & Massas WS (1993). Occupational risk factors associated with soft tissue disorders of the shoulder: a review of recent investigations in the literature. *Ergonomics*, **36**, 697–717.

Spence SH (1990). Psychopathology amongst acute and chronic patients with occupationally related upper limb disorders versus accident injuries of the upper limbs. *Australian Psychologist*, **24**, 293–305.

Sundelin G & Hagberg M (1989). The effects of different pause types on neck and shoulder activity during VDU work. *Ergonomics*, **32**, 527–37.

Taylor R & Pitcher M (1984). Medical and ergonomic aspects of an industrial dispute concerning occupational related conditions in data process operators. *Community Health Studies*, **8**, 172–80.

Thompson AR, Plewes LW & Shaw EG (1951). Peritendinitis crepitans and simple tenosynovitis: a clinical study of 544 cases in industry. *British Journal of Industrial Medicine*, **8**, 150–8.

Travell JG & Simons DG (1983). Myofascial pain and dysfunction. In *The Trigger Point Manual*, pp. 45–218. Baltimore: Williams & Wilkins.

Tyrer FH (1987). Organization of occupational health services. In: *Textbook of Occupational Medicine*, ed. J. K. Howard & F. H. Tyrer, pp. 21–45. Edinburgh: Churchill Livingstone.

Tyrer SP (1994*a*). Repetitive strain injury. *Journal of Psychosomatic Research*, **38**, 493–8.

Tyrer SP (1994*b*). Repetitive strain injury. Pain linked to repetitive work. *British Medical Journal*, **308**, 269–70.

Tyrer SP, Capon M, Peterson DM, Charlton JE & Thompson JW (1989). The detection of psychiatric illness and psychological handicaps in a British Pain Clinic population. *Pain*, **36**, 63–74.

Vender MI, Kasdan ML & Truppa KL (1995). Upper extremity disorders: a literature review to determine work-relatedness. *Journal of Hand Surgery*, **20A**, 534–41.

Webster BS & Snook SH (1994). The cost of compensable upper extremity cumulative trauma disorders. *Journal of Occupational Medicine*, **36**, 713–717.

Westgaard RH & Jansen T (1992). Individual and work-related factors associated with symptoms of musculoskeletal complaints. Different risk factors amongst sewing machine operators. *British Journal of Industrial Medicine*, **49**, 154–9.

Zigmond A & Snaith RA (1983). The hospital anxiety and depression scale. *Acta Psychiatrica Scandinavica*, **67**, 361–70.

10

Multiple Chemical Sensitivities

ABBA I. TERR

The concept of an illness with subjective wide-ranging symptoms triggered by exposure to numerous environmental chemicals, called multiple chemical sensitivities (MCS), has existed for at least 40 years, but it remains controversial. MCS bears a close resemblance to other current syndromes such as the chronic fatigue syndrome, myalgic encephalomyelitis and various chronic pain syndromes. These are also typically multisymptomatic, although they have a sentinel symptom – fatigue, pain or musculoskeletal discomfort – and there is no connection to environmental exposures.

MCS has also been compared with somatoform illness because the numerous somatic symptoms suggest physical illness involving many different body organs and systems, but without objective evidence of disease.

MCS may be confused with allergic, toxic, irritant or even infectious diseases because of its presumed association with the environment. Allergic diseases are characterized by inflammation and organ dysfunction usually localized to a particular tissue such as the nasal or bronchial mucosa or the skin, and established testing procedures can identify the specific immunological sensitivities. Toxic and irritant diseases are reliably dose dependent with objective evidence of pathology consistent with the chemical and/or physical properties of the environmental chemical and route of exposure. Building-related illnesses should also not be confused with MCS. Occupational asthma and hypersensitivity pneumonitis are allergic diseases in which well-validated tests determine the specific allergen and the immunological sensitivity of the patient. The sick-building syndrome, while its pathogenesis is not yet fully understood, occurs in buildings with inadequate or defective ventilation, causing reversible mucous membrane irritation. Legionnaire's disease is an example of an airborne infectious disease acquired in buildings harboring the microorganism.

A number of major medical organizations have taken the position that MCS is not a recognized clinical syndrome and its concepts are unscientific and lack validation. A recent workshop organized by the International Program on Chemical Safety of the World Health Organization recommended a new name – idiopathic environmental intolerances – because the term multiple chemical sensitivities makes an unsupported judgment on causation, does not refer to a clinically defined disease, is not based on accepted theories of underlying mechanisms or validated clinical criteria for diagnosis, and because the relationship between exposures and symptoms is unproven (United Nations Environmental Program, 1996).

History

The existence of MCS as a medical illness was first proposed in the 1950s by T. G. Randolph, who founded a movement known as clinical ecology, which postulates that a variety of diseases of uncertain etiology, including virtually all forms of psychiatric illness, are caused by the toxic properties of low levels of environmental chemicals (Randolph, 1962). He and others envisioned the mechanism of disease as a failure of human adaptation to twentieth century synthetic chemicals. The favored term for this condition for many years was 'environmental illness'. Seventy years earlier, however, G. M. Beard described the same clinical condition, which he in turn ascribed to certain items and activities introduced into nineteenth century living, specifically the telegraph, the sciences, industry, the periodical press and female education (Beard, 1881).

The currently popular name of MCS was suggested by Cullen (1987), who also proposed a definition that describes the condition as subjective. Other followers of Randolph have come forward with a number of alternative theories that generally focus on the immune system or the nervous system as the site of disease activity. As the number of cases has grown, investigators from many different medical specialties have critically examined these patients and the theories. There is now a strong consensus that the MCS phenomenon is best explained as a psychosocial one, and that the clinical features are similar to those of other currently popular, but controversial, syndromes. As patients with MCS attribute their symptoms and disability to environmental chemicals, this 'diagnosis' is increasingly being used as a cause of legal action against manufacturers and marketers of many common products, especially perfumes, pesticides and organic solvents, as well as those responsible for disposal of commercial toxic wastes.

Definition

The term MCS was invented by Cullen for patients with the condition believed to be caused by their work. His definition is as follows:

> an acquired disorder characterized by recurrent symptoms, referable to multiple organ systems, occurring in response to demonstrable exposure to many chemically unrelated compounds at doses far below those established in the general population to cause harmful effects. No single widely accepted test of physiologic function can be shown to correlate with symptoms. (Cullen, 1987)

Dickey uses the following definition (for environmental illness, the term widely used before Cullen):

> an adverse reaction to environmental insult or excitant in air, water, food, drugs, or our habitat – domiciliary, occupational, or avocational. (Dickey, 1976)

Definitions of MCS are inseparable from terminology, which in turn relates to theories of causation. Table 10.1 lists some of the names that are synonymous with MCS.

Case presentation

The following case history is typical of those with a diagnosis of MCS.

Case

A 42-year-old former dental technician was referred for evaluation of MCS and nickel allergy. She wore a mask and nasal prongs for oxygen. A metal brace, presumably containing nickel, was applied to her teeth four years earlier. She subsequently developed nausea, vomiting, diarrhea, headaches, muscle spasms, staggering gait, mouth sores and bleeding, ecchymoses, nose bleeds, tongue swelling, hives and daily 'convulsions'. The braces were replaced with plastic ones one year later, but these symptoms persisted, and much later improved. Since then she has reacted adversely to perfumes, cigarette smoke, cologne, hair spray, detergents, car fumes, smog, gasoline, oil, aerosols, turpentine, furniture polish and carpet cleaners. She has always been intolerant of most drugs.

Her nickel allergy was diagnosed prior to this illness on the basis of toothache and sore throat which were attributed to nickel in her amalgam fillings. These were removed.

Table 10.1. *Other names for multiple chemical sensitivities*

Specific adaptation syndrome
Environmental illness
Twentieth century disease
Universal allergy
Total allergy syndrome
Cerebral allergy
Chemically-induced immune deficiency
Chemical AIDS
Chemical hypersensitivity syndrome
Idiopathic environmental intolerances

She spent two months at an MCS treatment facility where her diagnoses were chemical sensitivity, migraine, neurotoxicity, immune suppression, nickel toxicity, malnutrition, malabsorption and somatic dysfunction. Extensive testing was carried out. Treatment consisted of 57 prescribed items, including sublingual antigen neutralization; sublingual histamine and serotonin; oxygen; celery extract; intravenous vitamin C (15 g daily), nutrients and magnesium sulfate; and elimination diets.

Her past history included 17 operations for pelvic inflammatory disease beginning at age 14 years and culminating in hysterectomy at age 20 years.

The physical and neurological examinations were unremarkable. She refused nickel allergy patch testing.

Her medical records for this illness include visits to 19 physicians, alternative practitioners, clinics and hospitals, and 11 dentists. None document objective physical findings for her numerous complaints, although she was successfully treated for superficial thrombophlebitis complicating her intravenous treatment for MCS.

Prior medical records showed many visits for headaches, repeated chest and abdominal pains, anxiety with hyperventilation, and numerous drug intolerances.

As exemplified by this case history, patients diagnosed with MCS are mostly adult women (Terr, 1986; Black et al., 1990). The most common complaints are cognitive difficulties and fatigue (Sparks et al., 1994*a*). Somatic symptoms are numerous, including a variety of pains, mucosal irritation, weakness, nausea, headache and paresthesias. Symptoms are related to incidents of known or perceived exposure to environmental chemicals, although the relationship of chemical to symptom is neither specific nor constant, and the connection is frequently made in retrospect (Terr, 1989). The environmental triggers may be specified chemicals such as formaldehyde, phenol, ethanol or ammonia, but usually they are familiar items of everyday occurrence, often identified as having a 'chemical odor'. New carpets, automobile exhaust fumes, perfume, pesticides, paints, solvents and household cleaners are cited frequently. Symptoms are also triggered by the ingestion of foods (Rea, 1978; Jewett et al., 1990), food additives, drugs, natural gas, *Candida albicans* (Crook, 1983), viruses, electromagnetic fields and even endogenous compounds, such as progesterone, histamine and serotonin.

Some patients report that their illness began with a specific exposure, in some cases occupational, to a certain chemical followed by reactions to numerous unrelated chemicals (Ashford & Miller, 1991; Cullen et al., 1992; Terr, 1989).

MCS is subjective with respect to both the complaints and their presumptive triggers. Physical examinations typically reveal no objective findings that can explain the patient's subjective complaints. Extensive laboratory testing is frequently used in an effort to identify a pathognomonic finding, but without success to date. No gross or microscopic pathology has been reported. There are no long-term prospective studies on the course, prognosis or outcome of MCS.

Epidemiology

No studies to date have been carried out to assess the prevalence of patients with the diagnosis of MCS in any community. The subjective nature of the condition makes case finding for epidemiological evaluation difficult if not impossible.

Economic costs

There are no published data on the economic costs of MCS, but they are undoubtedly staggering. Laboratory tests utilized currently by proponents of MCS, particularly quantitative measurements of lymphocyte subsets in the blood, panels of the levels of xenobiotic chemicals and nutrients in various body fluids, and brain single proton emission computerized tomography (SPECT) of the brain may cost the patient thousands of dollars. The recommended treatment generally involves little if any expense for drugs, but the prescribed environmental chemical avoidance program frequently entails prolonged, if not lifelong, work disability with its attendant loss of income to the patient and family.

The author is aware of hundreds of lawsuits in which one or more plaintiffs claim personal injury caused by the infliction of MCS by a variety of defendants, especially chemical manufacturers, pesticide applicators, industries and communities using chemical waste sites, and many others. As many as 5000 plaintiffs have been named in a single suit, damages claimed often reaching hundreds of millions of dollars. The cost of litigating even a single case is likely to be tens, if not hundreds, of thousands of dollars, even if the case is settled without a trial. Thus the MCS phenomenon today has an enormous impact on society in terms of both financial resources and loss of personal productivity.

Confirmations

In a series of case reports published in abstract form in the 1950s, Randolph introduced the concept of MCS, initially called cerebral allergy (Randolph, 1954*a*) and later named the specific adaptation syndrome (Randolph, 1956). He enumerated the environmental triggers (solvents, fuels, pesticides, exhaust fumes, gas and oil fumes, drugs, cosmetics, combustion products, foods and food additives), described the numerous symptoms, recommended 'neutralization' treatment with sodium bicarbonate (Randolph, 1954*b*), and suggested that psychiatric disease was in fact caused by environmental chemicals (Randolph, 1959). He later published several books on the subject and founded the field of clinical ecology (Randolph, 1962; Randolph & Moss, 1980). He and others (Willoughby, 1965; Lee et al., 1969; Morris, 1969) recommended provocation-neutralization testing.

Clinical descriptions of MCS have appeared subsequently in several texts (Dickey, 1976; Ashford & Miller, 1991; Rea, 1992). These anecdotal reports generally agree well with those originally provided by Randolph.

Claims that blood levels of immunoglobulins, complement components and lymphocyte subsets are abnormal are based on selected cases (Rea, 1977, 1978; McGovern et al., 1983*a*), although the published abnormalities are minimal and inconsistent (Terr, 1987). Many MCS proponents today measure blood, urine and fat tissue levels of environmental and natural chemicals, although there are no published data to evaluate these test results.

The claim that MCS is caused and exacerbated by endogenous hormones (especially progesterone), electromagnetic radiation, viruses, fungi, yeast (especially *Candida albicans*) and foods has no published confirmation.

Treatment by environmental chemical avoidance, elimination diets, rotational diets, neutralization therapy by injected or sublingual chemicals or oral administration of salts, immune system modulation, antifungal drugs, and vitamin and mineral supplements have been described and recommended on theoretical grounds (Crook, 1983; Ashford & Miller, 1991; Rea, 1992), but at this time none of these forms of treatment has yet been subjected to controlled clinical trials (Sparks, 1994*b*).

Contradictions

The basis for the diagnosis of MCS (or its various synonyms) has been examined by a number of investigators and found to be arbitrary and predicated solely on the fact or perception by the patient that a harmful environmental exposure had occurred and was responsible for subsequent symptoms (Terr, 1986, 1989; Brodsky, 1987; Grammer et al., 1990; Sparks et al., 1990; Selner & Staudenmayer, 1992; Simon et al., 1993; Staudenmayer et al., 1993*a*). The wide range of symptoms, the enormous variety of reported exposure items and the unlimited time span between exposure and symptoms raises fundamental doubt that a single pathophysiological process could be responsible, especially in the absence of any objective physical or laboratory abnormality or pathology. The clinical pattern of symptomatology was found by some investigators to be most consistent with a somatization process, while others uncovered objective evidence by standardized psychological testing for significant pre-existing and comorbid psychopathology. This is discussed more fully below.

Placebo-controlled blinded testing both by sublingual administration of food extracts (Jewett et al., 1990) and environmental booth challenges with chemicals (Selner & Staudenmayer, 1985; Staudenmayer et al., 1993*a*) have shown that responses by MCS patients are not reproducible when the patient is unaware of the nature of the challenge substance, demonstrating the importance of suggestion in this condition (Ferguson, 1990).

The anecdotal reports of immunological abnormalities in MCS have been discovered to be unfounded when immunological testing has been repeated in unselected series of patients with proper controls (Terr, 1986; Patterson et al., 1985; Simon et al., 1993).

Pathogenetic hypotheses

Theories of the etiology and pathogenesis of MCS are numerous and frequently change. They encompass physical, psychological and social concepts. They periodically change and each is controversial because scientifically rigorous experimental or clinical research is problematic owing to the subjective nature of the illness and lack of a precise definition.

Failure of adaptation theory

When originally proposed, the condition was viewed as a failure of evolutionary adaptation to the synthetic chemicals of Western industrialization (Randolph, 1956). The patient's symptoms were viewed as a newly discovered form of allergy to environmental chemicals. The increasing disability of these patients from an expanding number of environmental triggers was named 'spreading phenomenon', a term with no physiological explanation. The theory has never been tested, and it is inconsistent with current immunological knowledge.

Allergic theory

The presumptive allergy to environmental chemicals and foods was predicated on both IgE and IgG antibody-mediated models of symptom pathogenesis (Rea, 1978; McGovern et al., 1983*a*). There is no evidence of an immune-generated inflammatory response in these patients.

Autoimmune theory

An autoimmune theory based on either molecular mimicry (Rea, 1977) or toxic induction of immune dysregulation (Levin & Byers, 1987) does not fit a purely subjective condition without tissue pathology. Low autoantibody levels reported occasionally in MCS patients occur also in normal individuals.

Immunotoxic theory

Toxic immune dysregulation by environmental chemicals causing autoimmunity or immunodeficiency has been a prevalent concept among proponents of MCS (Bell, 1982; Levin & Byers, 1987). Presumably this would be expressed as adverse reactions to chemicals, foods and drugs. Support consists only of serum immunoglobulin and complement levels in selected cases (Rea, 1976, 1977, 1978; McGovern et al., 1983*b*), but even these are at best marginally abnormal. Other investigators find no consistent immunological abnormalities (Terr, 1986; Simon et al., 1993), and clinically MCS bears no resemblance to any recognized immunological disease.

It is unlikely that the diverse chemicals typically cited as causing MCS would have the same potential for immunotoxicity, especially as the healthy population overwhelmingly tolerates these everyday items without suffering disease.

Neurotoxic theory

A recent theory postulates that MCS is caused by chemical odor-induced olfactory nerve stimulation of the limbic system and hypothalamus resulting in autonomic nervous system activity. Disease progression is explained by 'limbic kindling', reminiscent of the 'spreading phenomenon' (Bell et al., 1992, 1996; Miller, 1992). To date there is no experimental proof of this theory.

Sociogenic theories

The theory that MCS is a belief system expressing an unfounded fear of chemicals and distrust of the conventional medical care system is based on patient interviews. The belief is strengthened by media reporting of environmental pollution and by a strong group dynamic among patients with this disorder that has been called a 'medical subculture' (Brodsky, 1983*a*).

Conditioned response theory

A theory that MCS is a behavioral conditioned response proposes that an initiating unpleasant or strong odor conditions the person to later responses to the same or different chemical exposures at lower doses (Shusterman et al., 1988). Even the perception of exposure can result in a conditioned response of behavioral, cognitive and somatic symptoms. There is no direct experimental proof of this theory to date.

Psychogenic theories

A high prevalence of current and past depression, anxiety, somatization, conversion, obsessive-compulsive and panic disorders have been found in MCS patients (Brodsky, 1983*b*; Stewart & Raskin, 1985; Black et al., 1990; Selner & Staudenmayer, 1992; Simon et al., 1993). The patients typically reject any suggestion that they are psychiatrically ill. The psychiatric model of MCS proposes that attributing illness to the environment is less threatening to the patient than is the need to face unpleasant internal conflicts and stresses. One study of an occupational epidemic of MCS supports this theory. A group of workers had transient irritation from phenol-formaldehyde fumes. Those with a pre-existing tendency to somatization later developed MCS, whereas those without such a history did not (Sparks et al., 1990).

The symptom complex of MCS has been compared to somatoform illness, panic disorder (Dager, 1987), mass hysteria and atypical post-traumatic stress disorder (Schottenfeld & Cullen, 1985). The condition has also been characterized as an adult manifestation of prior childhood abuse (Staudenmayer et al., 1993*b*). Several investigators have observed a high prevalence of several different psychiatric diagnoses among patient with MCS (Black et al., 1990). Clinical ecologists often recognize the presence of psychopathology in their patients, but they view this as the result and not the cause of the illness (Randolph, 1959).

Other theories

MCS has been ascribed to the effects of oxidative damage by environmental chemicals to unspecified tissues (Levine & Reinhart, 1983), a newly described form of hereditary coproporphyria (Hahn & Bonkovsky, 1997), and an overly sensitive state of the respiratory (Bascom, 1992) or nasal (Meggs & Cleveland, 1993) mucosa. There are no clinical or experimental data supporting any of these views.

Diagnostic and treatment approaches

Diagnosis

Many testing procedures have been recommended for MCS, but self-diagnosis satisfies the disease definition.

History

The diagnosis of MCS is usually made from the patient's history of subjective experiences as reported to the examining physician or by a standardized questionnaire that emphasizes common everyday environmental exposures.

Physical examination

Both proponents and critics agree that physical findings are absent in MCS.

Provocation testing

Provocation-neutralization is a procedure advocated by some physicians to document specific chemical sensitivities. The patient is given small amounts of highly diluted chemicals in solution to provoke symptoms, followed by further challenges to clear the symptoms ('neutralization'). Challenges are by intradermal or subcutaneous injections or by sublingual drops (Lee et al., 1969). The testing is performed without controls, and it has not been standardized (Grieco, 1982).

Laboratory tests

Measurements of the blood levels of immunoglobulins, complement components, immune complexes, autoantibodies and lymphocyte subsets have all been claimed to be useful in diagnosis. Some reports favor quantitative measurements of pesticides, organic solvents, amino acids, vitamins, minerals and other chemicals in the blood and other body fluids to confirm the diagnosis. Antibodies to certain chemicals such as formaldehyde and acid anhydrides are recommended, even in cases without known exposure to these chemicals.

Treatment

Many potential treatment modalities have been recommended, each based on one or more theories of MCS pathogenesis.

Environmental chemical avoidance

This is the mainstay of treatment recommended by physicians who diagnose MCS as a toxic or allergic disease. The list of products to avoid usually includes pesticides, solvents, perfumes, all scented products, exhaust fumes from cars and trucks, synthetic clothing, plastics, medications and any other item suspected to cause symptoms. Continued symptoms lead to more restrictions. In extreme cases the patient may be advised to exist virtually 'in a bubble'. Work disability is common.

Avoiding electromagnetic radiation and the removal of dental amalgams is sometimes advised.

No scientifically valid study of environmental avoidance therapy to show efficacy has yet been undertaken. On the contrary, there are many anecdotal reports of serious iatrogenic disability resulting from extreme 'chemical' restrictions (Terr, 1986).

Detoxification

Reducing the so-called 'body burden' of foreign chemicals is recommended in a rigid program of saunas, exercise, induced sweating, induced flushing with niacin and 'mobilization' of toxins from fat by administration of fatty acids (Root et al., 1985). There are no reliable data to show that toxins are removed by this method, or that it is safe.

Elimination diets

Elimination of specific food items such as sugar, wheat, corn, red meats and all additives is usually recommended, whether or not the patient has experienced any adverse effects from them. A rotary diet is commonly followed by MCS patients so that the same food is not eaten more often than once every four or five days.

None of these dietary recommendations for management of MCS is supported by proper clinical trials to establish efficacy and safety.

Neutralization therapy

Neutralization is a therapeutic extension of the diagnostic provocation-neutralization (Kailin & Collier, 1971). Sublingual drops or injections of extracts of foods or chemicals are self-administered prior to anticipated exposure, following exposure, during symptomatic experiences or on an ongoing routine basis. There have been no clinical trials to document efficacy and safety of neutralization therapy.

Anti-yeast medications

Physicians who subscribe to the theory of multisystem disease caused by a toxin from *Candida albicans* prescribe nystatin and/or ketoconazole and its congeners, along with a diet free from sugar and yeast.

Antifungal medications

A few practitioners diagnose 'mold allergy' as one cause of MCS, based not on evidence of allergy to mold spores, but rather on a theory that all molds from the air and in food can exacerbate MCS. Antifungal drugs such as amphotericin B may then be prescribed.

Vitamins, minerals and diet supplements

Multiple vitamin and mineral supplements, amino acids and antioxidants are frequently prescribed for a presumed but undocumented immune-enhancing effect.

Immune system stimulants

As a result of the persisting theory of MCS as an immune disorder, some clinicians have recommended intravenous gammaglobulin therapy for its presumed immunomodulatory effect, but to date there are no clinical trials showing benefit in MCS.

Psychotherapy

Psychopharmacology in MCS treatment is frequently recommended, although without specific data on results. Some practitioners justify their use in these patients by informing them that they are 'immune-modifying' drugs, although there is no evidence that such an action occurs clinically in this group of patients.

A strong patient–physician supportive relationship in the usual ambulatory setting where these patients are ordinarily seen by physicians is consistent with good medical practice and is especially recommended for MCS. Psychotherapy might be considered in certain individual cases.

Behavior modification

Intervention at the symptomatic phase of the patient's experience without altering the exposure is the antithesis of environmental avoidance therapy. The relationship of the environmental exposure to symptom production is viewed as an undesirable behavior pattern causing disability through unnecessary avoidances. The aim of behavior modification is symptomatic tolerance accomplished by a series of graded, controlled exposures to achieve behavioral tolerance ('desensitization'). It is labor intensive, time consuming and dependent upon the skill of a trained professional. A variety of methods appropriate to the symptomatology have been used, e.g. visualizations, breathing exercises and various forms of relaxation techniques. To date, success in MCS is limited to a few anecdotal reports.

Short-term inpatient supportive therapy

In an effort to address functional disabilities, a small number of patients were treated with brief inpatient non-judgmental supportive therapy to reduce anxiety and enhance the patient's ability to cope with the effects of illness. The result was temporarily successful, but within weeks following discharge, significant symptom exacerbation occurred (Haller, 1993).

Other treatment recommendations

A regular program of physical exercise, biofeedback and even massage and prayer have been mentioned as worthy of consideration. No information exists to analyze any of them for effectiveness.

Multiple treatment modalities

An eclectic counseling approach has been recommended with initial diet modification and environmental changes. If the patient sees that these modalities are ineffective, stress is explained as a possible cause of symptoms, and the patient is counseled in self-help with physician support. Those patients who continue to list environmental chemicals and foods as the primary stressors are considered treatment failures (Jewett, 1992).

Conclusion

The concept of an illness called MCS is currently popular among a small group of physicians who believe that exposure to low levels of numerous environmental chemicals can cause a disease with numerous symptoms but no objective physical or laboratory abnormalities. The condition has been known by many names, but it lacks a clear definition. Numerous theories have been offered to explain the condition. These encompass immunotoxic, allergic, autoimmune, neurotoxic, cytotoxic, metabolic, behavioral, psychiatric, iatrogenic and sociological mechanisms.

MCS has many features in common with other controversial syndromes such as the chronic fatigue syndrome. Patients with the diagnosis of MCS are frequently subjected to unproven and unnecessary diagnostic tests and untested therapeutic modalities. In spite of the lack of physical illness and the absence of pathology, patients often experience extreme disability because their symptoms are triggered by common environmental exposures. The phenomenon known as MCS needs to be evaluated critically by scientifically sound methods.

References

Ashford NA, Miller CS (1991). *Chemical Exposures: Low Levels and High Stakes.* New York: Van Nostrand Reinhold.

Bascom R (1992). Multiple chemical sensitivity: a respiratory disorder? *Toxicology and Industrial Health*, **8**, 221–8.

Beard GM (1881). *American Nervousness, its Causes and Consequences: a Supplement to Nervous Exhaustion (Neurasthenia).* New York: GP Putnam.

Bell IR (1982). *Clinical Ecology: a New Medical Approach to Environmental Illness.* Bolinas, CA: Common Knowledge Press.

Bell IR, Miller CS & Schwartz GE (1992). An olfactory-limbic model of multiple chemical sensitivity syndrome: possible relationships to kindling and affective spectrum disorders. *Biological Psychiatry*, **32**, 218–42.

Bell IR, Bootzin RR, Davis TP, Hau V, Ritenbaugh C, Johnson KA & Schwartz GE (1996). Time-dependent sensitization of plasma beta-endorphin in community elderly with self-reported environmental chemical odor intolerance. *Biological Psychiatry*, **40**, 134–43.

Black DW, Rathe A & Goldstein RB (1990). Environmental illness. A controlled study of 26 subjects with '20th century disease'. *Journal of the American Medical Association*, **264**, 3166–70.

Brodsky CM (1983*a*). Allergic to everything; a medical subculture. *Psychosomatics*, **24**, 731–42.

Brodsky CM (1983*b*). Psychological factors contributing to somatoform diseases attributed to the workplace: the case of intoxication. *Journal of Occupational Medicine*, **25**, 459.

Brodsky CM (1987). Multiple chemical sensitivities and other 'environmental illness'; a psychiatrist's view. *Occupational Medicine: State of the Art Reviews*, **2**, 695–704.

Crook WG (1983). *The Yeast Connection: A Medical Breakthrough.* Jackson, TN: Professional Books.

Cullen MR (ed.) (1987). The worker with multiple chemical sensitivities: an overview. *Occupational Medicine: State of the Art Reviews*, **2**, 655–61.

Cullen MR, Pace PE & Redlich CA (1992). The experience of the Yale Occupational and Environmental Medicine Clinics with multiple chemical sensitivities, 1986–1991. *Toxicology and Industrial Health*, **8**, 15–19.

Dager SR, Holland JP & Cowley DS (1987). Panic disorder precipitated by exposure to organic solvents in the workplace. *American Journal of Psychiatry*, **144**, 1056–8.

Dickey LD (ed.) (1976). *Clinical Ecology*. Springfield, IL: Charles C. Thomas.

Ferguson A (1990). Food sensitivity or self-deception? *New England Journal of Medicine*, **323**, 476–8.

Grammer LC, Harris KE, Shaughnessy MA, Sparks PJ, Ayars GH & Altman LC (1990). Clinical and immunological evaluation of 37 workers exposed to gaseous formaldehyde. *Journal of Allergy and Clinical Immunology*, **86**, 177–81.

Grieco MH (1982). Controversial practices in allergy. *Journal of the American Medical Association*, **247**, 3106–11.

Hahn M & Bonkovsky HL (1997). Multiple chemical sensitivity syndrome and porphyria. *Archives of Internal Medicine*, **157**, 281–5.

Haller E (1993). Successful management of patients with 'multiple chemical sensitivities' on an inpatient psychiatric unit. *Journal of Clinical Psychiatry*, **54**, 196–9.

Jewett DL (1992). Diagnosis and treatment of hypersensitivity syndrome. *Toxicology and Industrial Health*, **8**, 111–23.

Jewett DL, Fein G & Greenberg MH (1990). A double-blind study of symptom provocation to determine food sensitivity. *New England Journal of Medicine*, **323**, 429–33.

Kailin EW & Collier R (1971). 'Relieving' therapy for antigen exposure. *Journal of the American Medical Association*, **217**, 78.

Lee CH, Williams RT & Binkley EL (1969). Provocative testing and treatment for foods. *Archives of Otolaryngology*, **90**, 87–94.

Levin AS & Byers VS (1987). Environmental illness: a disorder of immune regulation. *Occupational Medicine State of the Art Reviews*, **2**, 669–82.

Levine SA & Reinhart JH (1983). Biochemical pathology initiated by free radicals, oxidant chemicals and therapeutic drugs in the etiology of chemical hypersensitivity disease. *Journal of Orthomolecular Psychiatry*, **12**, 166–83.

McGovern JJ, Lazaroni JA, Hicks MF, Adler CJ & Cleary P (1983*a*). Food and chemical sensitivity: clinical and immunologic correlates. *Archives of Otolaryngology*, **109**, 292–7.

McGovern JJ, Lazaroni JA & Saifer P (1983*b*). Clinical evaluation of the major plasma and cellular measures of immunity. *Orthomolecular Psychiatry*, **12**, 60.

Meggs WJ & Cleveland CH Jr (1993). Rhinolaryngoscopic examination of patients with the multiple chemical sensitivity syndrome. *Archives of Environmental Health*, **48**, 14–18.

Miller CS (1992). Possible models for multiple chemical sensitivity: conceptual issues and role of the limbic system. *Toxicology and Industrial Health*, **8**, 181–202.

Morris DL (1969). Use of sublingual antigen in diagnosis and treatment of food allergy. *Annals of Allergy*, **27**, 289–94.

Patterson R, Beltrani VS, Singal M & Gorman RW (1985). Creating an indoor environmental problem from a nonproblem: a need for cautious evaluation of antibodies against hapten-protein complexes. *New England Regional Allergy Proceedings*, **6**, 135–9.

Randolph TG (1954*a*). Sensory aspects of cerebral allergy. *Journal of Laboratory and Clinical Medicine*, **44**, 910.

Randolph TG (1954*b*). Sodium bicarbonate in the treatment of allergic conditions. *Journal of Laboratory and Clinical Medicine*, **44**, 915.

Randolph TG (1956). The specific adaptation syndrome. *Journal of Laboratory and Clinical Medicine*, **48**, 934.

Randolph TG (1959). Ecologic mental illness – psychiatry externalized. *Journal of Laboratory and Clinical Medicine*, **54**, 936.

Randolph TG (1962). *Human Ecology and Susceptibility to the Chemical Environment*. Springfield, IL: Charles C. Thomas.

Randolph TG & Moss RW (1980). *An Alternative Approach to Allergies*. New York: Lippincott and Crowell.

Rea WJ (1976). Environmentally triggered thrombophlebitis. *Annals of Allergy*, **37**, 101–9.

Rea WJ (1977). Environmentally triggered small vessel vasculitis. *Annals of Allergy*, **38**, 245–51.

Rea WJ (1978). Environmentally triggered cardiac disease. *Annals of Allergy*, **40**, 243–51.

Rea WJ (1992). Considerations for the diagnosis of chemical sensitivity. In *Biologic Markers in Immunotoxicology*, ed. D. W. Talmage. Washington DC: National Academy Press.

Root DE, Katzin DB & Schnare DW (1985). Diagnosis and treatment of patients presenting subclinical signs and symptoms of exposure to chemicals which bioaccumulate in human tissue. *Proceedings of the National Conference on Hazardous Wastes and Environmental Emergencies*, May 14–16, pp. 150–3.

Schottenfeld RS & Cullen MR (1985). Occupation-induced posttraumatic stress disorder. *American Journal of Psychiatry*, **142**, 198–202.

Selner JC & Staudenmayer H (1985). The practical approach to the evaluation of suspected environmental exposures: chemical intolerance. *Annals of Allergy*, **55**, 665–73.

Selner JC & Staudenmayer H (1992). Neuropsychophysiologic observations in patients presenting with environmental illness. *Toxicology and Industrial Health*, **8**, 145–55.

Shusterman D, Balmes J & Cone J (1988). Behavioral sensitization to irritants/odorants after acute exposure. *Journal of Occupational Medicine*, **30**, 565–7.

Simon GE, Daniell W, Stockbridge H, Claypoole K & Rosenstock L (1993). Immunologic, psychological and neuropsychological factors in multiple chemical sensitivity. A controlled study. *Annals of Internal Medicine*, **119**, 97–103.

Sparks PJ, Simon GE, Katon WJ, Ayars GH & Johnson RL (1990). An outbreak of illness among aerospace workers. *Western Journal of Medicine*, **153**, 28–33.

Sparks PJ, Daniell W, Black DW, Kipen HM, Altman LC, Simon GE & Terr AI (1994*a*). Multiple chemical sensitivity syndrome: a clinical perspective. I. Case definition, theories of pathogenesis and research needs. *Journal of Occupational Medicine*, **36**, 718–30.

Sparks PJ, Daniell W, Black DW, Kipen HM, Altman LC, Simon GE & Terr AI (1994*b*). Multiple chemical sensitivity syndrome: a clinical perspective. II.

Evaluation, diagnostic testing, treatment and social considerations. *Journal of Occupational Medicine*, **36**, 731–7.
Staudenmayer H, Selner JC & Buhr MP (1993*a*). Double-blind provocation chamber challenges in 20 patients presenting with multiple chemical sensitivity. *Regulatory Toxicology and Pharmacology*, **18**, 44–53.
Staudenmayer H, Selner ME & Selner J (1993*b*). Adult sequelae of childhood abuse presenting as environmental illness. *Annals of Allergy*, **71**, 538–46.
Stewart DE & Raskin J (1985). Psychiatric assessment of patients with '20th-century disease' ('total allergy syndrome'). *Canadian Medical Association Journal*, **133**, 1001–6.
Terr AI (1986). Environmental illness. A clinical review of 50 cases. *Archives of Internal Medicine*, **146**, 145–9.
Terr AI (1987). 'Multiple chemical sensitivities': immunologic critique of clinical ecology theories and practice. *Occupational Medicine State of the Art Reviews*, **2**, 683–94.
Terr AI (1989). Clinical ecology in the workplace. *Journal of Occupational Medicine*, **31**, 257–61.
UNEP-ILO-WHO (1996). Conclusions and recommendations of a workshop on 'multiple chemical sensitivities' (MCS). *Regulatory Toxicology and Pharmacology*, **24**, S188–S189.
Willoughby JW (1965). Provocative food test technique. *Annals of Allergy*, **23**, 543–54.

11

Psychopharmacology of Functional Somatic Syndromes

ARTHUR RIFKIN

The psychopharmocologist may assist the primary physician in treating some disorders that seem to stand between physical and mental conditions, such as fibromyalgia, chronic fatigue syndrome, migraine, irritable bowel syndrome, atypical facial pain and premenstrual dysphoric disorder. All of these conditions have shown some responsiveness to psychotropic drugs, as reviewed elsewhere in this volume. Our purpose here is to help the primary physician to use psychotropic drugs.

As with all treatments, the primary physician has to decide when to treat the patient, when to get a consultation and when to refer the patient to a consultant to provide ongoing care. First, let us define the various professionals in the field. A psychiatrist has medical training with additional training in the diagnosis and treatment of mental disorders. Psychiatry covers a vast field and no practitioner masters all aspects. The bedrock expertise of any psychiatrist is the diagnosis of mental disorders. Psychiatrists differ in their expertise in using different treatments.

Nonpsychiatrists often think that psychiatric diagnoses use vague, inexact criteria to diagnose vague, inexact disorders. This untruth comes, we believe, from a misunderstanding of the nature of evidence used to validate disorders. Those trained in medicine have generally learned to appreciate the value of 'hard' findings, i.e., those quantifiable through laboratory machinery or directly observable from imaging studies. Physicians accustomed to directly visualizing the heart or the gastrointestinal tract, for example, might consider psychiatric diagnoses 'soft' because they rely on the history and mental status to make diagnoses, without technology.

The physician himself is the only measuring instrument to detect most mental disorders. No laboratory test or imaging study provides much help, except to rule out medical disorders that mimic psychiatric disorders, or to detect the etiology of brain disorders that produce dementia or delirium.

If we know that the etiology of mental symptoms has a clear physical origin, such as hypothyroidism causing depression, or hypoglycemia causing anxiety and dizziness, the patient usually receives treatment most appropriately from a nonpsychiatric physician. The most common psychiatric disorders, such as mood and anxiety disorders, psychoactive substance abuse and syndromes of abnormal mood and anxiety that may accompany other medical disorders, depend for their diagnosis on the psychiatric interview, which consists in taking a history, inquiring about feelings and thoughts, and observing behavior. The assessment of what another person feels comes not only from what he/she says he/she feels (many people poorly report their feelings), but from the examiner's intuitive empathy.

From a laboratory test or imaging study to an intuitive empathic judgment seems, on the surface, to illustrate a slide from exact to inexact assessment. This common belief does not withstand close scrutiny. Diagnosis in medicine derives its validity from its usefulness. We can measure countless mental and physical features of a person, but most will not help us in doing what the physician must do: predict the cause of what bothers the patient, predict its course and predict its response to treatment. The value of the examination devolves ultimately to its aide in making these predictions. A diagnostic tool helps to the extent that it improves prediction. It matters not if the diagnostic tool is a laboratory test, an image or an intuitive feeling about what the patient feels. The most exact measurement of some bodily function may provide no useful information for diagnosis; the most subjective feeling the physician has may enable him or her to make the best predictive statement.

Too often the nonpsychiatric physician will try to diagnose a psychiatric disorder by eliminating medical disorders that might explain the symptoms. The patient with palpitations, chest pain, dyspnea and diaphoresis often has panic disorder, which the primary physician should diagnose by obtaining the specific symptoms of panic disorder, not just from ruling out cardiac or pulmonary disorders. The predictive value of correctly diagnosing panic disorder provides just as accurate and important information as diagnosing myocardial infarction or an arrhythmia that requires technical data.

The morbidity of some psychiatric disorders equals or surpasses that of many common medical disorders, and the success of treating these psychiatric disorders, likewise, equals or surpasses the efficacy of treating most common medical disorders. Psychiatric disorders do suffer a distinct disadvantage to many medical disorders: etiology remains unknown. Despite much effort to prove psychological or physiological etiologies, no effort has succeeded. This ignorance, however, does not detract from the usefulness of accurately diagnosing and treating psychiatric disorders. Without knowing the etiology of major depression, for example, treatment, nevertheless, usually succeeds. The history of medicine has many examples of successfully diagnosed and treated disorders in the absence of understanding the etiology.

The assessment of psychiatric symptoms does not require esoteric knowledge or procedures. Although some psychiatrists (and other mental health professionals) may use theories about unconscious conflicts or primal screams, and many other theories, the accepted diagnosis of psychiatric disorders depends on largely atheoretical descriptions of symptoms. To diagnose major depression, for example, we need not subscribe to any theory, whether psychoanalytical, cognitive, behavioral, etc., and drug treatment of major depression requires no adherence to a particular physiological theory of etiology.

The primary physician, in treating the disorders which this volume considers, should look with particular care for concomitant psychiatric symptoms and disorders. As the etiology and treatment of functional psychosomatic disorders remain unsatisfactory, we must not miss any psychiatric disorder for which we have good, proven treatments. Even if a clear psychiatric disorder does not seem present, some psychiatric symptoms usually occur and should concern the physician. Whether or not psychiatric symptoms occur, treatment with psychotropic drugs may help to alleviate symptoms.

Primary physicians vary in their abilities to diagnose and treat psychiatric disorders or psychiatric symptoms associated with other disorders. The decision when to refer a patient for psychiatric evaluation depends on this degree of psychiatric competence. The diagnosis and initial treatment of most common psychiatric disorders lies within the competence of any primary physician who takes the trouble to become familiar with the techniques of psychiatric interviewing and drug treatment. The primary physician should consider referral to a psychiatrist if the diagnosis seems unclear or if the initial drug treatment has failed.

Some psychiatrists focus on drug treatment and are called 'psychopharmacologists', which has no official status, unlike recognized subspecialties of child and adolescent psychiatry and geriatric psychiatry. The primary physician should expect from a psychiatric consultation a diagnostic assessment and recommendations about drug treatment. Whether the primary physician wishes to administer the drug treatment, with guidance from the psychiatrist, depends on his or her interest and knowledge. As with all areas of medicine, the subject matter contains enormous complexity and the physician choosing to focus on a narrow area acquires more experience in that area, but also loses something – familiarity with other areas and a lack of experience in treating the patient for a spectrum of disorders.

General principles of psychotropic drug treatment

Have a clear idea of the symptoms expected to change. This may include a full diagnostic entity, such as major depression or panic disorder, or psychiatric symptoms, such as anxiety associated with other disorders.

Plan a clear strategy and follow it, unless significant changes in symptoms or side-effects occur. Patients generally follow the lead of their physicians in what to expect from drug treatment, and what side-effects to tolerate. Patients placed in large, uncomfortable casts for a hip fracture do not usually refuse to continue such treatment because of side-effects, neither do patients receiving drugs for cancer despite, often, many uncomfortable side-effects. Yet, many patients refuse to tolerate even modest side-effects of psychotropic drugs in the mistaken belief that these drugs should work rapidly and without adverse reactions. When their physicians support this view, explicitly or tacitly, patients often stop the drug prematurely, lower the dose or refuse to raise it to therapeutic levels.

Given the serious dysphoria and disability from psychiatric symptoms, it serves the patient well to accept the mild to moderate side-effects of treatment. Many such side-effects remit with continued treatment, and most are far less bothersome than the disorder they may eventually relieve. The alternative approach leads to frequent changes of drugs and poor results from not receiving a drug treatment long enough at an optimal dose.

Most psychotropic drugs have a latency period of weeks before they show optimal results, and it may take weeks to gradually raise the dose to optimal levels. Ending the trial before that point not only prevents a probable remission, but it means the patient has endured the side-effects of the latency period for naught; a probable effective drug has falsely received the label of ineffective.

Education is the best way to get the patient to accept the delay of response and side-effects. Before beginning the trial, explain the latency, warn him or her of possible side-effects (without going through every possible but unlikely one, as the package insert does), and demonstrate by your equanimity that these side-effects do not indicate a serious concern. Sometimes, symptomatic treatment helps bothersome side-effects, such as bethanechol for dry mouth and other anticholinergic side-effects, and laxatives for constipation. Overconcern for the patient's nonserious side-effects that results in an inadequate dose or duration of a trial hardly benefits the patient.

Of course, some side-effects deserve more serious concern because of their severity or danger, and require reducing dosage or stopping the agent. Interactions with other drugs causes an ever-increasing complexity in using psychotropic drugs. Obtain a complete list of all drugs that the patient takes, and assure yourself that they do not interact. If they do, choose a different drug, or monitor carefully for symptoms of a significant interaction. Many interactions do not require complete avoidance of the two drugs, but merely careful monitoring. For example, some diuretics, such as thiazides, may decrease lithium clearance and require a reduction in the dose of lithium. Many drugs do not interact but cause additive side-effects, especially sedation.

Never stop diagnosing. Diagnosis requires constant assessment, and when necessary, revision. A drug may not work because of an incorrect diagnosis. As you get to know your patient better you may learn significant information, such as psychoactive substance abuse, or that the seemingly pervasive sad mood, with marked loss of interest, seems less so, especially when you seek confirmation from spouses and other informants.

Involve spouses and family members, or anyone else close to the patient, as much as is feasible. Contrary to common belief, most patients want these people to participate in their treatment. Often they feel, correctly or not, that these people think they do not have a real problem, that they even fake symptoms and they could get better if they just tried harder. Participating in treatment enables family members to lose these incorrect ideas, it provides a sense of a joint effort that decreases the patient's feeling of isolation, and it offers the physician an excellent source of information. At times the patient requests, openly or not, more privacy to relate information he or she has good reason to keep from the family. We should respect that.

If you use a psychiatric consultant, ask his or her advice about ongoing treatment. A one-shot consultation has less than perfect accuracy. Follow-up information improves this accuracy and helps you to refine your strategy.

Avoid a hostile relationship with the patient. Under the best of circumstances, treating these patients poses difficulties. The patient, and perhaps the physician, doubts whether he or she has a 'true' disorder. Symptoms usually remain chronic and require chronic treatment and possibly several courses of treatment to find the optimal one. The patient may turn his or her anger toward the physician. We physicians lack perfect control and understanding. If you find yourself chronically angry at your patient, refer him or her elsewhere; and if he or she expresses chronic anger toward you, suggest he or she changes physicians.

On the other hand, if the anger is not too severe or chronic, try sticking with the patient. Someone else will most likely have the same problem as you and it helps a patient to see that the physician does not run away and can redirect inappropriate anger. We do not treat symptoms but people. We do not dispense drugs through vending machines. Most psychiatric symptoms have a high placebo response (as do most medical conditions) which should temper our certainty that our drug has caused the changes we see, and should encourage us to stimulate hope and acceptance, probably the elements that foster the placebo response.

In the following sections we describe current knowledge about two drug treatment of depression, anxiety, pain and sleep disorders as these psychiatric syndromes often accompany the functional somatic syndromes described in this volume.

Treatment of depression

The many antidepressants available might bewilder the physician trying to choose rationally which ones to use, and in what order. The number available does not mean we understand the pathophysiology of depression and have designed drugs to counter such abnormalities. The first two antidepressants, imipramine and monoamine oxidase inhibitors (MAOIs), appeared on the basis of perspicacious serendipity. Imipramine has a similar structure to chlorpromazine. Its developers, in the late 1950s, hoped it would help schizophrenia. It turned out to not help schizophrenia but unexpectedly to work well against depression.

MAOIs came from the antitubercular drug iproniazid that appeared to alleviate depression in patients with tuberculosis. It proved too toxic for further use, but evidence suggested that other inhibitors of MAO could help depression. All further antidepressants came from studies on the observed behaviors in animals caused by these effective antidepressants and the increasing knowledge of their pharmacological properties, which mainly involved varying mechanisms of increasing the available norepinephrine and/or serotonin.

Tricyclic agents

These drugs (imipramine, amitriptyline, nortriptyline, desipramine, trimipramine, clomipramine, protriptyline), and later similar compounds (amoxapine, doxepin and maprotiline), share the same side-effects, with some differences of degree. All subsequent antidepressants have equal efficacy. That all antidepressants seem equally effective may stem from the fact that we can find new antidepressants only by mimicking the older ones. For the most part we cannot match the particular symptoms of depression to a choice of antidepressant, but there are with two exceptions: atypical depression and psychotic depression. 'Typical' depression, officially designated Major Depression in the USA's DSM-IV, consists of a persistent sad mood, loss of interest in usual activities, poor appetite, poor sleep, fatigue, excessive guilt, psychomotor retardation and/or agitation, poor concentration and a wish to die, or even commit suicide.

Atypical depression shares the cardinal symptoms of persistent sad mood and loss of interest, but the sad mood often seems in response to an upsetting situation, and the patients tend to oversleep, eat excessively, feel so much fatigue that they may say their limbs feel like lead, and seem particularly sensitive to felt rejection. Atypical depression responds better to MAOIs than to imipramine (Liebowitz et al., 1988). How new antidepressants compare with MAOIs in this regard remains uncertain. Many clinicians report that the selective serotonin reuptake inhibitors (see below) work as well as MAOIs for this disorder, and produce fewer side-effects.

Psychotic depression, i.e., major depression with delusions and/or hallucinations, responds better to a combination of an antidepressant and an antipsychotic than to either drug given separately. These examples of matching clinical syndromes to antidepressant medication might help the physician to choose an antidepressant to use in cases of depression associated with functional psychosomatic disorders.

Tricyclic agents, like all antidepressants, on average begin to work in the first or second week, but do not reach a peak effect until after four to six weeks. A patient may show no response for several weeks and then show a robust response. A recent analysis of many patients treated with an active antidepressant versus placebo shows that we cannot predict who will not respond by the sixth week unless he or she shows no response at all by the fourth week, or only a partial response by the fifth week (Quitkin et al., 1996). We recommend that these results guide physicians in deciding for how long to treat patients with functional psychosomatic disorders, although similar research has not yet been published for such patients.

The optimal dose of a tricyclic agent depends on the specific drug. Nortriptyline has a unique dosing relationship: a curvilinear response according to blood level. The best results occur between 50 and 150 ng/ml. This requires, usually, a dose of 50–125 mg/day, considerably less than the optimal dose for other tricyclic agents (with the exception of protriptyline, a rarely used drug) which require 150–300 mg/day. The most common errors in treating depression consist of trials that are too short and low doses. To minimize side-effects, raise the dose gradually, reaching full dosage by the end of the second or third week.

Tricyclic agents have varied side-effects, most, fortunately, more troublesome than dangerous. The side-effects stem from their varied pharmacological effects. These drugs bind to muscarinic acetylcholine receptors, which cause dry mouth, blurred vision, constipation and urinary hesitancy. Binding to histamine receptors probably causes the sedation and weight gain. Blockade of alpha-adrenergic receptors causes postural hypotension, the most frequent serious side-effect, resulting in, at times, fractures and, perhaps, myocardial infarction. The elderly pose the most serious risk. Of the tricyclic agents, nortriptyline shows the least propensity for causing postural hypotension.

These drugs slow cardiac conduction and prolong the PR and QRS intervals. Roose (1992) found that 9% of 41 depressed patients who had first-degree atrioventricular or bundle brand block (or both) prior to treatment with a tricyclic agent developed two-to-one atrioventricular block, compared with 0.7% of 151 patients who had normal electrocardiographs before treatment. Overdose with a tricyclic agent can cause severe arrhythmias, a serious drawback in using these drugs in suicidal patients.

Selective serotonin reuptake inhibitors (SSRIs)

These antidepressants inhibit the reuptake of serotonin, as do tricyclic agents (to varying extents), but have little effect on the noradrenergic system, histaminic receptors or muscarinic receptors and, therefore, cause side-effects less often. This class of drugs includes fluoxetine, fluvoxamine, paroxetine, sertraline and citalopram. Citalopram is not marketed in the USA and fluvoxamine is marketed in the USA only for obsessive-compulsive disorder. These drugs show equal efficacy to tricyclic agents, with fewer side-effects.

Another advantage over tricyclic agents for the SSRIs comes from the likelihood that the initial dose may be the optimally therapeutic dose, making gradual increases in dose unnecessary. The available data do not prove this conclusively (Rifkin, 1997), and we advise physicians to raise the initial dose of SSRIs for patients who have not responded after three weeks. The initial and maximum doses are: sertraline 50–200 mg/day; fluoxetine 20–80 mg/day; paroxetine 10–50 mg/day; fluvoxamine 50–300 mg/day.

The side-effects of SSRIs probably come from the serotonin agonist effects and consist of headache, dizziness, nausea, diarrhea, constipation, sleepiness (or insomnia), sweating, tremor, dry mouth, anxiety, restlessness and sexual dysfunction (mainly inhibition of ejaculation and orgasm, and erectile difficulties). As the side-effects from SSRIs usually prove less troublesome than those of tricyclic agents, and because the initial dose usually suffices, the SSRIs have replaced tricyclic agents as the most prescribed antidepressants. Concern that fluoxetine increases the risk for suicide and/or violence appears incorrect.

Other antidepressants

Trazodone inhibits serotonin reuptake, blocks the serotonin inhibitory autoreceptor and downregulates norepinephrine receptors (as do most antidepressants). It inhibits serotonin reuptake less than the selective agents already discussed. This drug, and all the others that follow in this section, show equal efficacy to the preceding antidepressants, and differ by the degree and type of side-effects. Trazodone lacks anticholinergic effects, does not cause atrioventricular block and has less toxicity in overdose than any of the tricyclic agents. It causes much sedation (some physicians use it as a hypnotic), does cause postural hypotension and, rarely, causes priapism. The usual therapeutic dose is 200–600 mg/day.

Bupropion does not affect serotonin or noradrenergic neurotransmission at doses commonly employed for the treatment for depressive disorders. We do not know its mechanism of action; it may involve stimulating dopamine receptors. It has a low likelihood of causing sedation, and does not cause anticholinergic side-effects, postural hypotension or arrhythmias. Its side-effects consist of restlessness, tremors, insomnia and nausea. Grand mal seizures occur at a rate of 0.4% at doses up to 450 mg/day, which has caused some concern, but the seizure rate of tricyclic agents is about 0.2%, which means one would have to treat 500 patients with bupropion rather than a tricyclic agent to notice a difference in the rate of seizures (1.0/0.002). The usual therapeutic dose is from 150 to 450 mg/day. We do not know whether the higher doses have greater efficacy. As with other nontricyclic agents, given our ignorance about dose–response relationships, if the initial dose does not work after three weeks, begin to raise the dose.

Venlafaxine inhibits the reuptake of serotonin and norepinephrine and weakly inhibits dopamine reuptake. It affects mainly serotonin, but less so than the SSRIs. Unlike other antidepressants, vanlafaxine induces a rapid downregulation of noradrenergic receptors. It does not affect adrenergic, muscarinic or histaminergic receptors. Its major side-effects are headache, decrease in sexual desire or ability, blurred vision and hypertension. At doses above 300 mg/day 13% of patients show elevated diastolic blood pressure. The initial dose is 75 mg/day, going up to 375 mg/day.

Nefazodone's mechanism of action is not known, but it inhibits neuronal reuptake of serotonin and norepinephrine, antagonizes the 5-HT_2 receptor, and antagonizes the $alpha_1$-adrenergic receptor. It does not affect the $alpha_2$-adrenergic, beta-adrenergic, cholinergic, dopaminergic or benzodiazepine receptors. The most common side-effects of concern are ataxia, blurred vision, postural hypotension, rash and tinnitus. The initial dose is usually 200 mg/day, and 300–600 mg/day is the range of most therapeutic doses.

MAOIs have less usefulness now that newer antidepressants have appeared that, generally, have fewer side-effects but they remain a well-studied class of drugs that show particular efficacy in atypical depression. These drugs inhibit the enzyme that metabolizes serotonin, norepinephrine and dopamine and interact with drugs or foods that increase these precursors of these neurotransmitters especially norepinephrine and dopamine. Of particular concern is interactions with cocaine, other antidepressants, levodopa, meperidine, sympathomimetic agents and foods rich in tyramine, such as cheeses, aged or cured meats, broad (fava) bean pods, yeast extracts, sauerkraut, soy sauce and soy bean condiments and tap beer. Wine and domestic bottled or canned beer are safe in moderation. These foods and drugs may precipitate a hypertensive reaction consisting of severe headache, stiff neck, sweating, diaphoresis and vomiting. Phenelzine and tranylcypromine have similar efficacy and side-effects. Postural hypotension constitutes the most common serious side-effect for which increasing fluid and salt intake often helps. For patients showing an excellent response, not seen with other antidepressants, but have postural hypotension unrelieved by these measure, the physician should consider using a mineralocorticoid such as fluorohydrocortisone, starting at 0.1 mg/day and increasing, if necessary, to 0.8 mg/day.

Moclobemide is a reversible MAOI available in Canada and the UK. Phenelzine and tranylcypromine are irreversible and it requires two weeks after the end of treatment to obtain enough new enzyme, and therefore this is the interval required before adding another antidepressant. Moclobemide only weakly inhibits the B-type of monoamine oxidase, the enzyme that metabolizes tyramine, so it causes only a weak tyramine reaction. In placebo-controlled trials, only nausea occurred significantly more often with moclobemide than with placebo. Of particular interest is that postural hypotension occurred in only 1%

of subjects. The initial dose is usually 300 mg/day, increasing to 600 mg/day if necessary.

Treatment of resistant depression

When a course of treatment with an antidepressant fails, the physician has the choice of switching to a different drug, or augmenting the first one. Two augmentation strategies have support from randomized controlled trials: lithium and triiodothyronine (T3) (Joffe et al., 1993). Response to augmentation occurs within two to three weeks, a shorter interval than occurs when stopping one antidepressant and starting another as the second trial takes up to 6 weeks. Most studies used lithium to blood levels of 0.6–1.0 mEq/l, or T3 to 10–50 κg/day. Lithium has side-effects of nausea, tremors, headache and polyuria. T3 rarely causes side-effects at these doses, but it may cause tachycardia, palpitations and restlessness.

Not all depressed patients will respond to the treatments so far outlined. In addition to reconsidering the diagnosis, clinicians should check that they have prescribed the standard antidepressant at optimal dosage for at least six weeks, that the patient has complied with the treatment, and should consider obtaining blood levels of the antidepressant (useful for imipramine and nortryptiline) to determine whether they have prescribed an optimal dose (Fava & Davidson, 1996). Depression in family members predicts a poorer response to treatment (Akiskal, 1982), as do a long duration of the current episode, a later age of onset, fewer prior episodes and fewer drug treatments (Deykin & Dimascio, 1972; Amsterdam et al., 1994). In reviewing the diagnosis in nonresponders, the clinician should consider the subtypes of depression that require different drug treatments, e.g., atypical depression and psychotic depression. Major depression with concomitant generalized anxiety disorder or panic disorder has a greater severity of depression (Manu et al., 1991), a slower response to antidepressants and a worse prognosis (Clayton et al., 1991; Fawcett, 1994; Fava & Davidson, 1996).

In summary, the physician faces a bewildering choice of drugs for depressed patients, and no one strategy or sequence of treatments has universal support. We favor: (1) using a nontricyclic agent as the first or second drug because they have fewer side-effects and less risk from overdose, (2) using augmentation before switching drugs, (3) using MAOIs for atypical depressive symptoms if a selective serotonin reuptake inhibitor has failed, (4) using nortriptyline as the tricyclic agent, and (5) considering electroconvulsive therapy if drugs fail. Above all, do not give up. If a patient has significant depressive symptoms, the physician should use the full panoply of treatments before considering the patient refractory to treatment.

Treatment of anxiety

We divide anxiety into several types. Generalized anxiety, also called anticipatory anxiety, is the fearfulness we normally feel in frightening situations either carried to an extent beyond what seems appropriate, or occurring without an apparent stimulus. It comprises fear, insomnia, restlessness, poor concentration, headache, palpitations, dyspnea, sweating, chest pain, feeling hot or cold, paresthesias and, when severe, fear of losing control, going 'crazy' or dying. This anxiety tends to wax and wane according to the situation.

Panic anxiety occurs abruptly, without an appropriate stimulus, and has greater severity than generalized anxiety. Panic attacks often drive patients to emergency rooms because it seems like a heart attack. Phobias produce anxiety in the feared situation. Persons with obsessive-compulsive disorder become anxious when they try to stop the obsessions or compulsions. Post-traumatic stress disorder causes anxiety from reliving the stressful event. Patients with functional somatic syndromes often display generalized anxiety and might benefit from anxiolytic drug treatment.

The benzodiazepines represent the mainstays of anxiolytics. The physician has a large number from which to choose. Those marketed as anxiolytics (alprazolam, chlordiazepoxide, clorazepate, diazepam, halazepam, lorazepam, clonazepam, oxazepam, prazepam) probably differ not at all from those marketed as hypnotics (estazolam, flurazepam, quazepam, temazepam, triazolam). All share the same efficacy and side-effects, with some differences in degree. They alleviate whatever symptom of anxiety predominates and often bring much relief. Their drawback comes from their side-effects and concern about addiction.

The benzodiazepines differ according to lipid solubility, rapidity of absorption, metabolism/elimination and potency. Prazepam has low lipid solubility which prevents a rapid action, but also tends to prevent a bothersome initial 'buzz' that some patients dislike. The most important difference among the benzodiazepines comes from differing half-lives that predict their duration of action. Of those commonly used for anxiety, alprazolam, chlordiazepoxide, lorazepam and oxazepam have shorter half-lives than clorazepate, diazepam, halazepam, clonazepam and prazepam. Short-lived anxiety suggests use of benzodiazepines with shorter half-lives, while with the longer lasting anxiety, benzodiazepines with longer half-lives could be used. These differences seem more useful in principle than in fact. Lorazepam and oxazepam are metabolized by hepatic conjugation, which is disturbed less by liver disease than is the oxidative hepatic metabolism used by the other drugs. A rough guideline to some relative potencies is: diazepam = 10, chlordiazepoxide = 20, lorazepam = 2, clonazepam = 0.5, alprazolam = 1, prazepam = 20, clorazepate = 15 and oxazepam = 30.

Adverse reactions to benzodiazepines consist of sedation, cognitive impairment and poor coordination. Patients differ markedly in their sensitivities to side-effects, and to differences in efficacy and side-effects among the benzodiazepines. For one patient 2 mg of diazepam may have the same effect as 20 mg in another; one patient may show much more sedation for the same degree of anxiety reduction on diazepam than on chlordiazepoxide, and the next patient might show the opposite. We cannot predict these responses, so the physician might have to try several benzodiazepines to find the optimal one.

Reports have appeared about behavioral disinhibition from benzodiazepines causing hostility, aggressiveness, rage reactions, paroxysmal excitement, irritability and behavioral dyscontrol (Dietch & Jennings, 1988). We believe this occurs rarely, if at all. Most reports describe patients who had such symptoms prior to using benzodiazepines, so the causative role of the benzodiazepine remains questionable. Placebo-controlled studies have not demonstrated that these symptoms occur more often in subjects treated with placebo. Yet, just as some people become more aggressive when intoxicated with alcohol, this could happen with any central nervous system depressant.

The fear of addiction discourages physicians and patients from using benzodiazepines. This is unfortunate. Addiction to benzodiazepines can occur, causing tolerance, withdrawal symptoms, poor functioning from excessive sedation, an inability to reduce or stop the drug, interpersonal difficulties from the effects of benzodiazepines, and dangerous behaviors (such as driving when intoxicated); so taking the drug becomes of paramount interest. The dependence and abuse of benzodiazepines are relatively uncommon compared with other addictive drugs and almost always occur in persons who use benzodiazepines not to alleviate anxiety, but for its euphoriant effect, to potentiate other drugs, or to alleviate the unpleasant effects of stimulating drugs. The patient seeking relief from anxiety rarely becomes addicted (Rifkin et al., 1989). Tolerance does not develop to the anxiolytic effect of benzodiazepines, but it does to their euphoriant effect. Long-term users of benzodiazepines for anxiety do not show increasing dosage. Therapeutic users dislike the sedative effect of benzodiazepines, and often dislike continuing them because they fear addiction.

Physical dependence can occur from therapeutic uses of benzodiazepines if the patient takes a benzodiazepine for a long time at a sufficiently high dose. This does not constitute addiction. It does mean that the patient should withdraw slowly, when the need for the drug has ended.

A difficult clinical problem comes from distinguishing withdrawal symptoms (and even rebound anxiety) from a resurgence of the anxiety from psychopathology upon reducing or stopping a benzodiazepine. The symptoms of withdrawal usually resemble those of anxiety. Withdrawal tends to occur more rapidly than clinical worsening, but often the distinction remains difficult. Returning the benzodiazepine regimen to a higher dose and then, when the symptoms have remitted, trying reduction again, but with a slower rate of withdrawal, usually suffices. Should anxiety return, even with a slower rate of withdrawal, especially if it returns after a delay of a week or more, this probably represents clinical worsening.

Benzodiazepine treatment should continue for as long as the anxiety continues. For some patients this means short-term treatment, for others long-term. Although the package inserts for benzodiazepines suggest an indication for only short-term treatment of anxiety, that should not deter the physician from long-term use. The risk of side-effects and addiction do not increase with the length of treatment.

Buspirone is another useful anxiolytic that differs considerably from the benzodiazepines. It does not bind to benzodiazepine receptors, but probably acts by several effects on the serotonin system. It appears as effective as the benzodiazepines for generalized anxiety, but its onset is much slower – one to two weeks. Unlike benzodiazepines, it does not cause sedation or cognitive impairment, does not have an additive effect with alcohol or other central nervous system depressants, and does not cause euphoria or sedation and, therefore, has no potential for abuse.

Clinical experience indicates that buspirone works best in subjects not treated with benzodiazepines. We do not know whether benzodiazepines interfere with buspirone's efficacy, or the subjects who had no previous exposure to benzodiazepines differed from those who did. Unlike benzodiazepines, which work rapidly and help brief, situational anxiety, buspirone works only after weeks of steady dosing. Buspirone occasionally causes the side-effects of nausea and dizziness. Research studies have not focused on establishing the optimal doses. Considering the relative absence of significant side-effects, physicians should use doses of up to 30–40 mg/day for six weeks as an adequate trial.

Antidepressants such as tricyclic agents, selective serotonin reuptake inhibitors and trazodone have shown usefulness for patients with generalized anxiety disorder (Kahn et al., 1986; Rickels et al., 1993). They, like buspirone, do not work quickly and episodically, as benzodiazepines do. Benzodiazepines, especially alprazolam and clonazepam, tricyclic agents, and SSRIs alleviate panic disorder. Tricyclic agents usually require a lower dose (e.g. 25–150 mg/day of imipramine or desipramine) than is needed for depression. Buspirone does not appear to be effective for this indication. Primary care physicians should consider using an SSRI as the first choice because they have fewer side-effects than benzodiazepines or tricyclic agents.

Treatment of disturbed sleep

Disturbed sleep accompanies many functional psychosomatic disorders and deserves attention. Sleep apnea, the most common serious primary sleep problem, presents with reports by the patient's bed companion of marked snoring and intermittent arousals. Such a history suggests referral to a sleep clinic for a definitive diagnosis.

Nonpharmacological measures should precede drug treatment of insomnia, such as: (1) eliminating stimulants such as caffeine; (2) avoidance of sleeping at other times; (3) vigorous exercise; (4) maintaining regular hours for sleep, including arising at the same time regardless of when the patient falls asleep; (5) avoidance of activities in bed, such as eating and watching TV; and (6) avoidance of long sleepless periods in bed, i.e., the patient should get out of bed and not return until sleepy.

Hypnotics usually help should these efforts at 'sleep hygiene' not work. Research shows that hypnotics stop working after several weeks (Kripke et al., 1987), although many patients do not report this, or they report renewed insomnia when stopping the hypnotic. This raises concerns that the patient has come to depend on the hypnotic. The physician should periodically try to reduce and then stop the hypnotic, but if this proves unsuccessful the drug should be resumed, as long as its benefits outweigh the side-effects.

Many drugs have hypnotic activity. All the benzodiazepines used for anxiety also serve as hypnotics. Some benzodiazepines have an indication for sleep, e.g., estazolam, flurazepam, quazepam, temazepam and triazolam. These hypnotic benzodiazepines show no different pharmacological features from anxiolytic benzodiazepines; the difference comes from the manufacturer's decision about which indication to study. Triazolam has a very short half-life (2–6 hours) which, theoretically, means it might help with the initial insomnia and cause less morning hangover than other benzodiazepines. As with anxiolytic benzodiazepines, the relationship of pharmacokinetics to clinical effects remains weak, and therapeutic responses vary a great deal.

Zolpidem, not a benzodiazepine, effectively treats insomnia without the risks of dependence and addiction. Low doses of antidepressants such as trazodone and amitriptyline help insomnia, as do sedating antihistamines. Chloral hydrate, barbiturates and barbiturate-like compounds seem less desirable as hypnotics because they cause more central nervous system depression when combined with alcohol and have great lethality from accidental or intentional overdoses.

All hypnotics may cause cognitive difficulties, sometimes subtle, especially in the elderly, where it may be mistaken for normal aging or even dementia. In such patients insomnia may cause fewer problems than its treatment. On the other hand, a restful night's sleep may bring considerable relief to patients suffering from chronic conditions. The physician need not hesitate to use them judiciously.

Insomnia may be a symptom of many disorders, mental and physical, so that the most effective treatment of insomnia in such instances is effective treatment of the disorder, e.g. depression, anxiety and pain cause insomnia. Yet, attempts to treat the underlying cause need not replace symptomatic treatment of insomnia with hypnotics, at least until remission of the underlying disorder.

Treatment of pain

Patients with chronic psychosomatic pain pose difficult therapeutic challenges. We should not neglect such pain as if it were less worthy of attention than from more physiologically understandable pain. Yet, we do not wish to cause unintended problems from side-effects. Most mild pain responds to analgesics such as acetaminophen, aspirin and other nonsteroidal anti-inflammatory drugs, but some patients may need doses that pose risks, such as liver and kidney disorders from large amounts of acetaminophen.

Opioids are the 'heavy hitters' of analgesia, starting with the more mild ones (codeine, oxycodone, propoxyphene and hydrocodone), to more pure opioid antagonists (morphine, methadone and hydromorphone). We usually avoid opioid analgesics for pain associated with functional somatic syndromes because of their side-effects (somnolence, nausea, constipation) and, especially out of concern for the risk of addiction and/or tolerance. Pentazocine, an opioid-type analgesic, should be avoided due to its risk of psychotomimetic effects. The risk of addiction to opioids used for analgesia is very low: 0.033% per 12 000 patients studied (Porter & Hick, 1980). Opioids may have the most favorable risk : benefit ratio for treatment of chronic pain. Nevertheless, in our practice it seems most conventional to try nonopioid analgesics first, and if they prove ineffective to consider psychotropic drugs.

Psychotropic medication may alleviate the pain of functional somatic syndromes. Tricyclic agents are widely used and appear to be effective in doses of 25–150 mg imipramine, amitriptyline or desipramine per day. Carbamazepine, an anticonvulsant agent, has shown efficacy especially for neurogenic pain, at doses of 200–1200 mg/day, in divided doses. Less studied for pain are the selective serotonin reuptake inhibitors, but there are some encouraging reports, such as the use of fluoxetine for fibromyalgia (Geller, 1989).

References

Akiskal H (1982). Factors associated with incomplete recovery in primary depressive illness. *Journal of Clinical Psychiatry*, **43**, 266–71.

Amsterdam JD, Maislin G & Potter L (1994). Fluoxetine efficacy in treatment-resistant depression. *Progress in Neuropsychopharmacology and Biological Psychiatry*, **18**, 243–61.

Clayton P, Grove W, Coryell W, Keller M, Hirschfeld R & Fawcett J (1991). Follow-up and family study of anxious depression. *American Journal of Psychiatry*, **148**, 1512–17.

Deykin E & Dimascio A (1972). Relationship of patient characteristics to efficiency of pharmacotherapy in depression. *Journal of Nervous and Mental Diseases*, **155**, 209–15.

Dietch JT & Jennings RK (1988). Aggressive dyscontrol in patients treated with benzodiazepines. *Journal of Clinical Psychiatry*, **49**, 184–8.

Fava M & Davidson KG (1996). Definition and epidemiology of treatment-resistant depression. *Psychiatric Clinics of North America*, **19**, 179–97.

Fawcett J (1994). Antidepressants: partial response in chronic depression. *British Journal of Psychiatry*, **165** (Suppl. 26), 37–41.

Geller S (1989). Treatment of fibrositis with fluoxetine hydrochloride (Prozac). *American Journal of Medicine*, **87**, 594–5.

Joffe RT, Singer W, Levitt AJ & MacDonald C (1993). A placebo-controlled comparison of lithium and triiodothyronine augmentation of tricyclic antidepressants in unipolar refractory depression. *Archives of General Psychiatry*, **50**, 387–93.

Kahn RJ, McNair DM, Lipman RS, Covi L, Rickels K, Downing R, Fisher S & Frankenthaler LM (1986). Imipramine and chlordiazepoxide in depressive and anxiety disorder. II. Efficacy in anxious outpatients. *Archives of General Psychiatry*, **43**, 79–85.

Kripke D, Hauri P & Roth T (1987). Sleep evaluation in chronic insomnia during short- and long-term use of two benzodiazepines, flurazepam and midazolam. *Sleep Research*, **16**, 99.

Liebowitz M, Quitkin F, Stewart J, McGrath P, Harrison W & Markowitz J (1988). Antidepressant specificity in atypical depression. *Archives of General Psychiatry*, **45**, 129–37.

Manu P, Matthews DA & Lane TJ (1991). Panic disorder among patients with chronic fatigue. *Southern Medical Journal*, **84**, 451–6.

Porter J & Hick H (1980). Addiction rate in patients treated with narcotics. *New England Journal of Medicine*, **302**, 303.

Quitkin FM, McGrath PJ, Steward JW, Taylor BP & Klein DF (1996). Can the effects of antidepressants be observed in the first two weeks of treatment? *Neuropsychopharmacology*, **15**, 390–4.

Rickels K, Downing R, Schweizer E & Hassman H (1993). Antidepressants for the treatment of generalized anxiety disorder: a placebo-controlled comparison of imipramine, trazodone and diazepam. *Archives of General Psychiatry*, **50**, 884–95.

Rifkin A (1997). Optimal doses of SSRIs. *Journal of Clinical Psychiatry*, **58**, 87–8.

Rifkin A, Doddi S & Karajgi BM (1989). Benzodiazepine use and abuse by patients at outpatients clinics. *American Journal of Psychiatry*, **146**, 1331–2.

Roose S (1992). Modern cardiovascular standards for psychotropic drugs. *Psychopharmacology Bulletin*, **28**, 35–434.

12

Psychotherapy of Functional Somatic Syndromes

GARY TAERK

Psychotherapy can be defined as all systematic interactions between a sufferer and a socially designated healer, in which the healer undertakes to relieve the sufferer's distress by symbolic communications (Frank, 1975). The role of psychotherapy in the treatment of bodily diseases depends on the extent to which psychological factors play a role in their etiology and course. As have been demonstrated in the previous chapters in this volume, psychological factors do play a significant role in the evolution of functional somatic syndromes and, as such, psychotherapy is an essential component in the comprehensive treatment of every patient who presents with a functional somatic syndrome.

It is generally assumed that patients who present with functional somatic symptoms are poor candidates for psychotherapy. Bodily preoccupation and the tendency to experience one's self in physical terms can be serious impediments to psychotherapeutic work. Such individuals have difficulty distinguishing somatic from psychological distress and therefore have difficulty identifying and communicating emotional experiences. As such, they present special challenges to the clinician.

Commonly, patients are concerned that their symptoms are caused by organic disease. The tendency to somatize is fundamental to understanding functional somatic syndromes and the psychotherapeutic options available to the clinician. Somatization can be understood from a variety of perspectives. Psychodynamically, it has been regarded as a drive derivative, a defensive displacement or a wish for nurturance and support. Relational theorists have attributed somatization to a developmental arrest resulting from the lack of responsiveness of parental figures in helping their infants to differentiate somatic from psychological experience. When such responsiveness is not available, infants may learn to respond somatically to situations in which it would be more appropriate to respond socially (Rodin, 1984). This development may contribute to the tendency toward somatization in adults who have been described as alexithymic (Taylor, 1977). Also, it has been suggested that these individuals lack the capacity to modulate psychological and physiological stimuli (Taerk & Gnam, 1994), and as a result form immature, enmeshed or symbiotic relationships to compensate for this defect. Self-psychologists have tended to view somatization as a regressive self-state induced by narcissistic injury, expressed as physical symptoms.

Cognitive-behavioral theorists suggest that somatization results from a misinterpretation or misattribution of bodily sensations. Such cognitions tend to be self-perpetuating. The more one believes that one has a disease the greater is the focus on the body and the more symptoms are perceived (Wessely & Sharpe, 1995). The resulting behavioral and physiological changes may contribute to this process. This preoccupation may also be associated with a reluctance to consider psychological explanations for the symptoms and to accept a psychotherapeutic approach.

As this tendency is to experience their distress in physical terms, care must be taken in engaging patients in psychological therapies. Understanding, explanation and reassurance go a long way to establishing the trust required to elicit the patient's cooperation in considering psychotherapeutic treatments. The initial assessment and explanation given to the patient is a general psychological treatment of great importance and potential efficacy. It is a skill that should be possessed by all doctors (Sharpe et al., 1995). Becoming embroiled in arguments with the patient over whether symptoms originate in the mind or the body will further alienate the patient. Figure 12.1 outlines the psychotherapeutic option to consider in the overall treatment of patients with functional somatic syndromes.

Cognitive-behavioral therapy

Cognitive-behavioral therapy is considered to be the treatment of choice for a wide range of functional somatic syndromes. It is brief, effective and cost efficient and can be practiced by family physicians, internists and nonmedical professionals, as well as psychiatrists. For a more complete description of cognitive-behavioral therapy the interested reader should refer to Beck et al. (1979) and Hawton et al. (1989).

It is psychotherapy which aims to diminish the perpetuating psycho-

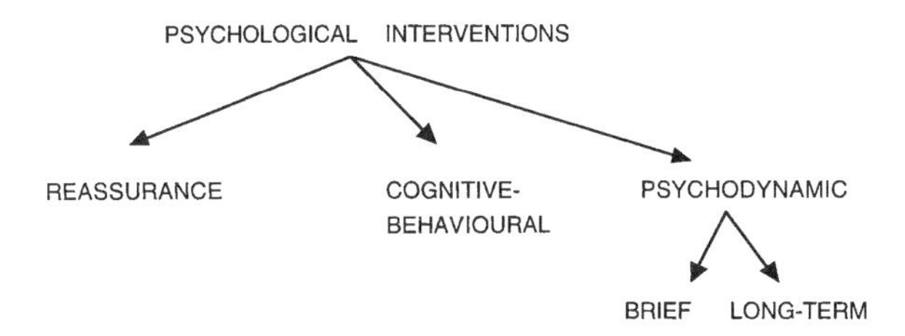

Figure 12.1. Psychotherapeutic options in the treatment of patients with functional somatic syndromes.

logical factors in a patient's illness by changing maladaptive and dysfunctional attitudes and the behaviors that follow from these mistaken beliefs. It has been shown to be effective in the treatment of chronic fatigue syndrome (Sharpe et al., 1996; Wessely *et al.*, 1991), irritable bowel syndrome (Greene & Blanchard, 1994), premenstrual syndrome (Kirkby, 1994) and chronic pain syndromes (Pearce, 1983; Farquar et al., 1990; Dworkin et al., 1994).

Central to cognitive theory is the view that a patient's cognitions are of primary importance in determining his or her behavior and his or her emotional and physiological state. Patients with functional somatic symptoms commonly hold dysfunctional beliefs. Just as the thinking of patients suffering from depressive disorders is typically dysfunctional in that it tends to a distorted and excessively negative view of the self, the world and the future, patients with functional somatic syndromes commonly hold similar dysfunctional beliefs concerning their physical health and functioning. They tend to attribute bodily sensations to physical disease rather than to emotional or trivial causes (Sharpe, 1995).

Like thinking, behavior can also be regarded as either functional, if it is helpful in resolving problems, or dysfunctional, if it tends to perpetuate them. Dysfunctional behaviors include the inactivity of patients with various functional somatic syndromes. In chronic fatigue syndrome, nonischemic heart chest pain, repetitive strain injury and other pain-related syndromes, symptoms worsen with minimal physical or mental exertion. Accordingly, patients and their doctors commonly assume that the best therapy is rest. Wessely & Sharpe (1995) pointed out how this behavior can lead to physiological changes in the form of deconditioning and progressive weakness, muscular atrophy, pain and fatigue when activity is resumed. A vicious cycle develops leaving patients discouraged and hopeless.

Sharpe (1995) also emphasized the role of interpersonal factors in giving rise to cognitions that may reinforce preoccupation with disease and symptom maintaining behaviors. The attitudes of relatives, friends

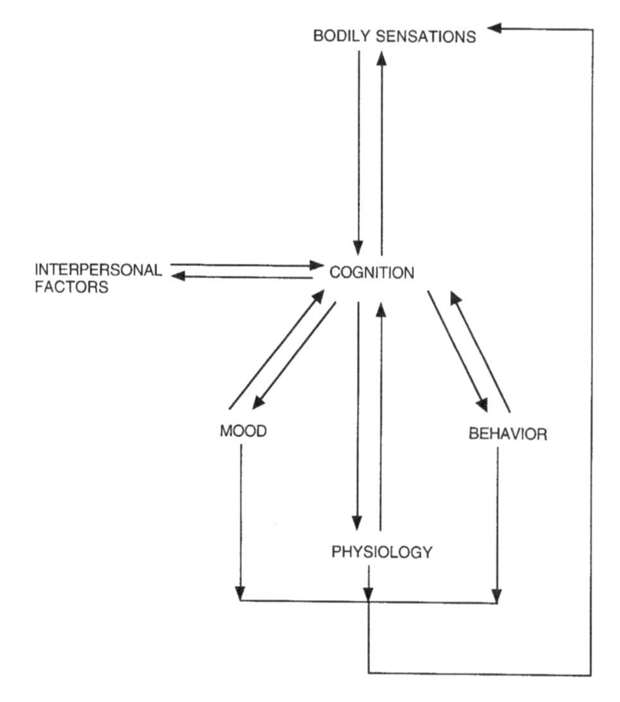

Figure 12.2. A cognitive-behavioral model of functional somatic syndromes. (From *Treatment of Functional Somatic Symptoms* ed. R. Mayou, C. M. Bass & M. Sharpe, Oxford University Press, 1995, p. 128, by permission of Oxford University Press.)

and medical practitioners often contribute to emotional distress and unintentionally perpetuate patients' distorted views of their symptoms. Sharpe has combined the components of cognition, behavior, emotion and physiology to form a cognitive behavioral model of functional somatic syndromes (Figure 12.2).

Reformulating the illness

Deconstructing the patient's perception of his or her condition and developing a new, shared formulation of the illness is crucial to the success of cognitive-behavioral therapy in the treatment of functional somatic syndromes. Chronic fatigue syndrome will be used to demonstrate this technique.

In chronic fatigue syndrome, patients often view their condition as resulting from an external agent, usually a simple infection from a virus. Instead, a more complex model is proposed to the patient. For instance, it is plausible that in chronic fatigue syndrome an initial infective trigger or depressive episode may begin a cycle in which the patient's beliefs and fears concerning symptoms and activity fuel avoidant behavior. The initial symptoms of fatigue and myalgia, which are unpleasant and uncontrollable, together with the attribution of symptoms to a persistent untreatable virus may lead to a state akin to 'learned helplessness' (Seligman, 1975) and hence foster disability and depression. Avoidance behavior sustains symptoms by decreasing activity tolerance and increasingly sensitivity to any stimulation. Re-exposure to activity causes more symptoms and more fear. The result is a vicious circle of symptoms, avoidance, fatigue, demoralization and depression, the clinical picture of chronic fatigue syndrome (Wessely & Sharpe, 1995). A similar role for avoidance in perpetuating symptoms has been implicated for chronic pain syndromes, fibromyalgia and nonischemic chest pain.

Treatment requires attention to illness beliefs, mood disorder and behavioral avoidance. Accordingly, therapeutic success should result from reducing avoidance behavior, decreasing helplessness, and improving mood.

According to Wessely & Sharpe (1995), the cognitive behavioral treatment of chronic fatigue syndrome consists of the following steps:

(1) *Assessment*
Exclude physical disease
Assess cognitions and behavior
(2) *Engagement in treatment*
Agree formulation of illness
Agree realistic and valued goals
(3) *Cognitive components*
Education about chronic fatigue syndrome
Modify attribution for symptoms
Challenge excessive perfectionism
Problem solving
(4) *Behavioral components*
Graded increase in activity
Relaxation
(5) *Other ingredients*
Antidepressant medication

Wessely & Sharpe (1995) make a number of important observations regarding the cognitive-behavioral model in relation to functional somatic syndromes in general and the chronic fatigue syndrome in particular:

(1) The aim of treatment is to reduce functional disability, which is to be achieved through increasing activity before symptoms diminish. Conventional approaches wait for symptoms to diminish first.

(2) The model does not contradict the evidence of an organic origin to symptoms; it is based instead on the assumption that the factors that initiate an illness are not necessarily the same as those that perpetuate it.
(3) The purpose of cognitive-behavior psychotherapy is not to replace extreme organic assumptions with extreme psychological ones but to generate a model that encompasses a variety of factors and to demonstrate to the patient that they can influence the course of the illness.

Robbins & Kirmayer (1991) have demonstrated the correlation between various functional somatic syndromes noting the overlap in the symptomatology of chronic fatigue syndrome, nonischemic chest pain and fibromyalgia in terms of muscle pain, breathlessness and fatigue. It is perhaps not surprising that controlled trials of cognitive-behavioral therapy have been shown to be effective in decreasing the perception of pain, diminishing autonomic symptoms and in decreasing limitations and disruptions of life, in nonischemic chest pain and in fibromyalgia as well.

Case 1

A 23-year-old college student presents to his primary care physician complaining of tightness in his chest, shortness of breath and nausea on mild exertion. A medical work-up proved to be negative. The patient was given reassurance that he was free to resume normal activity. Three months later he returned to his physician continuing to report symptoms and disability despite the reassurance he had received. A 10-week course of once weekly cognitive-behavioral therapy was instituted by the primary care physician with the result that at six-month follow-up, the patient was free from symptoms. This fitness-conscious student was against putting any 'unnatural chemicals' into his body and was probably fearful about the meaning of having a mental disorder. Accordingly, it was decided to treat his problem initially at least as one based on a misapprehension of normal physiological processes. As such, a cognitive-behavioral approach to his problem was developed. As treatment progressed it became apparent that the family context was important in the creation of his physical concerns. His father had a 10-year history of mysterious chest pain when the patient was a child. The father's frequent middle of the night trips to the emergency department disrupted family life to the point that the patient became convinced that his father might die at any instant during his childhood. He took it upon himself to be vigilant of any signs of cardiac disease in his father and thereby to protect the father and keep him alive.

Bass & Mayou (1995) reported that, although many patients with benign cardiac symptoms have an excellent recovery following medical assessment and reassurance, a minority do less well and describe continuing symptoms, disability and worry about their disease. This minority requires extra help. This help may include any or all of the following:

(1) More detailed explanation of the noncardiac origins of their symptoms.
(2) Correction of their idiosyncratic and dysfunctional interpretations of somatic perceptions.
(3) Reintroduction of graded activity.
(4) Relaxation exercises and the learning of slow-paced breathing.

The college student described in case 1 is not atypical of many patients presenting with functional somatic syndromes. There is overlap in the symptomatology with other conditions such as anxiety or panic disorder. A decision must be made as to the diagnosis and therefore the route of treatment.

Psychodynamic psychotherapy

Psychodynamic theories

Early psychoanalytical theories viewed psychosomatic illnesses as resulting from repressed instinctual drives. The resulting internal tension was converted along somatic rather than motor pathways into bodily symptoms. Treatment was aimed at bringing repressed psychosexual conflicts or trauma into consciousness so that the energy associated with their repression could be properly discharged. Classical Freudian drive theory advocated interpretation of unconscious conflict and abreaction of the associated memories. Although elegant in its conception this formulation often failed to bring about the expected alleviation of symptoms.

More recently psychoanalytical theory has placed object relations rather than sexual and aggressive drives as the central building blocks in psychological development, particularly in the development of the capacity for physiological as well as psychological self-regulation. This theory has interesting implications for understanding functional somatic syndromes. The term functional implies a disturbance of physiological function rather than anatomical structure. Functional disorders probably involve physiological disruptions that are too complex or subtle to be reflected in gross structural defects and may involve abnormal processes occurring in structurally intact organ systems. Findings of abnormal physiology, biochemistry and immune response do not correlate with easily discernible organ damage, although many of these patients exhibit evidence of dysregulated biological systems such as motility disturbances in irritable bowel syndrome (Tilbe & Sullivan, 1990), sleep rhythm abnormalities in fibromyalgia (Moldofsky, 1989), and alterations in immune functioning (Klimas et al., 1990), muscle metabolism (Byrne & Trounce, 1987), cognitive functioning (Wessely et al., 1991) and hypothalamic pituitary-adrenal axis functioning (Demitrack et al., 1991) in chronic fatigue syndrome.

From birth the child is part of a system of self and mutual regulation within the infant–caregiver dyad (Taylor, 1982*a*,*b*). Severe misattunements by the caregiver in this early regulatory system gives rise to a faulty capacity for self-regulation in the infant with regards not only to psychological states but also to internal physiological states. The child experiences difficulty in differentiating physical from psychological distress, has difficulty calming and soothing itself and remains vulnerable to states of psychological and physiological dysregulation. In other words, both a physiological and a psychological vulnerability exists in patients with functional somatic syndromes as a result of problems in early object relations. Furthermore, it could be proposed that this vulnerability results from a poorly developed capacity for regulating internal states in response to various physical and psychological stressors (Taerk & Gnam, 1994).

To compensate for this deficiency in modulating dysphoric states such individuals may attach themselves to idealized others who can provide tension-regulating functions such as calming and soothing, only to fall ill when an attachment disruption occurs or is threatened. The particular functional syndrome that emerges when general susceptibility is increased is presumed to be determined by biological, psychological and social factors. The relationship between these various factors in the development of functional somatic syndromes might be represented in the model given in Figure 12.3.

Emphasizing the importance of faulty object relations in the development of functional somatic syndromes, Guthrie (1995) has conceptualized psychodynamic psychotherapy as acting to repair the resulting defects through the medium of the intense, personal and intimate doctor–patient relationship. She observes that psychodynamic object relations theory postulates that a significant degree of psychological and physical distress is either caused or exacerbated by relationship problems in the patient's life. These difficulties might include the loss of

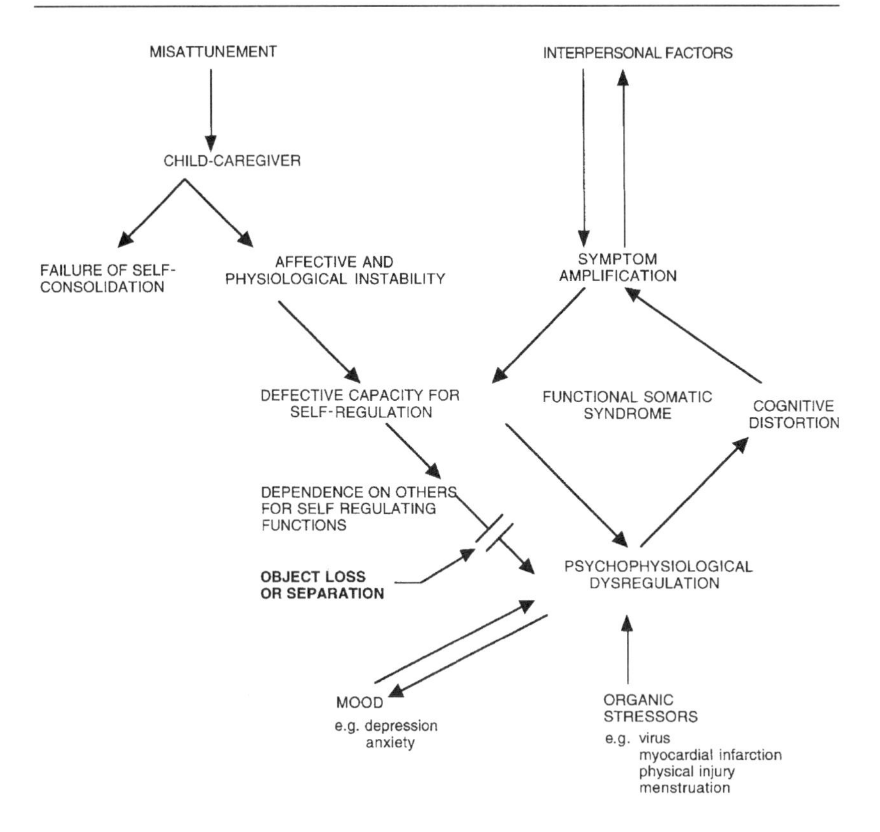

Figure 12.3. A multifactoral model which hypothesizes an increased susceptibility to the development of functional somatic syndromes in individuals with difficulties in early object relations. (Reproduced from the *Journal of General Hospital Psychiatry* (1994), **16**, by permission of Elsevier Science, Inc.)

someone close, the inability to form satisfactory relationships or unhappiness resulting from dissatisfaction with current relationships. As a result of the intensity of the relationship between the doctor and patient, the problems in the patient's life are mirrored or recur in the relationship that the patient forms with the doctor. Analysis of the transference helps the patient to understand the relation of physical symptoms to psychological events, and helps to clear up distortions in the patient's object relationships (Case 2).

This leads to a reduction in symptom formation in at least two ways. In the first place the understanding of the patient's distortions and misperceptions which become available to both doctor and patient in the course of the analytical work enables the patient to overcome disruptions in important relationships caused by these recurrent misperceptions and thereby enables the patient to develop more constant, reliable and satisfying object relationships outside the therapy. These relationships provide regulating functions previously unavailable to the patient and this, in turn, makes the recurrence of symptoms less likely.

Secondly, through the repair of inevitable disruptions in the doctor–patient relationship (transference) a bond (self-object bond) is established and maintained with the doctor which provides vital regulating functions to the patient that evoke, maintain and positively affect the sense of self. These functions include attunement to affective states, validation of subjective experience, affect containment, tension regulation, soothing sustaining and organizing, and recognition of uniqueness and creative potential (Bacall & Newman, 1990). Over time the regulating functions of the self-object are internalized so that the patient can provide these regulating functions for him or her self.

Brief dynamic psychotherapy

Guthrie (1995) pointed out that patients with functional somatic symptoms are seen to lie on a continuum. At one end are those individuals with good enough care during childhood who develop somatic symptoms at certain times in their lives in relation to particular problems, but essentially form healthy and mutually supportive relationships. Recognition and change in the individual results in improvement in the relationship and resolution of the symptoms. These individuals respond to a time-limited psychodynamic approach. Guthrie pointed out that brief dynamic psychotherapy has the advantage of being easily learned and can be practiced by a wide range of health professionals.

Guthrie (1991) studied 102 outpatients with chronic symptoms of irritable bowel syndrome. The criteria for participation included patient's who were unresponsive to conventional medical treatment, with at least a one-year history of abdominal pain, distension and abnormal bowel habit associated with normal hematology, rectal biopsy and colonoscopy. Following randomization, the treatment group received seven sessions of brief dynamic psychotherapy and the control group five sessions of supportive listening. Both groups continued with their medical treatment unchanged. Bowel symptomatology was independently assessed by a gastroenterologist blind to the treatment condition. At the end of the trial period, the treatment group showed significantly greater improvement than the control group in terms of both gastroenterological and psychological symptoms. Following the end of the trial, patients in the control group, who were still severely distressed by their symptoms, were offered dynamic psychotherapy. These patients also showed a significant improvement in their bowel and psychological symptoms following therapy. Baseline predictors of good outcome included symptoms of anxiety and depression and the recognition that stress affected their symptoms.

Case 2

Ms D is a 43-year-old divorced mother of three girls (aged 13, 11 and 10 years) who entered treatment on referral from her family physician because of incapacitating bowel symptoms which were affecting her ability to work effectively. She works as a bank manager. In spite of glowing evaluations she avoids pursuing promotions because she will end up having to chair meetings and give presentations. Prior to meetings in which she expects to be called upon to speak she often gets violent stomach cramps and diarrhea. She finds it especially difficult whenever her female supervisor is going to be present at a meeting or when she has to make a request of the supervisor in private. Her supervisor has a distinctly different philosophy and style from that of the patient. Ms D views the supervisor as a 'real tight ass' who cannot appreciate Ms D's more relaxed management approach.

She is the only female child in a family of four children. Her mother is described as a cold, formal woman who had especially high expectations of the patient, scholastically and socially. Ms D remembers working hard at school to win her mother's praise. In fact Ms D now believes her choice of husband was an attempt to please her mother as her husband, although quite a successful businessman, had little in common with the patient.

Her husband also had high expectations of the patient. She felt she was never able to please him. For instance, she related that he 'put her into high heels' immediately after their marriage because he felt she was too short. He criticized her for dressing in too casual a manner in front of his business associates. He was particularly angry with her for giving up a promising business career in order to stay home and raise their children. When she complained about his lack of involvement in the life of the family, he would tell her that she was a 'nagging bitch'. She could not shake the feeling that she was responsible for the break-up of her marriage one year previously. She felt terribly unsure of herself. Whatever confidence she had prior to the nine year marriage was now gone.

Her parents' marriage was filled with tension. Mother constantly belittled father, who had working-class roots, as being a poor provider and beneath her socially. Ms D often felt that her mother turned to her and her accomplishments for solace from her disappointing marriage.

Ms D seems to have a split view of her father. Prior to his retirement she saw him as dismissive and belittling of her, more interested in his sons. Afterwards, in his later years, she came to pity him as a pathetic individual plagued as he was after retirement by anxiety attacks which rendered him dependent on diazepam to get through the day. She worries that she is becoming like him and that a similar fate awaits her as she gets older.

At times prior to meeting with me, she will report having gastrointestinal symptoms similar to those she experiences at work. These seem to occur when she anticipates having to ask me something which she believes I will find bothersome, such as changing an appointment time or telling me about an upcoming vacation which she fears will disrupt my schedule. She will agonize about my anticipated reaction to the point of wanting to quit therapy before I kick her out for being such a nuisance.

I came to see here as an individual who has difficulty maintaining self-cohesion in the face of the fear of not achieving desperately needed mirroring responses from authority figures, i.e., women like her mother and her supervisor and men like her husband and me. This fear of individuals she admires renders her unable to internalize tension-regulating functions that idealizable figures might potentially provide.

Psychotherapy with Ms D involved the repeated working through of her anxiety which occurred prior to encounters with her mother, her supervisor and the doctor. She became better able to engage in relationships with authority figures as a result of the understanding she acquired in therapy. Consequently after six months of weekly psychotherapy, her bowel symptoms diminished to the point where she could accept a promotion and the benefits in terms of increased job satisfaction and the increase in self-esteem that accompanied it.

Long-term psychodynamic psychotherapy

At the other end of the spectrum are those individuals with a history of severe emotional deprivation during childhood, who have great difficulty in making and sustaining relationships as adults. The relationships they form are either chaotic, fragile or more typically symbiotic. These symbiotic or enmeshed relationships are often characterized by a carer as an invalid. Engel (1955), followig his work with patients suffering from bowel disease, recommended that patients with psychosomatic illnesses who fit this profile should be treated with a long-term supportive relationship by their primary care physician, internist or psychiatrist and furthermore that the treatment relationship never be completely terminated. Instead the physician should be available to help with advice and support both medically and psychologically at times of crisis. The physician assumes the role of a dependency figure for the patient but discourages regression by avoiding interpretations of underlying conflicts and limiting the frequency of meetings except around medical issues.

As clinicians have widened the scope of analytical therapy to include the treatment of patients with severe character pathology (Kernberg, 1975; Kohut, 1977), these individuals may be helped to overcome their conditions with long-term psychodynamic psychotherapy. In a prior publication, Taerk & Gnam (1994) described two cases of long-term intensive psychoanalytical psychotherapy with chronic fatigue syndrome patients in which the intimate relationships of fatigue symptoms to disturbances in object relationships, particularly within the transference, was demonstrated. Improvement in symptoms was noted when these relationships were seen and understood by the patient and the importance of the therapist–patient bond as a facilitating medium for clinical improvement was also understood. Krystal (1979) suggested an initial phase in which the therapist helps the patient to name an emotional experience, followed by a more conventional psychodynamic approach.

Case 3[1]

Ms M was a 29-year-old single woman who lived alone and worked as an intensive care nurse at a major pediatric hospital at the time she was diagnosed as suffering from chronic fatigue syndrome. At her request she was referred by the family medical service of a university teaching hospital after exhaustive medical evaluations failed to reveal organic factors contributing to her incapacitating fatigue and multiple somatic symptoms. Her family physician suggested that she might benefit from an antidepressant, which she grudgingly accepted but discontinued within one week due to intolerable side-effects. She was so angered by the implicit suggestion that she was depressed that she relied exclusively thereafter on the prescriptions of unconventional alternative 'practitioners', which involved stringent diets and high doses of vitamins. She became desperate when she only partially improved and with embarrassment arranged for psychiatric evaluation after reading an article relating cancer patients recovery to psychological factors.

[1] A version of this case was published in *General Hospital Psychiatry* (1994), **16**, 322–3, and is reprinted by permission of Elsevier Science, Inc.

Ms M frequently stressed that she had doubts about psychiatry and wondered whether the therapist is 'just another doctor who thinks the problem is all in my head'. In early sessions she repeatedly apologized for complaining about her life. She suspected that the therapist was skeptical about the legitimacy of her need for therapy. Over several sessions it emerged that this suspicion reflected the general lack of supportive validating relationships in her life and the resulting failure to develop a genuine sense of entitlement to empathic responsiveness from those around her. Her mother had been depressed throughout Ms M's childhood because of her father's frequent trips and had relied on Ms M for comfort and support. Her relationship with her current boyfriend also left her feeling exploited and unfulfilled.

Ms M's identity was consolidated by her function as a caregiver for her mother, a role which enabled her to maintain vital ties to the family and gave her a sense of self-worth. She therefore had difficulty trusting that the therapist would be genuinely interested in her. Much of the early therapeutic work focused on allowing Ms M to freely express her worries. These were initially related to her physical condition but gradually shifted to her emotional life, particularly her feelings related to two catastrophic events, namely the car accident 10 years previously that rendered her sister paraplegic and the death of her brother from cancer 18 months before beginning therapy. In both instances Ms M recalled having to comfort her mother and having no one with whom to share her own grief. She remembers feeling tremendous resentment when forced to catheterize her newly disabled sister because her mother's hand shook with anxiety.

Her brother was a particularly significant figure in her life. He was the only person who listened to her and accepted her. In turn, she intensely idealized him and his accomplishments. She remarked that she knew who she was when she was with her brother and in his presence felt good about herself. Following his death she fell ill with the chronic fatigue syndrome. She revealed that she had rarely spoken about her brother since his death and had not had the opportunity to grieve for him.

Over the initial nine months of twice weekly treatment there was a gradual improvement in her fatigue symptoms. She reported an increase in energy and a reduction in muscle pain; however, there was a noticeable deterioration at the time of the therapist's first vacation. Although Ms M claimed to be unperturbed by the announced two week break, she began experiencing fatigue as the vacation approached. When the therapist returned Ms M related how she had been unable to work for several of the days the therapist was absent. This pattern repeated itself several times but was gradually recognized and understood as a reawakening of the loss of the brother and the regulatory functions he provided.

Ms M was also embarrassed by the need for the therapist which was revealed. This shame was worked through as well, as Ms M gradually became aware that the therapist was able to accept her self-object needs and consequently she became more tolerant of her self. This in turn led Ms M to expect more from her male partner and to move into a more mutual kind of relationship with him rather than having to always be the caregiver. Moreover, she became encouraged through the relationship with the therapist to rely on her boyfriend for comforting and understanding of her affective experiences.

After 18 months, when therapy was terminated, Ms M displayed much freer access to dreams and fantasy and her somatic preoccupation diminished. She was able to resume a more active work schedule and abandoned her severe dietary restrictions.

Medication as an adjunct to psychotherapy

For many patients who will be treated psychotherapeutically, the psychiatric symptoms accompanying functional somatic syndromes are so debilitating that psychotropic medication will be a necessary and welcome component of the comprehensive treatment approach taken by their physician. Anxiety states and depressive episodes in particular frequently require immediate relief in order to allow and encourage the patient to participate in the psychotherapeutic relationship.

Case 4

Mr K is a 36-year-old high school teacher who was referred for psychiatric assessment because no organic cause had been discovered to account for his extreme fatigue and nausea on exertion. He had been a dedicated jogger for the past several years but had gradually become aware of an increasing lack of stamina and feelings of nausea beginning shortly after starting out on his daily three mile run. This turn of events was especially disturbing to Mr K as he feared he would lose the strength and endurance he had taken years to acquire. He valued his physical prowess because he had grown up fearful of any physical activity owing to his overly protective rather phobic mother. His mother's anxiety often prevented him from joining in the roughhousing activities of other boys and had left him feeling isolated and insecure in his masculinity. Mr K was becoming afraid to jog for fear he would pass out from fatigue or have to vomit from his nausea. He was becoming frightened as well that he would become so exhausted that he would not be able to work and support his family.

Mr K had married his physiotherapist wife 10 years previously. He saw himself as quite reliant upon her for her strength and coping abilities. Shortly before the onset of his symptoms, she had begun to develop vague neurological symptoms which he suspected and which were later confirmed to be caused by multiple sclerosis. As evidence of her condition mounted Mr K found himself becoming more and more focused on his own deterioration until he became housebound and unable to work. Whenever he attempted to go to his office he became extremely anxious and on two separate occasions had to call for his wife to come and take him home because he was having a full-blown panic attack.

Although Mr K was eager to explore the relationship of his past experiences to the current state of affairs and to understand the relationship of his symptoms to his wife's illness, it became clear that Mr K needed some immediate relief from his panic states to even get to the physician's office. He agreed to begin a course of fluoxetine 40 mg daily and to continue his twice weekly psychotherapy. Within a month he was able to return to work and was generally free from panic symptoms and within 18 months was back to his jogging. At that time he expressed his desire to stop the medication but continues the psychotherapy. Two years later he terminated treatment feeling much improved and better prepared to cope with the uncertainty and responsibilities that lay ahead in his family situation.

Conclusion

Doing psychotherapy with patients suffering from functional somatic syndromes presents formidable challenges. Patients are often distrustful of physicians in general, who have failed to relieve their suffering and who have tended to dismiss the severity of their complaints. Care must, therefore, be taken in establishing a trusting relationship. Becoming embroiled in arguments with the patient over whether symptoms originate in the mind or the body will further alienate the patient. An approach which integrates psychological, biological and social factors in syndrome development avoids the anachronistic mind-versus-body debate that too often develops in the course of treating patients with functional somatic syndromes. If the physician can conceptualize the syndrome as being multifactorial in origin, he or she is free to listen to the patient's symptoms empathically and to respond with concern and respect for the person and his or her suffering.

Using the integrated model of functional somatic syndromes presented above (see Figure 12.3), treatment interventions can be instituted at various points in the system depending on the presenting complaint, as well as the needs, wishes, psychological make-up and financial resources of a particular patient. These interventions might include explanation, reassurance, cognitive behavioral therapy, antidepressants, anxiolytics and so forth. Psychodynamic treatment seems to be most beneficial to those patients who experience anxiety and depression as part of the syndrome and who believe that stress affects their symptoms (Guthrie, 1991).

The treatment of functional somatic syndromes requires the coordinated efforts of a variety of health professionals so as to minimize duplication of medical investigations, decrease costs to the health care system and most importantly to bring effective treatment to the patients as swiftly as possible. This will decrease the morbidity resulting from symptom chronicity. Those centers which specialize in the treatment of functional somatic syndromes stress an integrated psychobiological approach with early involvement of psychiatric consultants.

This chapter has attempted to outline the various psychotherapeutic techniques that have proved to be effective in the treatment of functional somatic syndromes. As well, it is hoped that the reader has gained an understanding of the psychological factors involved in the development and maintenance of these syndromes and has thereby gained an appreciation of the rationale behind the various treatment options presented.

References

Bacall HA & Newman MK (1990). *Theories of Object Relations: Bridges to Self Psychology*. New York: Columbia University Press.

Bass CM & Mayou R (1995). Chest pain and palpitations. In *Treatment of Functional Somatic Symptoms*, ed. R. Moyou, C. M. Bass & M. Sharpe, pp. 328–49. New York: Oxford University Press.

Beck AT, Rush AJ, Shaw BF & Emory G (1979). *Cognitive Therapy of Depression.* New York: Guilford Press.

Byrne E & Trounce I (1987). Chronic fatigue and myalgia syndrome: mitochondrial and glycolytic studies in skeletal muscle. *Journal of Neurological and Neurosurgical Psychiatry*, **50**, 743–6.

Demitrack MA, Dale JK & Straus SE (1991). Evidence for impaired activation of the hypothalamic-pituitary-adrenal axis in patients with chronic fatigue syndrome. *Journal of Clinical Endocrinological Metabolism*, **73**, 1224–33.

Dworkin SF, Turner JA, Wilson L, Massoth D, Whitney C, Huggins KH, Burgess J, Sommers E & Truelove E (1994). Brief group cognitive-behavioural intervention for temporomandibular disorders. *Pain*, **59**, 175–87.

Engel GL (1955). Studies of ulcerative colitis. III. The nature of the psychological processes. *American Journal of Medicine*, **19**, 231–56.

Farquar CM, Rogers V, Franks S, Pearce S, Wadsworth J & Beard RW (1990). A randomized controlled trial of medroxyprogesterone and psychotherapy for the treatment of pelvic congestion. *British Journal of Obstetrics and Gynaecology*, **6**, 1152–62.

Frank JD (1975). Psychotherapy of bodily disease. *Psychotherapy and Psychosomatics*, **26**, 192–202.

Greene B & Blanchard EB (1994). Cognitive therapy for irritable bowel syndrome. *Journal of Consulting and Clinical Psychology*, **62**, 576–82.

Guthrie E (1991). Brief psychotherapy with patients with refractory irritable bowel syndrome. *British Journal of Psychotherapy*, **8**, 175–88.

Guthrie E (1995). Treatment of functional somatic symptoms: psychodynamic treatment. In *Treatment of Functional Somatic Symptoms*, ed. R. Mayou, C. M. Bass & M. Sharpe, pp. 144–60. New York: Oxford University Press.

Hawton KE, Salkovskis P, Kirk J & Clark DM (1989). *Cognitive Therapy for Psychiatric Problems: A Practical Guide*. Oxford: Oxford University Press.

Kernberg OF (1984). *Severe Personality Disorders*. New Haven, CT: Yale University Press.

Kirkby RJ (1994). Changes in premenstrual symptoms and irrational thinking following cognitive-behavioral coping skills training. *Journal of Consult Clinical Psychology*, **62**, 1026–32.

Klimas NG, Salvato FR & Morgan R (1990). Immunologic abnormalities in the chronic fatigue syndrome. *Journal of Clinical Microbiology*, **28**, 1403–28.

Kohut H (1971). *The Analysis of the Self.* New York: International Universities Press.

Krystal H (1979). Alexithymia and psychotherapy. *American Journal of Psychotherapy*, **33**, 17–31.

Moldofsky H (1989). Nonrestorative sleep and symptoms after a febrile illness in patients with fibrositis and chronic fatigue syndromes. *Journal of Rheumatology*, **16**, (Suppl. 19), 150–3.

Pearce S (1983). A review of cognitive-behavioural methods for the treatment of chronic pain. *Journal of Psychosomatic Research*, **27**, 431–40.

Rodin G (1984). Somatization and the self. *American Journal of Psychotherapy*, **38**, 257–63.

Robbins JM & Kirmayer L (1991). Attributions of common somatic symptoms. *Psychological Medicine*, **21**, 1029–45.

Seligman MEP (1975). *Helplessness*. San Francisco: Freeman.
Sharpe M (1995). Cognitive behavioural therapies in the treatment of functional somatic symptoms. In *Treatment of Functional Somatic Symptoms*. ed. R. Mayou, C. M. Bass & M. Sharpe, pp. 122–43. New York: Oxford University Press.
Sharpe M, Bass CM & Mayou R (1995). An overview of the treatment of functional somatic syndromes. In *Treatment of Functional Somatic Symptoms*, ed. R. Mayou, C. M. Bass & M. Sharpe, pp. 66–86. New York: Oxford University Press.
Sharpe M, Hawton K, Simkins S, Suraway C, Hackmann A, Klimes I, Peto T, Warrell D & Seargroatt V (1996). Cognitive behaviour therapy for the chronic fatigue syndrome: a randomized controlled trial. *British Medical Journal*, **312**, 22–6.
Taerk G & Gnam W (1994). A psychodynamic view of the chronic fatigue syndrome. *General Hospital Psychiatry*, **16**, 319–25.
Taylor GJ (1977). Alexithymia and the countertransference. *Psychotherapy and Psychosomatics*, **28**, 141–7.
Taylor GJ (1992*a*). Psychosomatics and self-regulation. In *The Interface of Psychoanalysis and Psychology*, ed. J. W. Barron, M. N. Eagle & D. Wolitsky, pp. 464–88. Washington, DC: American Psychological Association Press.
Taylor GJ (1992*b*). Psychoanalysis and psychosomatics: a new synthesis. *Journal of the American Academy of Psychoanalysis*, **20**, 251–75.
Tilbe K & Sullivan S (1990). The extracolonic manifestations of the irritable bowel syndrome. *Canadian Medical Association Journal*, **142**, 539–40.
Wessely S & Sharpe M (1995). Chronic fatigue, chronic fatigue syndrome and fibromyalgia. In *Treatment of Functional Somatic Symptoms*, ed. R. Mayou, C. M. Bass & M. Sharpe, pp. 285–312. New York: Oxford University Press.
Wesseley S, Butler S, Chalder T & David A (1991). The cognitive behavioural management of the post-viral fatigue syndrome. In *Post-viral Fatigue Syndrome*, ed. R. Jenkins & J. Mowbray, pp. 305–34. New York: John Wiley.

13

Determination Of Disability Claimed By Patients With Functional Somatic Syndromes

PETER MANU

The evaluation of disability of patients with functional somatic syndromes has received only scant attention. A MEDLINE search of the literature published from 1983 through 1996 identified 7265 publications focusing on the nine syndromes discussed in this volume; the evaluation of disability was discussed in only 51 (0.7%). The situation is equally dismissive when seen from the vantage point of the scientific reports on disability evaluations for which MEDLINE lists 4560 publications: here, the 51 papers represent only 1.1% of the body of work. The distribution of these publications among the nine functional somatic syndromes (Table 13.1) indicates that only the disabilities claimed by patients with fibromyalgia and chronic fatigue syndrome (CFS) have been the object of sustained scientific attention and are discussed in detail in this chapter.

Clinical epidemiology

The only approximation of the period prevalence of occupational disability among patients with CFS and fibromyalgia is contained in a recent study of patients examined at the Chronic Fatigue Clinic of the University of Washington (Bombardier & Buchwald, 1996). The variable measured was employment status at the time of the initial examination and at follow-up 1.7 years (average) later. On both

Table 13.1. *MEDLINE citations (1983–96) of evaluation of disability of patients with functional somatic syndromes*

Syndrome	Total citations	Disability citations
Fibromyalgia	1047	33
Chronic fatigue syndrome	1139	12
Repetitive strain syndrome	37	2
Temporomandibular syndrome	1820	2
Irritable bowel syndrome	1066	1
Multiple chemical sensitivities	112	1
Premenstrual syndrome	1245	0
Interstitial cystitis	380	0
Atypical chest pain	251	0

occasions, patients were asked whether, during the past 3 months, they were able to remain at work on a full-time or part-time basis. The initial cohort consisted of 236 patients with a chief complaint of chronic fatigue who fulfilled criteria for CFS (147 patients, 81% women), fibromyalgia (28 patients, 89% women) or both (61 patients, 90% women). The duration of illness averaged five years. Retention in the study was high, with 232 patients providing follow-up data. Overall, two-thirds of the patients (67.4%) reported significant occupational disability; 40.7% felt unable to work at all. At follow-up, the unemployment rate (38.4%) was only marginally different; however, the employment rate increased from 32.6% to 42.6%. The change was due to the fact that a substantial proportion of patients who had remained at work on a part-time basis had returned to full-time employment. Using as a benchmark the notion that about 5% of adults in the US claim to be unable to work (Pope & Tarlov, 1991), the study concludes that there is considerable work disability among individuals with CFS and fibromyalgia.

The effect of sex on the point prevalence of occupational disability among patients with CFS was studied well in an Australian cohort (Lloyd & Pender, 1992). The average age was 34 years, and most patients were included in the range 25–54 years of age, which corresponded to an average adjusted unemployment rate in Australia of 12% for men and 39% for women. Before CFS, 27% of male patients and 48% of female patients had been unemployed. During the chronic fatigue illness, the rate of unemployment rate rose to 64% for men and 81% for women. The net increases were similar for males (37%) and females (34%).

Challenges created by the disability claims made by patients with functional somatic syndromes

The difficulties center around the need to confirm the patient's perception of disability created by clinical conditions whose severity cannot be measured by specific tests. Most of the time, the primary care physician supports the claim of disability by finding that the patient fulfills the diagnostic criteria for the condition and by noting the persistence of subjective reports of symptoms that may affect the patient's work potential. In both CFS and fibromyalgia, the common disabling symptoms consist of cognitive deficits and exercise intolerance (White et al., 1995; Bombardier & Buchwald, 1996). These symptoms lead to a number of major difficulties in determining the patient's ability to function. First, the subjective nature of these complaints raises the possibility of a discrepancy between self-reported and observed disability. Secondly, given the well-established association between psychiatric disorders and CFS and fibromyalgia, the potential for improvement after psychopharmacological and psychotherapeutic intervention must be given careful consideration. In addition to expert psychiatric evaluation and treatment, benefit-granting agencies are entitled to require that the principal disabling symptoms (e.g., cognitive deficits and exercise intolerance) be quantified through scientifically valid and reproducible testing. Thirdly, the contribution of pain to the creation and maintenance of the alleged disability must be carefully addressed, in a manner consistent with the American Medical Association's position that 'chronic pain and pain behaviors are not, per se, impairments, but they should trigger assessments of the ability to function and carry out daily activities' (AMA, 1993).

The discrepancy between self-reported and observed disability

Empirical research addressing this question has found a striking discordance between *self-assessed* and *observed* functional disability in patients with fibromyalgia (Hidding et al., 1994). The study compared patients given the diagnosis of fibromyalgia (1) with age- and sex-matched patients diagnosed to have rheumatoid arthritis and (2) with healthy control subjects. Six occupational therapists and six physicians with expertise in assessing disabilities participated as observers in the study. The observers were not told about the inclusion of the healthy control subjects and were unaware about the rheumatological diagnoses.

Patients with fibromyalgia and rheumatoid arthritis completed a questionnaire on disability at home that asked them to rate on visual analog scales their ability to perform the following seven activities; turn a key in a lock, put a book on the floor and pick it up, sit down and get up from a chair, tie shoelaces, write, climb up and down stairs, and lie down in bed and get out of bed. A retest of the self-reports was carried out ten days later. Five days after the self-reports the patients and the healthy control subjects actually performed the seven activities and were recorded on videotape. The videotapes were then assessed in random order by each of the 12 observers individually. Just like the patients, the observers recorded their assessment of functional disability on visual analog scales.

All observers assessed the healthy control subjects as having no evidence whatsoever of disability. Patients with fibromyalgia were found to have only modest degrees of disability, in striking contrast to the patients' own assessment of having severe disabilities for all seven activities. Overall, the fibromyalgia patients' self-reported disability was more than twice that noted by the independent observers. In contrast, for rheumatoid arthritis the discrepancy between self-report and observed scores reached statistical significance for only one activity.

The role of disabling psychiatric disorders, cognitive deficits and exercise intolerance

To illustrate this challenge, the disability created by CFS will be examined. A multisymptomatic illness, CFS is by definition associated with significant reduction in premorbid levels of occupational and social activities (Fukuda et al., 1994). Without exception, the CFS patients examined in a specialized clinic setting since 1986 have indicated that the main areas of disability involved their cognitive deficits (primarily difficulties with attention, concentration, executive function and memory impairment) and a reduction in physical endurance, rather than myalgia, sore throat or tender lymph nodes.

The Social Security Administration's guide (SSA Publication 64-603) for providing medical evidence for individuals with CFS was the starting point. The document directs the physician to show that the CFS exists according to medically acceptable findings and makes clear that symptoms alone cannot be the basis for a finding of disability. Patients with CFS, however, create significant problems for public and private institutions that adjudicate claims for total disability because the condition is defined exclusively in subjective terms. The complete reliance on symptoms stands in contrast to the main goal of a process meant to identify and measure the dysfunction that prevents the continuation of gainful employment. The critical importance of this issue was recognized in 1992 and 1994 at the last two national meetings of the American Association for Chronic Fatigue Syndrome. The position statements presented at the first of these meetings recommended tests of sustained activity, motor strength, stamina and neurocognitive function (Loveless et al., 1994). A workshop presented at the second of these meetings indicated that cardiopulmonary exercise testing, psychometric testing and psychiatric evaluation should be performed to document physical and neurocognitive losses (Harrison, 1995; Stevens, 1995). The empirical research basis for these recommendations can be found in studies demonstrating abnormalities in the cognitive function of CFS patients through the use of standard neuropsychological tests that measure information-processing speed, attention, language, perception, reasoning, problem-solving, sensory function and motor coordination (Grafman et al., 1993; Sandman et al., 1993; DeLuca et al., 1995). Similarly, changes in the physical performance of CFS patients have been provided by testing isometric and dynamic strength, exercise endurance and cardiopulmonary fitness (Riley et al., 1990; Maffuli et al., 1993; Sisto et al., 1996).

A construct was then used for the evaluation of cardiac functional capacity (Wenger, 1991) to infer that the determination of disability produced by CFS must: (1) establish a causal relationship between CFS and the inability to work; (2) demonstrate CFS-related cognitive and physical impairments; and (3) determine that the claimant has reached a critical reduction in the ability to perform work-related activities.

Two steps are required to establish a causal relationship between CFS and the alleged inability to return to work. The first is to ensure that the claimant's symptoms are sufficient for the CFS diagnosis and that a thorough medical work-up has excluded other conditions that can produce persistent tiredness. The second is to obtain a careful psychiatric examination to determine whether the claimant has a mental disorder that excludes CFS (e.g. bipolar affective disorder, delusional disorder). The psychiatric evaluation also serves the purpose of identifying and treating disabling mental disorders allowed to coexist with CFS (e.g. major unipolar depression, panic disorder).

The determination that the claimant qualified for total disability status as a result of CFS should therefore answer the following questions. Does the claimant have CFS? Have common comorbid psychiatric disorders been carefully evaluated and treated by a psychiatrist? Is there objective evidence of significant cognitive impairment? Is there objective evidence of a critical reduction of physical strength and endurance? These four questions were used as criteria for the evaluation of 92 successful claims for total disability referred for an independent assessment by claims managers from five private insurance companies.

The average age of the study group was 39.6 years (standard deviation 8.4 years). The patients had been placed on total disability for an average of 2.3 years (standard deviation 1.9 years). Of the 92 patients,

86% were women and 99% were white. The majority (72%) of patients had had managerial (32%), or clerical or sales (40%) jobs. Other traditional 'white-collar' occupations (25%) included teachers, attorneys, writers, nurses and engineers. Only three patients (3%) had been employed in 'blue-collar' jobs (two assembly line workers and one cook). The three most common therapeutic interventions were antidepressants (70%), rest (62%) and vitamins (50%).

The physicians recommending total disability status for these 92 patients were trained in internal medicine (28%), infectious diseases (26%), family medicine (21%), psychiatry (7%) and other specialty fields (18%). In some instances the physician's specialty was unusual for the task of providing care for adults suffering from an illness with the clinical complexity of CFS. For example, a pathologist diagnosed 'CFS secondary to Epstein–Barr virus' in a patient with major depression and panic disorder and an ear, nose and throat specialist requested total disability benefits for 'CFS and *Candida*-related complex' in a patient with previously diagnosed dysthymia and substance use disorder. The majority of physicians expressed strong convictions with regard to the etiology of CFS. The most commonly held beliefs were that CFS was produced by an immune dysfunction (36%) or a viral infection (26% of physicians).

The analysis of the data indicated that no case had been fully assessed and that one in three patients (34%) fulfilled none of the four criteria.

A substantial number (36%) of patients did not satisfy the standard definition of CFS, because of specified exclusionary clauses or insufficient symptoms (Fukuda et al., 1994). One example is that of a patient with 14 psychiatric hospitalizations in the past five years for major depression with psychotic features and multiple personality disorder. The CFS definition is clear in excluding patients with psychotic depression. Another example is that of a patient with a history of cocaine dependence diagnosed to have CFS and depression starting several weeks after cocaine detoxification. The CFS diagnosis cannot be given to patients where substance use disorder is active within two years before the onset of fatigue. A third example is that of a patient whose weight ranged from 148 kg to 156 kg during the year prior to the CFS diagnosis; the patient's height was 1.66 m. The height and average weight computed a body mass index of 55, well above the limit of 45 considered exclusionary by the CFS definition. Finally, other patients were excludable because they had clinical and laboratory evidence of physical disorders sufficient to explain their chronic fatigue illness, such as hypothyroidism, multiple sclerosis, obstructive sleep apnea and metastatic ovarian adenocarcinoma.

The degree to which the other disability evaluation criteria were met were even worse. Only 33% of patients had been referred for psychiatric evaluation. Despite the fact that all patients claimed total disability on the basis of exercise intolerance and cognitive deficits, only 14% had their strength and endurance objectively measured and only 13% underwent neuropsychological testing. These data are similar to the experience published with regard to a cohort of 111 patients with chronic low back pain; only 12% were found to have evidence of significant objective impairments (Strang, 1985).

The role of psychiatric disorders

The magnitude of the psychiatric morbidity of patients receiving disability benefits for a primary diagnosis of functional somatic syndrome can be easily demonstrated. In our group of 92 consecutive successful disability claims for CFS, 79% of patients had sufficient symptomatic evidence for at least one current psychiatric disorder. As expected, mood disorders constituted the most likely diagnoses; 59% of patients had had at least one episode of major depression during their fatigue illness, 7% were dysthymic and 3% suffered from bipolar disorder. Panic disorder (18%) and somatization disorder (15%) also had a high frequency in this group. Of interest is also the fact that the psychiatric morbidity of this group of disabled patients includes conditions not reported in other clinical studies of CFS, such as conversion disorder (4%), post-traumatic stress disorder (3%) and dissociative disorders (3%). The findings support data recently collected in Australia showing that among chronic fatigue syndrome patients there is a statistically homogeneous subgroup characterized by more disability and a higher current psychiatric morbidity (Hickie et al., 1995). As demonstrated throughout this volume, a high psychiatric morbidity can be expected among patients with any functional somatic syndrome, underscoring the fact that a competent psychiatric evaluation is necessary in all cases in which these illnesses show an unfavorable progression or when the patients are claiming total disability.

Evaluation of cognitive ability

Neuropsychological disturbances, particularly poor memory and difficulty with tasks that require sustained attention and concentration, are commonly reported among the disabling symptoms of patients with CFS (Grafman, 1996) and fibromyalgia. Because of its use in clinical practice and litigation, primarily for the diagnosis of dementing illnesses and adjudication of claims following traumatic closed-head injuries, neuropsychological testing is widely available, has high reliability for deficit detection and allows the assessment of motivation to perform poorly, an important issue given the effect of financial incentives on symptoms and disability (Binder & Rohling, 1996). The neuropsychological evaluation, in conjunction with subjective measures of functional ability, is the premier way to determine cognitive disability. It typically examines motor coordination and strength, sensory functions, information-processing speed, attention, language, perception, reasoning and problem-solving, memory, mood state and personality. When job-specific requirements are taken into consideration, performance on individual neuropsychological tests can be significantly correlated with occupational function (Grafman, 1996). Motivation will affect performance, but experienced neuropsychologists will be able to assess its impact by evaluating the consistency and pattern of performance across many measures. Malingering can be detected through a specific test of the validity of memory complaints. The patient is told that 15 different items will be presented for memorization. These are in fact grouped items that require the recall of only three categories. Patients have ten seconds to view the items. Recall of fewer than nine items indicates malingering or advanced dementia.

The CFS patients referred for disability evaluation will have marked complaints of cognitive deficits, particularly in the domains of memory, attention and concentration, and problem-solving. A majority of patients will also have marked complaints of emotional distress. The first challenge for the neuropsychologist evaluating CFS patients is the recognition of disease-specific deficits (e.g. decreased response speed and difficulty remembering well-structured information) in a context in which many tests of memory and cognitive processing are within normal limits and remain accurate over time (Grafman, 1996). The second challenge is to correlate the subjective and objective evidence of disabling mental fatigue with the results of the evaluation of mood state and personality scales measuring anxiety, depression and somatization. A careful analysis of these data sets can help to sort out confounding variables, most notably the decreased effort and alertness due to a depressive disorder, which may affect performance on cognitive tasks (Altay et al., 1990; Grafman et al., 1993; Sandman et al., 1993; DeLuca et al., 1995; Grafman, 1996).

The following two case presentations illustrate the role of neuropsychological evaluation in establishing job-specific disability produced by CFS.

Case 1

A 41-year-old software engineer with a 10-month history of exhaustion, poor memory, pain over his body, confusion and nausea had performed well prior to this illness in a demanding managerial position, while at the same time pursuing an advanced degree in business administration.

The estimate of the premorbid function indicated a Full-scale IQ of 118, Performance IQ of 114 and a Verbal IQ of 119. The mental status examination indicated that the claimant was not in the demented or borderline range. He scored in the depressed range on a standard scale, but did not express depressive tendencies during the interview. The test of malingering tendencies was performed within the normal range. Performance on the Boston Naming Test was within normal limits, indicating that language deficits did not contribute to the complaint of memory difficulty. Tests of memory indicated a number of significant abnormalities. First, the patient overestimated his ability; he expected to recall 10 words and actually recalled 6 of 12 words. Secondly, his reaction time during an Item Recognition subtest was very slow, reflecting serious psychomotor compromise. Accuracy was maintained by a process which obtained correct results by a two-fold delay in reaction time. Thirdly, his memory for a simple story was in the 56th percentile, indicating a substantial loss in the ability to listen and recall a paragraph. Fourthly, the delayed memory for patterns was relatively impaired (74th percentile) for both visual and verbal information.

The examining neuropsychologist concluded that the claimant could not perform his supervisory software engineering job because his decision speed was greatly compromised, he suffered general intellectual impairment (especially in the visual/spatial and analytical domains), he exhibited focal (verbal) memory deficits and he overestimated his ability to recall information.

Case 2

A 37-year-old woman had a 11-month history of disabling chronic fatigue syndrome. She held a master's degree in business administration and was employed in an executive position by a large financial corporation. Her symptoms included cognitive impairment, including difficulty concentrating on written material (must re-read material because she could not process information), an inability to focus, word-finding difficulty, deteriorating spelling and poor memory (especially for names). A comprehensive evaluation of functional capacity for the physical demands of the job found her able to work at the sedentary level for a 4-hour day.

Her premorbid IQ placed her in the Above Average range

> of intellectual functioning. Although she performed adequately on many cognitive tasks, there were several specific deficits. They were most clearly demonstrated during the Wisconsin Card Sort Test (WCST). The WCST was devised to study abstract behavior and the ability to shift tests. The patient must determine the principles involved in organizing symbols into categories such as color, shape or number. In this case, the claimant placed in the 5th percentile for categories completed, 6th percentile for perseverative and nonperseverative errors and in the 1st percentile for the conceptual level of her responses. She also demonstrated deficits on a test of motor coordination (Grooved Pegboard). There was no emotional overlay and her current treatment was not considered to account for the cognitive problems.
>
> The neuropsychologist concluded that the claimant was unable to perform her supervisory job as a financial analyst because of cognitive inflexibility, impaired short-term visual memory and an inability to form abstract concepts.

Recent field experience supports the use of neuropsychological testing for the evaluation of disability, as shown in a recent publication describing the cognitive deficits of CFS patients (Marcel et al., 1996). The 29 patients included in the study were recurrently housebound or bedridden and felt unable to work full-time. Their mean age was 39.6 years and they had an average of 14.3 years of education. Their fatigue illness had an average duration of 5.7 years. An age- and sex-matched control group comprised 25 healthy subjects with an average of 16.3 years of education. Patients and control subjects were administered a battery of standardized neuropsychological tests and a set of tasks adapted for administration by computer to better measure speed and the accuracy of response. The primary differences between patients and control subjects were found on tests of memory and learning. Immediate recall was clearly impaired, as demonstrated by significant differences on the Wechsler Memory Scale (Russell, 1975) and also on a word list learning task and a pattern memory task. Other domains significantly impaired were those of language, spatial ability, and set shifting and conceptualization. The differences retained their significance when the degree of psychiatric symptomatology and psychoactive treatments were covaried, reinforcing the clinical validity of these assessments for the evaluation of disability claimed by CFS sufferers.

Evaluation of exercise tolerance

The evaluation of physical capacity must take into account the fact that exercise tolerance is the result of combined normal performance of the respiratory, cardiovascular and musculoskeletal systems. The method of testing consists of an integrated cardiopulmonary exercise study protocol which confirms the presence of the alleged impairment, quantifies its severity and pinpoints the system responsible (Hansen & Wasserman, 1996).

Prior to testing, a history and physical examination, a resting electrocardiogram, a chest radiograph and a spirometric evaluation of pulmonary function are obtained. The testing uses a 20-minute exercise protocol to evaluate the functional status during four stages: rest, constant low intensity exercise (e.g. 3–4 minutes of treadmill walking at zero grade inclination), incremental exercise to tolerance (7–10 minutes during which the grade of incline is increased 1–3% every minute), and recovery. Exercise is stopped by the investigator if the patient develops chest pain, significant arrhythmia, marked changes in blood pressure, lightheadedness or pallor. If the patient stops exercising prematurely, the test can be repeated after a short rest period. Data collected during the exercise testing of disability claimants is compared with the normative values for a sedentary working population, with appropriate corrections for age, sex and body height (Hansen & Wasserman, 1996).

The main variable measured during integrated exercise testing is oxygen uptake, measured in l/min or ml/min per kg. The measurement reflects the fitness of the cardiovascular system and the size of the muscle mass involved in the task. The goal here is to determine the level of effort at which the blood pressure, heart rate, ventilation and output of carbon dioxide are maintained constant without increasing the oxygen debt or producing lactic acidosis. A related variable is the lactic acidosis threshold, because levels of effort that produce lactic acidosis require rest periods for recovery. In a normal person, the onset of lactic acidosis occurs when the patient reaches 45–60% of his or her peak oxygen uptake. A lactic acidosis threshold that occurs at less than 40% of the predicted peak of oxygen uptake is abnormal and reflects circulatory dysfunction or deconditioning. Two other measurements have clinical significance: the oxygen uptake/work rate relationship, which may discover an oxygen diffusion defect at the capillary level; and the oxygen uptake/heart rate relationship, which helps to define subtle decreases of the maximal cardiac stroke volume or the inability to exercise to higher levels because of systemic disease. Other measurements address pulmonary mechanics, ventilation/perfusion mismatching, analysis of the S-T segment depression on electrocardiogram and the changes in the arterial oxygen saturation (Hansen & Wasserman, 1996).

In addition to documenting poor exercise tolerance, integrated cardiopulmonary exercise testing is extremely useful in defining its possible cause. Abnormalities of the heart, pulmonary vasculature and peripheral small vessels have already been mentioned. In addition, testing is useful in assessing the work intolerance created by obesity (increased oxygen uptake requirements at all work levels), obstructive lung disease, restrictive lung disease, anemia, cigarette smoking, adrenergic blockade and defects in bioenergetics (muscle pain during maximal exercise without elevation of blood lactate values). Of great importance is the ability of the integrated testing to detect poor effort in situations in which the disability claimant had stopped exercise. The finding of a low peak oxygen uptake, a high heart rate reserve, a high breathing reserve and a normal lactic acidosis threshold are among the variables indicating that the claimant has not performed at his or her true potential. Testing anxiety is characterized by bizarre or irregular ventilatory pattern and an elevated heart rate at rest; these manifestations are usually overridden by the requirements of the increased work rate (Hansen & Wasserman, 1996).

The integrated cardiopulmonary exercise assessment can be complemented by direct measurements of muscular strength. A recent study has used such an approach to evaluate eight athletes with postviral fatigue syndrome (Maffulli et al., 1993). Prior to their illness they routinely competed at regional or national level and had been training an average of 80 minutes a day, for six days a week. They were part of a longitudinal study of healthy athletes prior to the index viral infection. Selection for postillness evaluation was based on the fact that, one month after the clinical resolution of the viral infection, they were still complaining of profound chronic fatigue. The infectious agent was the Epstein–Barr virus in four cases, cytomegalovirus in three and Coxsackie virus in one. In addition to the maximal oxygen uptake and the anaerobic threshold, measurements included the maximal voluntary isometric contraction of the elbow flexor and knee extensor muscles. Data were collected prior to illness and at 1, 3, 7, 10 and 13 months after the viral illness. The results indicated that although maximal oxygen uptake has returned to normal 13 months after the viral illness, the anaerobic threshold was still significantly reduced. Moreover, strength endurance was still significantly reduced by the end of the study, e.g. subjects were able to maintain maximal isometric contraction of the arm muscles for a preinfection average of 46 seconds, but only 29 seconds at one year after infection.

The study confirms the fact that serial observations of exercise tolerance are reliable means for documenting changes difficult to quantify during standard physical examinations. Such testing protocols can be safely employed for patients with CFS. Despite a low fitness level, one such group demonstrated the ability to withstand a maximal treadmill exercise test without a major exacerbation of either fatigue or other symptoms of their illness (Sisto et al., 1996).

Additional clinical data supporting the role of integrated cardiopulmonary testing in assessing the functional capacity of CFS patients have been published recently (Make, 1997). The investigator measured the muscle strength and exercise tolerance of CFS patients and two control groups, healthy subjects and patients with a primary diagnosis of mood disorder. Isokinetic testing indicated that the fatigability, endurance and recovery of the elbow and knee muscles of CFS patients were similar to the values recorded in the control groups. CFS patients showed significant reduction in the maximal work and oxygen consumption compared with healthy control subjects and depressed patients.

The role of chronic pain in the initiation and maintenance of disability

Most disability rating systems in the USA, including those used by the Social Security Administration, the Department of Veterans' Affairs and the American Medical Association, take the consistent position that chronic pain cannot be considered impairment or the cause of impairment (Aronoff, 1996). Nevertheless, an attempt to measure pain must be part of the evaluation when pain is considered among the disabling symptoms by the patient or the supporting attending physician. A number of self-report instruments have been developed to assess pain severity and its associated symptoms and consequences (Aronoff, 1996). For example, the West Haven–Yale Multidimensional Pain Inventory (Kerns et al., 1985) evaluates the patient's ability to participate in common daily activities and the response of others to the patient's communication of pain; the Vanderbilt Pain Management Inventory (Brown & Nicassio, 1987) addresses the patient's coping style, and the McGill Pain Questionnaire (Melzack, 1975) measures the intensity and the affective and sensory components of the pain experience. An important task for the disability evaluator is to determine whether the allegedly disabling chronic pain symptom belongs to a functional somatic syndrome (CFS or fibromyalgia) or is the defining complaint of a discrete chronic pain syndrome. Patients with chronic pain syndrome (also called somatoform pain disorder when no anatomical cause or pathophysiological explanation are found) have an intense preoccupation with pain (and not with tiredness or cognitive difficulty), use pain as a symbolic means of communication, show passivity, have strong dependency needs, are unable to deal appropriately with anger and hostility and have a developmental history remarkable for emotional neglect, a high incidence of alcoholism in the family, childhood trauma and early adult responsibilities (Aronoff, 1996). These characteristics are only occasionally identified among patients with CFS and fibromyalgia. Extreme caution in making a diagnosis of disabling CFS or fibromyalgia is appropriate when the claimant has had multiple pain-related surgeries without beneficial results, is involved in pain-related litigation (workers' compensation or personal injury), has evidence of major psychopathology and a history of overuse of health care services (Aronoff, 1996). In these cases, the disability evaluation should become the responsibility of a multidisciplinary team in a specialized pain center.

Conclusion

The scientific evidence and clinical experience support a paradigmatic shift in the evaluation of disability of patients with functional somatic syndromes. After the identification and treatment of the pain component, the determination that a claimant qualified for total disability status as a result of a functional somatic syndrome should attempt to answer the following four questions. Does the claimant have the syndrome in question? Have common comorbid psychiatric disorders been carefully evaluated and treated by a professional with expertise in pharmacology and psychotherapy? Is there objective evidence of cognitive impairment? Is there objective evidence of a critical reduction in muscle strength and endurance? This framework can lead to standardized and quality-controllable sequential processes that will determine the severity of the dysfunction, define the goals of vocational and social rehabilitation and enable specific changes in the work environment and job requirements to be addressed.

References

Altay HT, Toner BB, Brooker H, Abbey SE, Salit IE & Garfinkel PE (1990). The neuropsychological dimensions of postinfectious neuromyasthenia (chronic fatigue syndrome): a preliminary report. *International Journal of Psychiatry and Medicine*, **20**, 141–9.

American Medical Association (1993). *Guides to the Evaluation of Permanent Disability*, 4th edn. Chicago, IL: American Medical Association.

Aronoff GM (1996). Pain. In *Disability Evaluation*, ed. S.L. Demeter, G. B. J. Andersson & G. M. Smith, pp. 529–42. St. Louis, MO: American Medical Association, Mosby-Year Book.

Binder LM & Rohling ML (1996). Money matters: a meta-analytic review of the effects of financial incentives on recovery after closed-head injury. *American Journal of Psychiatry*, **153**, 7–10.

Bombardier CH & Buchwald D (1996). Chronic fatigue, chronic fatigue syndrome and fibromyalgia. Disability and health-care use. *Medical Care*, **34**, 924–30.

Brown GK & Nicassio PM (1997). Development of a questionnaire for the assessment of active and passive coping strategies in chronic pain patients. *Pain*, **31**, 53–64.

DeLuca J, Johnson SK, Beldowicz D & Natelson BH (1995). Neuropsychological impairment in chronic fatigue syndrome, multiple sclerosis, and depression. *Journal of Neurology, Neurosurgery and Psychiatry*, **58**, 34–43.

Fukuda K, Straus SE, Hickie I, Sharpe MC, Dobbins JG, Komaroff A and the International Chronic Fatigue Study Group (1994). The chronic fatigue syndrome: a comprehensive approach to its definition and study. *Annals of Internal Medicine*, **121**, 953–9.

Grafman J (1996). Neuropsychological assessment of patients with chronic fatigue syndrome. In *Chronic Fatigue Syndrome: An Integrative Approach to Evaluation and Treatment*. ed M.A. Demitrack & S.E. Abbey, pp. 113–29. New York: Guilford Press.

Grafman J, Schwartz V, Dale JK, Scheffers M, Houser C & Strans SE (1993). Analysis of neuropsychological functioning in patients with the chronic fatigue syndrome. *Journal of Neurology, Neurosurgery and Psychiatry*, **56**, 684–9.

Hansen JE & Wasserman K (1996). Integrated cardiopulmonary exercise testing. In *Disability Evaluation*, ed. S. L. Demeter, G. B. J. Andersson & G. M. Smith, pp. 318–37. St. Louis, MO: American Medical Association, Mosby-Year Book.

Harrison AL (1995). Development and evaluation of claims involving chronic fatigue syndrome (CFS) under the Social Security disability provisions. *Journal of Chronic Fatigue Syndrome*, **1**, 131–3.

Hickie I, Lloyd A, Hadzi-Pavlovic D, Parker G, Bird K & Wakefield D (1995). Can the chronic fatigue syndrome be defined by distinct clinical features? *Psychological Medicine*, **25**, 925–35.

Hidding A, van Santen M, De Klerk E, Gielen X, Boers M, Geenen R, Vlaeyen J, Kester A & van der Linden S (1994). Comparison between self-report measures and clinical observations of functional disability in ankylosing spondylitis, rheumatoid arthritis and fibromyalgia. *Journal of Rheumatology*, **21**, 818–23.

Kerns RD, Turk DC & Rudy TE (1985). The West Haven–Yale Multidimensional Pain Inventory. *Pain*, **23**, 345–56.

Lloyd AR & Pender H (1992). The economic impact of the chronic fatigue syndrome. *Medical Journal of Australia*, **157**, 599–601.

Loveless MO, Lloyd A & Perpich R (1994). Summary of public policy and chronic fatigue syndrome: a perspective. *Clinical and Infectious Diseases*, **18** (Suppl. 1), S163–S165.

Maffuli N, Testa V & Capasso G (1993). Post-viral syndrome: a longitudinal assessment in varsity athletes. *Journal of Sport Medicine and Physical Fitness*, **33**, 392–9.

Make B (1997). Muscle strength and exercise tolerance in chronic fatigue syndrome. *Journal of Chronic Fatigue Syndrome*, (in press).

Marcel B, Komaroff AL, Fagioli L, Kornish RJ & Albert MS (1996). Cognitive deficits in patients with chronic fatigue syndrome. *Biological Psychiatry*, **40**, 535–41.

Melzack R (1975). The McGill Pain Questionnaire. *Pain*, **1**, 277–99.

Pope A & Tarlov A (1991). Disability in America: toward a national agenda for prevention. Washington, DC: Institute of Medicine, National Academy Press.

Riley MS, O'Brien CJ, McCluskey DR, Bell NP & Nichols DP (1990). Aerobic work capacity in patients with chronic fatigue syndrome. *British Medical Journal*, **301**, 953–6.

Russell EW (1975). A multiple scoring method for the assessment of complex memory functions. *Journal of Consulting and Clinical Psychology*, **43**, 800–9.

Sandman CA, Barron JL, Nackoul K, Goldstein J & Fidler F (1993). Memory deficits associated with chronic fatigue immune dysfunction syndrome. *Biological Psychiatry*, **33**, 618–23.

Sisto SA, LaManca J, Cordero DL, Bergen MT, Ellis SP, Drastal S, Boda WL, Tapp WN & Natelson BH (1996). Metabolic and cardiovascular effects of a progressive exercise test in patients with chronic fatigue syndrome. *American Journal of Medicine*, **100**, 634–40.

Stevens SR (1995). Using exercise testing to document functional disability in CFS. *Journal of Chronic Fatigue Syndrome*, **1**, 127–9.

Strang JP (1985). The chronic disability syndrome. In *The Evaluation and Treatment of Chronic Pain*, ed. G. M. Aronoff. Baltimore, MD: Urban & Schwartzenberg.

Wenger NK (1991). Ability, disability and the functional capacity of patients with cardiovascular disease. *Transactions of the Association of Life Insurance and Medical Directors*, **74**, 78–91.

White KP, Harth M & Teasell RW (1995). Work disability evaluation and the fibromyalgia syndrome. *Seminars in Arthritis and Rheumatism*, **24**, 371–81.

14

Functional Somatic Syndromes: Exploring Common Denominators

PETER MANU

As the preceding chapters have amply demonstrated, the search for answers to the questions raised by the existence and clinical importance of functional somatic syndromes has proceeded with increasing intensity and sophistication in the past decade. In addition to uncovering many individualizing dimensions of these syndromes, the research has also identified a number of methodologies that can be applied across the spectrum of these functional illnesses to investigate similarities and discrepancies. In this chapter, major research directions in the study of each of the nine syndromes are described and an attempt is made to highlight the following overlapping dimensions: biological markers of serotonergic responsivity in chronic fatigue syndrome and premenstrual syndrome; physical and psychological trauma in patients with fibromyalgia and irritable bowel syndrome; cognitive and sensory deficits of patients with premenstrual syndrome, multiple chemical sensitivity and repetitive strain injury; magnetic resonance and isotopic imaging and the psychological profiles of patients with temporomandibular joint dysfunction syndrome and atypical chest pain; biological dimensions, such as the genetic transmission of fibromyalgia and the experimental production of cellular abnormalities associated with interstitial cystitis. Finally, Gulf War illness is described, which has now been characterized as a collection of symptom-clusters overlapping with many of the functional somatic syndromes described in this volume.

Chronic fatigue syndrome: serotonergic responsivity; cognitive behavior therapy

The fact that a substantial proportion of chronic fatigue syndrome (CFS) patients have concurrent symptoms sufficient for a diagnosis of major depression has prompted the investigation of the serotonin function with the new method of *d*-fenfluramine challenge. The method is based on the serotonin-releasing effect of *d*-fenfluramine and on the serotonin effect on prolactin levels. The effect is highly specific and well-tolerated by patients. Blunted serotonergic responsivity, as indicated by lower prolactin levels after fenfluramine challenges, have been consistently demonstrated in depressed patients (Mann et al., 1995; Cleare et al., 1996). A controlled study comparing CFS with healthy subjects showed no difference in baseline and fenfluramine-induced responses between the two groups. Although about half of the CFS group had been given a diagnosis of depressive disorder, there was no correlation between the response to fenfluramine challenge and the severity of the depressive symptomatology (Yatham et al., 1995). A superior research design was employed by a group of investigators from the Maudsley Hospital and King's College Hospital, London (Cleare et al., 1995). The subjects were 10 patients with CFS (mean age 35 years) and 15 patients with major depression (mean age 39 years); each clinical group was closely matched with a similar-sized group of healthy control subjects. The CFS participants did not have evidence of a comorbid depressive disorder. Prolactin levels were measured at baseline and hourly for 5 hours after the oral administration of 30 mg of *d*-fenfluramine. To explore the relationship between serotonin-mediated neurotransmission and the function of the hypothalamic-pituitary-adrenal axis the authors performed concomitant serum cortisol assays. Analyses of the data were appropriately controlled for the phase of menstrual cycle, age, sex and weight.

Prolactin responses were lowest for the group of patients with major depressive disorder and highest for the CFS group. As expected, the depressed group had considerably lower prolactin levels after fenfluramine challenge compared with healthy control subjects. Statistically significant differences were also observed in the direct comparisons of the postchallenge prolactin levels between CFS patients and both control subjects and depressed patients. Compared with the CFS group, cortisol levels were significantly higher in the depressed group. A strong inverse correlation was observed between postchallenge prolactin and baseline cortisol levels. The healthy control responses fell halfway between the two study groups. The interpretation of the data was based on the clinical differences between the two groups of patients. According to the selection criteria used to assemble the study cohort, anorexia, insomnia and agitation were prominent among this group of depressed patients, but were not shown by the CFS patients, who in turn were much more likely to complain of hypersomnia and hyperphagia. The findings emphasize the role of serotonergic transmission in the modulation of general arousal, motor activity, feeding and sleep, and may explain why the nondepressed CFS patients responded poorly to treatment with selective serotonin reuptake inhibitors (Vercoulen et al., 1996). Of much interest is the finding that the enhancement of the prolactin response to fenfluramine observed in CFS has also been demonstrated in drug-naive schizophrenic patients (Abel et al., 1996), raising the possibility that drugs known to influence serotonergic activity in schizophrenia may be useful in carefully selected individuals with CFS.

The potential for progress in the psychopharmacology of CFS is just one piece of good news; another is the recent work that has established the role of cognitive-behavioral therapy for patients with this functional somatic syndrome (Deale et al., 1997). This contribution was needed to arbitrate contradictory results produced by previous studies, i.e. lack of significant clinical change in an Australian population (Lloyd et al., 1993) as contrasted with the encouragingly stable betterment noted in a British study (Sharpe et al., 1996) already reviewed in this volume. The research team recruited patients from a well-established specialized clinic operating at King's College Hospital, London. After a comprehensive medical and psychiatric evaluation, the 60 patients were randomly assigned to 13 sessions of either relaxation therapy or cognitive-behavioral therapy. All patients were seen individually and detailed session-by-session treatment manuals were used throughout the four to six months of therapy. The relaxation group received instruction regarding progressive muscle relaxation and visualization and were taught rapid relaxation skills; these techniques were then practiced twice daily at home. The cognitive-behavioral therapy used a structured, collaborative and negotiated protocol to convince patients that they could increase activities without exacerbating their symptoms. Daily targets, sleep routines and cognitive strategies were carefully monitored to obtain increased endurance and reduced periods of rest. The main outcome measures were functional ability, severity of fatigue and degree of psychological distress. The improvement criterion was met if the patients were able to carry out moderate activities, without limitations at the six-month follow-up.

The 30 patients entered in the trial of cognitive-behavioral therapy had a mean age of 31 years and had had an illness duration of 3.4 years. The majority of patients were receiving disability benefits (53%) and had past (30%) or current (37%) psychiatric diagnoses. Most patients (57%) attributed their symptoms to a physical illness. The patients in the relaxation group were somewhat older (mean age 38 years), but similar in all of the other characteristics with the cognitive-behavioral group. Three patients withdrew from cognitive-behavioral therapy and four from relaxation (two patients found the relaxation exercises too tiring).

At the six-month follow-up, 17 (63%) of the 27 patients who had received cognitive-behavioral therapy, but only four (15%) of the 26 patients who completed the relaxation therapy program, were no longer 'fatigue cases'. A total of 70% of the patients who completed the cognitive-behavioral therapy trial were improved, compared with 19% of those who had been enrolled in the relaxation therapy trial. Moreover, the magnitude of the improvement was substantially larger in the cognitive-behavioral group, as indicated by a change in the physical functioning score from an average of 24 to 85; the improved relaxation patients moved their average score from 33 to 70. Thus, a small group of patients in the cognitive-behavioral group appears to have gained in terms of physical ability, but remained fatigued and symptomatic. Detailed analyses indicated that both groups made linear progress during the first half of the treatment period, but only the cognitive-behavioral group continued its improvement afterwards. Illness attribution style and psychiatric diagnosis did not influence the outcome. Patients who made new claims for disability benefits during the trial did not improve. Altogether, these data indicate that supervised graded activity and cognitive restructuring produces substantial subjective improvement and restoration of functional status. It is also clear that this response was not due to a placebo effect or to the support provided by an empathic and knowledgeable caregiver.

Fibromyalgia: genetic factors; influence of trauma

A genetic factor responsible for the family aggregation of fibromyalgia has recently been demonstrated among patients attending the rheumatology clinic of the University Hospital, Beer Sheva, Israel (Buskila et al., 1996). The investigation focused on 20 complete nuclear families identified through a previously diagnosed mother. All 58 (60% males, median age 17 years) offspring agreed to a comprehensive interview and a complete physical examination. Main variables were age, sex, tenderness assessment (manual palpation and dolorimetry), symptoms, quality of life and physical functioning. The authors hypothesized that family aggregation would result in a significantly higher prevalence of fibromyalgia compared with the demonstrated 2% prevalence of the syndrome in the general population (Wolfe et al., 1995).

Sixteen offspring (28%) were found to have fibromyalgia; sex-specific frequencies were 39% for females and 20% for males. The prevalence of the syndrome in the 9–15 years age group was 33% for females and 50% for males. For females between the ages of 30 and 46 years the age-specific prevalence increases to 66%; offspring males in the same age group have a prevalence of 25%. In the general population, the prevalence for this age group is 3.4% for females and 0.5% for males. The presence of a genetic component rather than environmental or psychological influences was demonstrated by the fact that there were no significant differences in measures of global well-being, physical functioning, anxiety and depression between offspring with and without the syndrome and between offspring who were still at home and those who lived independently of their affected parent. These data confirm previous work (Pellegrino et al., 1989) that the idiopathic fibromyalgia has a genetic component of the autosomal dominant type, with complete penetration in women (observed prevalence approaching the expected 50%) and either weaker expressivity or decreased penetrance in males. Given the equally high prevalence among boys and girls, a greater likelihood of persistent remission may explain the lower prevalence of the syndrome among middle-aged male offspring. As an explanation for the observed family aggregation, the monogenic mode of inheritance appeared to be clearly superior to a polygenic multifactorial model which would have predicted only a 5% crude prevalence among first-degree relatives.

Given the strong family aggregation of fibromyalgia, it appears useful to examine the sporadic cases in which environmental factors appear decisive in initiating the illness. Fortunately, a group of pain researchers have recently published the results of an investigation between idiopathic and post-traumatic fibromyalgia (Turk et al., 1996). The initial study cohort comprised 153 consecutive fibromyalgia patients referred by community rheumatologists to the Pain Evaluation and Treatment Institute, University of Pittsburgh Medical Center. All patients met standard diagnostic criteria; 46 reported that their fibromyalgia symptoms were related to injury due to a work-related accident (19 patients), a motor vehicle accident (18 patients) and other physical trauma (nine patients). The control group was assembled by randomly selecting 46 patients with idiopathic onset of fibromyalgia who were matched for age and duration of pain with the members of the trauma onset group. The measurements included a comprehensive and standardized physical examination and diagnostic tests, a multidimensional pain inventory, a psychometric assessment of depressive symptomatology and a self-report measure of level of functioning or disability. The financial compensation status was ascertained and treated as a covariate in subsequent analyses.

The degree of physical abnormalities, depressive symptomatology and the level of support were similar in the two groups. Patients with posttraumatic onset reported significantly higher affective distress, perceived disability and pain severity and claimed a much lower general activity level. The patterns of response to pain were also substantially different; the primary profiles of 'dysfunction' and 'interpersonal distress' were found in 82% of the post-traumatic onset patients, but in only 38% of the idiopathic onset group. On the other hand, a significantly larger proportion of patients with idiopathic onset of fibromyalgia were found to be 'adaptive copers', a state characterized by low levels of affective distress and a greater sense of control over their lives. In aggregate, these substantial differences indicate that the clinical definition of fibromyalgia identifies at least two distinct populations. At this time, it seems prudent to recommend the recognition of these subgroups for clinical and research classifications and to study the effect of traumatic onset, claimed disability and status of financial compensation on symptom severity, response to treatment and quality of life.

Irritable bowel syndrome: association with chronic pelvic pain and childhood sexual abuse; cognitive behavior therapy

The overlap between chronic pelvic pain and irritable bowel syndrome was recently evaluated by a team of researchers from the University of Washington (Walker et al., 1996). The setting of the study was an urban gastroenterology outpatient clinic and the population consisted of 60 sequential patients given the diagnosis of irritable bowel syndrome. A control group included 26 patients with well-documented inflammatory bowel disease. Highly structured interviews were used to assess maltreatment in childhood (physical, emotional and sexual abuse), a lifetime history of chronic pelvic pain that had to be distinguishable from the history of bowel distress, and past and current psychiatric disorders.

Chronic pelvic pain was reported by 14% of inflammatory bowel group and by 35% of patients with a diagnosis of irritable bowel syndrome. The presence of chronic pelvic pain in patients with irritable bowel was associated with a significantly higher likelihood of childhood sexual abuse, current panic disorder and a lifetime history of dysthymia and somatization disorder.

These data support the growing evidence of a relationship between gastrointestinal illness and a history of physical and sexual abuse. The issue was comprehensively addressed by a task force organized by the Functional Brain–Gut Research Group of the American Gastroenterology Association (Drossman et al., 1995). The authors recognized the primacy of the abuse history and psychosocial disturbance and proposed several explanatory models, including enhanced visceral sensitivity, psychophysiological changes and psychodynamic effects. The enhanced visceral sensitivity model postulates that the traumatic stimulation of the anus and vagina in childhood leads to neural changes that decrease the activation thresholds of visceral nociceptors and amplify the perception of abdominal and pelvic pain. The psychophysiological model assumes that psychological distress produces the activation of autonomic pathways and direct central nervous system to enteric nerve endings pathways, resulting in increased intestinal motility and abdominal discomfort. Finally, the psychodynamic model is based on the observation that childhood sexual abuse results in the labeling of the anus/rectum or vulva/vagina as 'dirty' and 'bad'. These feelings call for punishment through physical suffering in the abdomen, pelvis or the genitourinary area. The task force emphasized that abdominal and pelvic pain are only two of the symptoms of a postabuse syndrome that includes pelvic dyssynergia (a form of obstructive defecation resulting in severe constipation), sexual dysfunction, unexplained vomiting, eating disorders and morbid obesity. Abnormal illness behaviors are the norm and are expressed, according to this meta-analysis, in claims of disability clearly disproportionate to the objective clinical data, requests for multiple diagnostic procedures and surgeries, and intense and chaotic attachments to health care providers.

Given the etiological importance of psychological distress in patients with irritable bowel syndrome, attention has been recently focused on efforts to change somatic attribution and maladaptive cognition. Economic imperatives have directed the investigation of interventions for groups, rather than individual patients. Short-term, uncontrolled trials of cognitive-behavioral group therapy have shown encouraging results (Wise et al., 1982; Blanchard & Schwarz, 1987). A recent study, performed in the Outpatient Internal Medicine Clinic of the University of Nijmegen, Nijmegen, The Netherlands, has finally addressed the issue in a controlled, long-term design (Van Dulmen et al., 1996).

The subjects were patients with irritable bowel syndrome with a duration of at least three months and the absence of any recognizable gastrointestinal pathology. Patients were entered sequentially into the treatment group (25 subjects) and the 'waiting' control group (20 patients). During the study period no somatic treatments were employed. The cognitive-behavioral therapy was administered in eight 2-hour group sessions over a period of three months and attempted to correct the dysfunctional and unfounded attribution and to help the patient to understand his or her thinking, feeling and behavior reaction to the presence of symptoms. Progressive muscle relaxation was practiced during each session. The group members were encouraged to mutually recognize maladaptive coping styles. Clinical outcome measures were assessed by the patients four times daily and included avoidance behavior, duration of abdominal pain, flatulence, belching, nausea, heartburn, abdominal rumbling and details of defecation. In addition, data were collected with regard to coping strategies and psychological well-being. After the completion of this phase of the study, the patients from the control group received the same course of group therapy and the entire sample was followed up for an average of 2.25 years.

The study and control groups were well matched; at baseline, there were no demographic, clinical, behavioral and psychological differences. After three months, direct comparison between the treated and control groups after the cognitive-behavioral intervention showed significant improvement, i.e., reduction, in duration and severity of abdominal pain and a substantial decrease in avoidance behaviors. The secondary gastrointestinal complaints and the level of psychological well-being improved in the treated and control subjects. The reductions in the number, severity and duration of the abdominal complaints correlated strongly with psychological well-being. The long-term follow-up data indicated the stability of improvement for daily duration of pain and the secondary symptoms of painful defecation, flatulence and abdominal rumbling. Patients were also using more successful coping strategies than before intervention; they were worrying less, were thinking that the pain would decrease and were getting angry less frequently. Although cognitive-behavioral therapy did not have a direct effect on psychological well-being, the improved level of somatic comfort (physical health) had a persistent positive influence on mental health.

Premenstrual syndrome: serotonergic deficiency; cognitive deficits

A prominent biological abnormality of patients with premenstrual syndrome is serotonergic deficiency. This abnormality has been inferred from work demonstrating an alteration of platelet serotonergic activity (Ashby et al., 1988), decrease in neuroendocrine responses after tryptophan infusion (Bancroft et al., 1991) and aggravation of symptoms after acute tryptophan depletion (Menkes et al., 1994). A powerful way of confirming serotonergic deficiency is to study the magnitude of serotonin release in the brain of the affected subjects. Experimentally this can be done by infusing the serotonin-releasing agent fenfluramine and measuring one of its specific central nervous system effects, i.e. prolactin level. A convincing placebo-controlled study of the fenfluramine challenge was recently published by investigators from Columbia University and its affiliated New York State Psychiatric Institute (FitzGerald et al., 1997). The study group included nine drug-free (mean age 27 years) patients meeting the standard criteria for premenstrual dysphoric disorder as evidenced by the analysis of daily rating forms for two menstrual cycles. All patients had a past history of either major depression or dysthymia, but none of them was in the midst of a depressive episode at the time of the study. A control group comprised 11 healthy women (mean age 33 years). All participants were physically healthy, had regular menses and were studied in the luteal phase. The baseline prolactin levels were similar in the two groups when measured on the preplacebo day and the prefenfluramine day. The net prolactin response to fenfluramine challenge was significantly lower in the premenstrual syndrome group compared with control subjects. The difference retained its significance by analysis of covariance when data were controlled for age, body weight and the pharmacokinetics of fenfluramine. The findings are important because they strengthen an important explanatory model for the clinical presentation of the premenstrual syndrome, indicate that the serotonergic abnormalities persist after the remission of a comorbid depressive disorder, and suggest efficacy for long-term therapeutic trials with selective serotonin reuptake inhibitors.

Attention has been directed recently at the cognitive deficits often reported by patients with premenstrual syndrome (Morgan et al., 1996). This deficit is expressed in a cluster of symptoms that includes an inability to think clearly, memory loss, distractibility, impaired concentration and mental slowness, and contributes to the functional disability claimed by some of these sufferers. The authors, a multidisciplinary team from the University of California at Los Angeles, used a commendably rigorous approach to selecting their study participants, using daily prospective ratings over two months of the following 13 symptoms; breast pain, edema or weight gain, headache, fatigue, sleep disturbance, increased appetite, avoidance of social activity, decreased work efficiency, depression, anxiety, irritability, mood swings and difficulty in concentrating. Inclusion in the study requires at least a 30% increase in symptoms from the follicular to the luteal phase and substantial subjective impairment for at least one week during the late luteal phase with resolution shortly after the onset of menstruation. A control group was assembled from subjects whose two-month daily ratings showed negligible symptoms throughout the menstrual cycle. All subjects in the study ($n = 30$) and control groups ($n = 31$) complied with the following: they had had regular menstrual cycles for the previous six months; they had not taken psychotropic medications, hormones, illegal drugs or vitamin supplements for one month before the study; they were not pregnant; they had no evidence of psychopathology on clinical interviews performed during the follicular phase; and they had no abnormalities on gynecological and general physical examination. The measures included a self-report assessment of depressive symptoms and a complete neuropsychological evaluation. Urinary hormone detection kits or basal body temperatures were used to determine the follicular and luteal phases in the test month. Half of the subjects in each group were tested in the luteal phase.

Study and control subjects were similar with respect to age (29.6 versus 27.1 years), educational level, proportion of singles (64% versus 72%) and parity status. The premenstrual syndrome group was 96.2% white and included no African-American women; the control group included 41% whites, 31% Asians and 14% African-American women. In the late luteal phase, premenstrual syndrome patients were significantly more depressed than control subjects and significantly more depressed than they had been during the follicular phase. In contrast, cognitive testing demonstrated no impairment among the premenstrual syndrome patients and no difference in selective sustained attention, visual and verbal memory, comprehension and cognitive flexibility compared with control subjects. The executive functions of the frontal lobe were intact. The authors reasonably interpreted their findings to indicate that the cognitive complaints of premenstrual syndrome patients represent altered self-perception and contradict the socially mediated expectations of the subjects and the current social stereotypes.

Interstitial cystitis: stress-induced mast cell activation

There is substantial evidence that mast cell activation plays an important role in the production of abnormalities associated with interstitial cystitis (IC). Ho et al. (Chapter 6) have analyzed the evidence that suggests that the mast cell may form the anatomical basis of the pathogenic effector mechanism of this syndrome. Our contributors have also presented the evidence linking emotional stress to the worsening of symptoms reported by patients with IC. Is there a relationship between stress and mast cell activation in the bladder? An answer has been recently provided by a very elegant animal model developed at Tufts University, New England Medical Center, Boston (Spanos et al., 1997).

To determine whether the effect of stress was mediated through a change in the hypothalamic-pituitary-adrenal axis or through a change in sensory neuropeptides, the animals were pretreated with anti-corticotropin-releasing factor (a mediator of hypothalamic activity) and capsaicin (a substance that destroys sensory nerve endings). The animals were Sprague-Dawley rats that had been treated with capsaicin one day after birth and polyclonal anti-corticotropin-releasing hormone seven weeks later. A control group was injected with suitable placebos. The stress applied was nontraumatic immobilization in which rats were kept for a period of 30 minutes. Control animals were kept in their laboratory cage. At the end of the period the bladders were rapidly removed and prepared for light and electron microscopy. All mast cells were independently counted and examined by two individuals who were unaware of the experimental conditions. Mast cell activation was judged by decreased cellular staining and extrusion of granular content.

Activation was demonstrated in 76% of the bladder mast cells of stressed animals compared with only 37% of the mast cells in the control group. Pretreatment of animals with polyclonal antiserum to corticotropin-releasing factor did not affect the stress-induced mast cell activation, which was noted for 81% of the cells. On the other hand, in animals treated neonatally with capsaicin, the immobilization stress was followed by a decrease in the proportion of activated mast cells (48%). The results indicate, with a high level of confidence, that stress contributes to mast cell activation in the bladder and that this process is likely to involve the local sensory nerve endings. In the authors' view, this role of the bladder neural system is mediated by neuropeptides such as substance P and calcitonin gene-related peptide, which are known to produce mast cell degranulation and neurogenic inflammation. The link to human pathology is suggested by the authors' previous work, which has demonstrated increased substance P-positive nerve fibers in the submucosa of patients with IC (Pang et al., 1995).

Temporomandibular joint pain and dysfunction syndrome: magnetic resonance imaging; association with depression

The interest in documenting a pathological process originating in the temporomandibular joint (TMJ) of patients with this syndrome has recently centered on the postulated relationship between pain and evidence of high signal intensity on magnetic resonance imaging (MRI) taken to indicate the presence of joint effusion (Schellhas & Wilkes, 1989; Westesson & Brooks, 1992). If this were true, it would be reasonable to assume a significant correlation between the presence of radiological abnormalities and the level of pain. To test this assumption, researchers from Kyoto University, Japan, studied a consecutive clinical series of 19 women with a chief complaint of painful hypomobility of the TMJ (Murakami et al., 1996). The severity of pain was assessed by clinicians through palpation of the joint and masticatory muscles and the measuring of the jaw opening. The pain was also rated by patients, who used visual analogue scales and pain questionnaires. Magnetic resonance images were interpreted by three examiners who were unaware of the patients' symptomatology and patients were assigned to two groups according to the absence or presence of high signal intensity into the upper or lower joint compartment deemed to represent joint effusion.

Nine of the 19 patients had normal magnetic resonance images of their painful TMJ. The intergroup comparisons (negative versus positive magnetic resonance study) showed good matching for age (41 years versus 37 years) and degrees of jaw opening (32 mm versus 31 mm). The severity of all the symptoms of TMJ syndrome (resting pain, opening pain, chewing pain, preauricular pain, cheek pain, temple pain and toothache) as well as the total pain scores were similar in the two groups. MRI appears to offer no support to the hypothesis that the pain experienced by patients with this functional somatic syndrome is correlated with a definable inflammatory process.

In the absence of definite anatomical changes, the TMJ pain and dysfunction syndrome has been studied extensively to determine its relationship to psychopathology and abnormal illness behavior. The best documentation has been provided with respect to the association with depressive symptomatology and a lifetime history of major depressive disorder, an association already discussed by Greco et al. (Chapter 7). Given the methods employed, we can only say that patients with this syndrome, like patients with other chronic pain syndromes, are prone to experiencing depressive symptoms of dysphoria, sleep disturbance, anhedonia, hopelessness and helplessness. Recent work performed by researchers from the University of Oulu, Finland, has expanded the search for this association at the level of an entire community (Vimpari et al., 1995).

The initial study cohort of 55-year-olds included all 1012 inhabitants of a medium-sized town, 780 (435 women, 247 edentulous) of whom agreed to participate. The subjects were questioned with regard to past medical history, use of drugs, health behavior, lifestyle, socioeconomic factors, symptoms of temporomandibular syndrome (joint sounds, jaw fatigue, jaw stiffness on waking or on mandibular movement, difficulties in opening the mouth, locking or luxation, and temporomandibular and masticatory muscle pain), and symptoms of depression. Clinical examinations were performed by two dentists, two physicians and a nurse. The examination data were used to classify patients according to a four-category clinical dysfunction index ranging from symptom-free to severe dysfunction.

Symptoms of temporomandibular pain and dysfunction syndrome

were reported by 10.5% of dentate and 15.4% edentulous participants. The symptoms produced moderate or severe dysfunction in 3.8% of dentate and 7.3% of edentulous individuals. Overall, 12.3% of subjects had clinically significant levels of depressive symptomatology (point prevalence 10.7% for dentate and 15.6 for edentulous participants). Dentate subjects (men and women) and edentulous women who were depressed had significantly more symptoms of temporomandibular syndrome and were significantly more impaired by them than non-depressed individuals. The data suggest an overlap with fibromyalgia, because the level of temporomandibular dysfunction was related to pain in other muscle groups, predominantly the shoulders and upper portion of the arms.

Noncardiac chest pain: diagnostic value of psychological profile; perfusion imaging for rapid triage

The psychological characteristics of patients with noncardiac chest pain have been recently integrated in a predictive diagnostic model by a group of investigators from the Erasmus University, Rotterdam, The Netherlands (Searlie et al., 1996). The study cohort comprised consecutive patients referred for evaluation to the Outpatient Cardiology Clinic with a chief complaint of chest pain. Exclusion criteria were a history of psychiatric illness, medical events (such as myocardial infarction or coronary artery bypass surgery) from the time of referral to the onset of study, and age younger than 18 or older than 75 years. After comprehensive diagnostic evaluation, 67 patients were entered in a noncardiac pain group and compared with 47 patients whose chest pain was a symptom of well-documented cardiac disease. The assessments focused on measuring the severity of depressed and anxious mood, perceived level of energy, agoraphobia, social anxiety, somatization, hypochondria, fear of bodily injury, obsessive-compulsive behavior, hyperventilation, interpersonal sensitivity and anger. Logistic regression analysis was used to determine the contribution of these variables to the accurate prediction of the noncardiac explanation of the chest pain syndrome.

The noncardiac chest pain group included significantly younger subjects (mean age 48 versus 61 years) and a higher proportion of women (57% versus 23%), single (33% versus 4%) and lifetime non-smoker patients (43% versus 18%) than the cardiac chest pain group. With regard to psychological characteristics, the patients with non-cardiac chest pain showed evidence of considerably more severe anxiety, somatization, obsessive-compulsive behavior, psychoneuroticism and hyperventilation. A predictive model that included the presence of abnormal scores for anxiety, hyperventilation, hypochondria, medical information seeking and functional disability was derived and classified correctly 75% of the subjects. After corrections for age and sex, the only variables required to predict a noncardiac diagnosis in patients with chest pain were hyperventilation and anxiety.

The extent to which these findings will find applicability in practice will depend on the availability of equally reliable screening tests for the cardiac cause of chest pain. Recently published data encourage us to think that the emergency use of resting myocardial perfusion imaging might fulfill this desiderate (Tatum et al., 1997). The data were collected by investigators from the Medical College of Virginia, Richmond, who analyzed 1187 consecutive patients seen in the emergency department of an urban tertiary hospital with a chief complaint of chest pain. All patients underwent rapid clinical examination and had an electrocardiogram and on the basis of history, chest pain characteristics. The presence of electrocardiographic ischemic changes was assigned to five levels of risk for acute myocardial injury or unstable angina. This screening process identified 282 patients who had no history of coronary artery disease or diagnostic electrocardiographic changes and had presented with a short duration of typical symptoms or a prolonged duration of atypical symptoms. This group underwent immediate myocardial perfusion imaging with technetium-99m sestamibi. The results were considered normal if there were no perfusion defects, no regional wall motion or thickening abnormality and normal systolic function. All patients were closely followed for at least 72 hours; long-term follow-up data were obtained through scripted telephone interviews and other means.

Of the 282 patients with an initial clinical diagnosis of probable nonischemic chest pain, 29 (10%) were admitted on the basis of abnormal resting perfusion findings. Two of these patients had a diagnosis of myocardial infarction and seven underwent myocardial revascularization, for a total of 28% cardiac endpoints. In contrast, among the 253 patients with normal resting perfusion imaging, there were no cardiac events during the first 72 hours and only 3.2% cardiac endpoints within 30 days of the index evaluation. These cardiac endpoints consisted of revascularizations for coronary abnormalities detected on further diagnostic testing. Thus, nuclear imaging appears very valuable for the initial assessment of patients with atypical chest pain; whether a negative result precludes the need for additional cardiac evaluation in selected patients will surely be investigated in the near future.

Repetitive strain injury: sensory dysfunction in focal hand dystonia

The clinical presentation of repetitive strain injuries (RSI) is usually dominated by complaints of pain. Tyrer (Chapter 9) has described the diffuse tenderness of the muscles involved in the action claimed to have caused the syndrome, usually the small muscles of the hands, the flexor and extensor muscles of the forearms, and the neck and shoulder muscles. In a variant of the syndrome, the main complaint is excessive fatigue and lack of coordination when performing a specific task. This condition, formerly identified as writer's cramp, is called focal dystonia of the hand (Sheehy & Marsden, 1982) and has recently been the object of a well-controlled study to define its neurological deficits (Byl et al., 1996).

The investigation was carried out by an interdisciplinary team from the University of California, San Francisco, who assembled a 60-member study cohort. Fifteen subjects had focal dystonia of the hand, characterized by: specific motor skill impairment with respect to trajectory, timing or force; abnormal involuntary movements during specific motor tasks such as typing, writing or playing a musical instrument; and degraded movements producing functional impairment. Additional requirements were persistence of the abnormalities despite resolution of any traumatic, inflammatory, neuropathic or myopathic processes and the loss of motor skills not explained by a decrease in practice or task performance. A comparison group included 15 patients with clinical evidence of tendinitis of the fingers or wrists resulting in a specific diagnosis, such as De Quervain's tendinitis, epicondylitis and flexor carpi ulnaris tendinitis. A second comparison group comprised 30 healthy control subjects, 15 of whom were musicians. The goal was to determine the presence of sensory dysfunction, as measured by tests of localization of tactile stimuli, kinesthesia, graphesthesia, manual form perception and motor accuracy on blindfolded subjects. Test–retest correlation coefficients were satisfactory, but indicated worse performance on localization and improved performance on graphesthesia that were considered to be within the expected procedural variability.

Patients with focal dystonia performed less accurately and took more time to complete manual form perception, graphesthesia and motor accuracy tests than patients with tendinitis and control subjects. Of interest was the fact that on most tests the patients with focal dystonia, but not those with tendinitis, demonstrated functional deterioration of the affected hand as well as the hand not affected by the repetitive strain. The findings support brain imaging (Tempel & Permutter, 1993) and electromyographic data (Cohen & Hallett, 1988), indicating that unilateral sensory training produces changes in the motor areas of both hemispheres. Such changes may mean that the functional disability associated with RSI is central in origin; the postulated mechanism includes rapid stimulation of the central control units followed by sensory and motor confusion. A clinical implication of this conjecture would suggest that improvement is more likely to follow a change in activity rather than an attempt to overcome the sensory deficits by increasing practice time.

Multiple chemical sensitivities: cognitive ability

Symptoms of poor memory, difficulty with attention and concentration and decreased accuracy and speed of decision-making and problem-solving are prominent among patients given the diagnosis of multiple chemical sensitivities (MCS). Recent work performed at Johns Hopkins University, Baltimore (Bolla, 1996), has described the results of objective testing of neurocognitive function of these patients in a very well-controlled study. The subjects were self-referred for clinical evaluation to the Occupational and Environmental Neurology Clinic after documented exposures to pesticides or chemical solvents at home or at work. Of the 35 patients, 16 were diagnosed to have MCS. The remaining 17 patients had neurological symptoms, but indicated no recurrent or worsened symptoms after exposure to chemicals and were designated as a control group. A second control group comprised 126 healthy adult volunteers. A standard battery of neuropsychological assessments was performed by a suitably trained examiner who was not aware of the diagnostic category of the chemically exposed subjects (K. I. Bolla, personal communication). In addition, the study investigated the presence of 16 symptoms commonly reported by workers exposed to chemicals.

The two chemically exposed groups were similar to each other with regard to age, sex distribution, years of education and number of symptoms thought to be related to the chemical exposure. The healthy control group was older than both patient groups. Vocabulary scores (verbal intelligence) were used to estimate the premorbid intellectual ability; data indicated similar ability for the patients with MCS and healthy control subjects. The chemically exposed group without MCS had a significantly lower vocabulary score. The neuropsychological test data, properly adjusted for age and vocabulary score, indicated no significant differences between the MCS group and the healthy control group with respect to memory, verbal learning and executive and psychomotor functioning. The patients with chemical exposure who did not receive a diagnosis of MCS performed the poorest on visual reaction time and the tests of executive and psychomotor functions.

Thus, objective neuropsychological testing does not bear out the cognitive deficits claimed by patients with the syndrome of MCS, confirming previous work that was either uncontrolled (Fiedler et al., 1992) or that did not involve chemically exposed individuals who failed to meet the criteria for the syndrome (Simon et al., 1993).

Gulf War illness: one syndrome or many?

The USA authorities deployed 697 000 military personnel in the Persian Gulf area to participate in Operation Desert Shield. The first troops arrived on 8 August 1990. The armed combat started on 16 January 1991 and consisted in a 39-day air war followed by a 4-day ground war. Combat casualties were few and the repositioning of the force back to Europe and the USA was completed by 31 July 1991. All veterans of this war had access to free care either through the facilities of the Department of Defense (DOD) for those still on active duty or through the hospitals and clinic of the Department of Veterans' Affairs (VA). The health status of these veterans is well known and data are available from two major sources: the VA Persian Gulf War Registry and the DOD Persian Gulf Health Surveillance System. According to a governmental interagency group, there are at least 17 000 ill or concerned veterans enrolled in these programs and at least 3000 of them have had unexplained illnesses as of June 1994 (Persian Gulf Veterans Coordinating Board, 1995). About half of these veterans had been enrolled in the reserves or National Guard units, a group comprising only 17% of the troops deployed to the area of conflict. The interagency group indicated that the symptoms commonly reported by the ill or concerned veterans include fatigue (17%), rash (17%), headache (14%), arthralgias or myalgias (14%), neuropsychological complaints (11%), dyspnea (8%), sleep disturbance (5%), diarrhea and other gastrointestinal complaints (4%) and cough (4%). No consistent physical signs or laboratory abnormalities have been identified, which suggests that these illnesses may constitute a functional somatic syndrome. The interagency group has pointed out that complaints have been voiced by only 33 British veterans of the conflict and by none of the troops of other combatant nations (Saudi Arabia, France, Egypt, Syria and Morocco) or by the local population. The same interagency group has described in detail the main pathogenetic hypotheses, which assume that the Gulf War illnesses have been produced by chemical and biological warfare, nerve agent prophylaxis (with pyridostigmine bromide) and immunizations (with botulinum toxoid and anthrax), infectious diseases (leishmaniasis, Q fever, brucellosis, sandfly fever, West Nile fever, Crimean-Congo hemorrhagic fever and dengue) or environmental hazards (oil fire smoke containing metals and volatile organic compounds, pesticides, depleted uranium, paint fumes containing isocyanate and various fuels and decontaminating solutions). None of these hypotheses has been confirmed in controlled studies of affected and healthy veterans (Persian Gulf Veterans Coordinating Board, 1995).

A definition was proposed by Haley et al. (1997), based on a recent summary of military surveys, registry data and review of selected cases (Persian Gulf Veterans Coordinating Board, 1994). Patterned after the definition of the CFS (Fukuda et al., 1994) the diagnosis requires: (1) presence in the theater of operations between 8 August 1990 and 31 July 1991; (2) no other medical or psychiatric illness (as diagnosed by a physician) that could cause the symptoms; (3) at least five of the following eight signs or symptoms – fatigue, arthralgia or low back pain, headache, intermittent nonbloody diarrhea, neuropsychiatric complaints (forgetfulness, difficulty with concentration, depression, memory loss and easy irritability), sleep disturbance, low-grade fever and weight loss.

The most recent analysis was published by a group of researchers coordinated through the Epidemiology Division, University of Texas Southwestern Medical Center at Dallas (Haley et al., 1997). The investigators chose as their study population members of the Twenty-Fourth Reserve Naval Mobile Construction Battalion called to active duty for the Persian Gulf War. The contacts were made in November 1994 with all veterans, ill and well, active and retired, who lived in Alabama, Georgia, Tennessee, South Carolina and North Carolina. The subjects gave informed consent and completed instruments designed to record and measure 22 symptoms and 51 unambiguous symptom factors that were clinically meaningful. For example, the symptom memory impairment was the basis for the following symptom factors: memory problems, short term; memory problems, long term; memory problems, unable to find where car is parked. The psychological profile and presence of psychopathology were assessed with the Personality Assessment Inventory (Morey, 1991). Two-stage factor analysis was used to identify syndromes.

Of the 606 Gulf War veterans contacted, 249 (41%) participated in the survey. Participants were sociodemographically similar to nonparticipants, but were more likely to be unemployed and to report a serious illness since their return from the war. Of 175 (70%) participating veterans reported to have serious health problems since the war, 160 had consulted physicians for their problem and 115 were certain that their health problem was the result of exposures received during the war. Only one veteran felt that his health problems were not related to the period of active military duty in the Persian Gulf. The analysis identified 6 syndromes in 63 (25%) participants: confusion-ataxia, arthro-myo-neuropathy, impaired cognition, phobia-apraxia, fever-adenopathy and weakness-incontinence. The first three of these syndromes involved strongly clustered symptoms. The last three syndromes overlapped frequently with the clusters of confusion-ataxia or arthro-myo-neuropathy.

The most disabling syndrome was confusion-ataxia, which was present in 21 of the cases. These individuals reported not knowing where they are or what they are doing, getting disoriented when trying to locate their car in a parking lot, stumbling often and feeling as if the room were spinning. In addition to getting confused, these veterans had problems with reading, writing and spelling. The study of their psychological profiles indicated substantial abnormalities as indicated by the Somatic Complaints Scale, a composite measure of conversion, somatization and general health concerns. The scale indicated significant abnormalities in only one (1.5%) veteran without health problems and in 71% of those with the confusion-ataxia syndrome. They had received a diagnosis of depression, post-traumatic stress disorder or liver disease and had experienced substantial levels of occupational disability, reflected by a 45% unemployment rate. A logistic regression analysis indicated that veterans with this syndrome were 12.5 times more likely to be out of work than those reporting no health problems.

The 22 veterans with the syndromes of arthro-myo-neuropathy had in common myalgias and arthralgias, fatigue and tingling or numbness of the extremities. The authors were laudably attentive to separating fatigue from excessive sleepiness. The symptom fatigue reflected items such as: too weak in hands, arms or legs to complete work; entire body too weak to do usual work; wearing out too quickly to finish work; and having too little energy to start work. Half of these veterans scored abnormally high on the Somatic Complaints Scale.

The impaired cognition syndrome was identified in 12 veterans who had in common memory deficits, distractibility and fatigue, which was defined as excessive daytime sleepiness without muscle exhaustion. Again commendable is the effort to define the individual features of the main symptom, variably expressed as: feeling too sleepy to do usual work; feeling very sleepy most of the day; having to take frequent naps; and nodding off to sleep while working or driving. In addition, these individuals complained of depression, insomnia, slurred speech, difficulty in thinking and migraine-like headaches. Abnormal scores on the Somatic Complaints Scale were recorded in only 25% of these cases.

The other three syndromes represented weaker clusters of symptoms. The phobia-apraxia syndrome associated panic-like symptoms (chest discomfort, dizziness, nausea and tingling sensations in tight places or situations from which escape would have been difficult) with difficulty in motor control and coordination (e.g. when brushing teeth or combing hair). The fever-adenopathy syndrome was characterized by low-grade elevation in temperature and swollen lymph nodes. The weakness-incontinence syndrome consisted of urinary or fecal incontinence and tingling or numbness of the face, tongue and lips. A component of this syndrome was also dyspareunia in the sexual partner. The Somatic Complaints Scale indicated abnormal psychological profiles in 65% of veterans with phobia-apraxia and 60% of those with fever-adenopathy syndromes. The abnormal profiles did not indicate traditional psychiatric disorders associated with combat experience, such as post-traumatic stress disorder and did not reflect malingering or factitious disorder. Nonetheless, they were considered to reflect heightened concerns over specific cognitive, motor or sensory deficits and to measure the psychological reactions to their presence.

The evidence presented in this study suggests that Gulf War illness comprises more than one syndrome. Data are not yet available to determine whether one or more of these syndromes denote specific neurotoxic consequences of exposure to one or more extrinsic factors, the manifestations of an emerging functional somatic illness, or atypical variants of CFS or MCS.

References

Abel KM, O'Keane V & Murray RM (1996). Enhancement of the prolactin response to *d*-fenfluramine in drug-naïve schizophrenia patients. *British Journal of Psychiatry*, **168**, 57–60.

Ashby CR, Carr LA, Cook CL, Steptoe MM & Frank DD (1988). Alteration of platelet serotonergic mechanism and monoamine oxidase activity in premenstrual syndrome. *Biological Psychiatry*, **24**, 223–33.

Bancroft J, Cook A, Davidson D, Bennie J & Goodwin G (1991). Blunting of neuroendocrine responses to infusion of L-tryptophan in women with perimenstrual mood changes. *Psychological Medicine*, **21**, 305–12.

Blanchard EB & Schwarz SP (1987). Adaptation of a multicomponent treatment program for irritable bowel syndrome to a small group. *Biofeedback and Self-Regulation*, **12**, 63–9.

Bolla KI (1996). Neurobehavioral performance in multiple chemical sensitivities. *Regulatory Toxicology and Pharmacology*, **24**, S52–S54.

Buskila D, Neumann L, Hazanov I & Carmi R (1996). Familial aggregation in the fibromyalgia syndrome. *Seminars in Arthritis and Rheumatism*, **26**, 605–11.

Byl N, Wilson F, Merzenich M, Melnick M, Scott P, Oakes A & McKenzie A (1996). Sensory dysfunction associated with repetitive strain injuries of tendinitis and focal hand dystonia: a comparative study. *Journal of Orthopedics in Sport and Physical Therapy*, **23**, 234–44.

Cleare AJ, Bearn J, Allain T, McGregor A, Wessely S, Murray RM & O'Keane V (1995). Contrasting neuroendocrine responses in depression and chronic fatigue syndrome. *Journal of Affective Disorders*, **35**, 283–9.

Cleare AJ, Murray RM & O'Keane V (1996). Reduced prolactin and cortisol responses to *d*-fenfluramine in depressed compared to healthy matched control subjects. *Neuropsychopharmacology*, **14**, 349–54.

Cohen L & Hallett M (1988). Hand cramps: clinical features and electromyographic patterns in focal dystonia. *Neurology*, **38**, 1005–12.

Deale A, Chalder T, Marks I & Wessely S (1997). Cognitive behavior therapy for chronic fatigue syndrome: a randomized controlled trial. *American Journal of Psychiatry*, **154**, 408–14.

Drossman DA, Talley NJ, Leserman J, Olden KW & Barreiro MA (1995). Sexual and physical abuse and gastrointestinal illness. Review and recommendations. *Annals of Internal Medicine*, **123**, 782–94.

Fielder N, Maccia C & Kipen H (1992). Evaluation of chemically sensitive patients. *Journal of Medicine*, **34**, 529–38.

FitzGerald M, Malone KM, Li S, Harrison WM, McBride PA, Endicott J, Cooper T & Mann JJ (1997). Blunted serotonin response to fenfluramine challenge in premenstrual dysphoric disorder. *American Journal of Psychiatry*, **154**, 554–6.

Fukuda K, Straus SE, Hickie I, Sharpe MC, Dobbins JG, Komaroff A & the International Chronic Fatigue Study Group (1994). The chronic fatigue syndrome: a comprehensive approach to its definition and study. *Annals of Internal Medicine*, **121**, 953–9.

Haley RW, Kurt TL & Horn J (1997). Is there a Gulf War syndrome? Searching for syndromes by factor analysis of symptoms. *Journal of the American Medical Association*, **277**, 215–22.

Lloyd A, Hickie I, Brockman A, Hickie C, Wilson A, Dwyer J & Wakefield D (1993). Immunologic and psychologic therapy for patients with chronic fatigue syndrome: a double blind, placebo controlled trial. *American Journal of Medicine*, **94**, 197–203.

Mann JJ, McBride PA, Malone KM, DeMeo M & Keilp J (1995). Blunted serotonergic responsivity in depressed inpatients. *Neuropsychopharmacology*, **13**, 53–64.

Menkes DB, Coates DC & Fawcett JP (1994). Acute tryptophan depletion aggravates premenstrual syndrome. *Journal of Affective Disorders*, **32**, 37–44.

Morey LC (1991). *The Personality Assessment Inventory: Professional Manual*. Odessa, FL: Psychological Assessment Resources.

Morgan M, Rapkin AJ, D'Elia L, Reading A & Goldman L (1996). Cognitive functioning in premenstrual syndrome. *Obstetrics and Gynecology*, **88**, 961–6.

Murakami K, Nishida M, Bessho K, Iizuka T, Tsuda Y & Konishi J (1996). MRI evidence of high signal intensity and temporomandibular arthralgia and related pain. Does the high signal correlate with pain? *British Journal of Oral and Maxillofacial Surgery*, **34**, 220–4.

Pang X, Marchand J, Sant GR, Kream RM & Teoharides TC (1995). Increased numbers of substance P positive nerve fibers in interstitial cystitis. *British Journal of Urology*, **75**, 744.

Pellegrino MJ, Waylonis GW & Sommer A (1989). Familial occurrence of primary fibromyalgia. *Archives of Physical Medicine and Rehabilitation*, **70**, 61–3.

Persian Gulf Veterans Coordinating Board (1994). *Summary of the Issue Impacting upon the Health of Persian Gulf Veterans*, Version 2.2. Washington, DC: Persian Gulf Veterans Coordinating Board.

Persian Gulf Veterans Coordinating Board (1995). Unexplained illnesses among Desert Storm veterans. *Archives of Internal Medicine*, **155**, 262–8.

Schellhas KP & Wilkes CH (1989). Temporomandibular joint inflammation: comparison of MR fast scanning with T1- and T2-weighted imaging techniques. *American Journal of Neuro Radiology*, **10**, 589–94.

Searlie AW, Duivenvoorden HJ, Passchier J, Ten Cate FJ, Deckers JW & Erdman RAM (1996). Empirical psychological modeling of chest pain: a comparative study. *Journal of Psychosomatic Research*, **40**, 625–35.

Sharpe M, Hawton K, Simkin S, Surawy C, Hacjman A, Klimes I, Peto T, Warrell D & Seagrott V (1996). Cognitive behavior therapy for the chronic fatigue syndrome: a randomized controlled trial. *British Medical Journal*, **312**, 22–6.

Sheehy MP & Marsden CD (1982). Writer's cramp: a focal dystonia. *Brain*, **105**, 461–80.

Simon G, Daniell W, Stockbridge H, Claypoole K & Rosenstock L (1993). Immunologic, psychological and neuropsychological factors in multiple chemical sensitivity. *Annals of Internal Medicine*, **119**, 97–103.

Spanos C, Pang X, Ligris K, Letourneau R, Alferes L, Alexacos N, Sant G & Teoharides TC (1997). Stress-induced bladder mast cell activation: implications for interstitial cystitis. *Journal of Urology*, **157**, 669–72.

Tatum JI, Jesse RI, Kontos MC, Nicholson CS, Schmidt KI, Roberts CS & Ornato JP (1997). Comprehensive strategy for the evaluation and triage of chest pain patients. *Annals of Emergency Medicine*, **29**, 116–25.

Tempel LW & Permutter JA (1993). Abnormal cortical responses in patients with writer's cramp. *Neurology*, **43**, 2252–7.

Turk DC, Okifuji A, Starz TW & Sinclair JD (1996). Effects of type of symptom onset on psychological distress and disability in fibromyalgia syndrome patients. *Pain*, **68**, 423–30.

Van Dulmen AM, Fennis JFM & Bleijenberg J (1996). Cognitive-behavioral group therapy for irritable bowel syndrome: effects and long-term follow-up. *Psychosomatic Medicine*, **58**, 508–14.

Vercoulen JH, Swanink CM, Zitman FG, Vreden SG, Hoofs MP, Fennis JF, Galama JM, van der Meer JW & Bleijenberg G (1996). Randomised, double-blind, placebo-controlled study of fluoxetine in chronic fatigue syndrome. *Lancet*, **347**, 858–61.

Vimpari SS, Knuutila ML, Sakki TK & Kivela SL (1995). Depressive symptoms associated with symptoms of the temporomandibular joint pain and dysfunction syndrome. *Psychosomatic Medicine*, **57**, 439–44.

Walker EA, Gelfand AN, Gelfand MD, Green C & Katon WJ (1996). Chronic pelvic pain and gynecological symptoms in women with irritable bowel syndrome. *Journal of Psychosomatic Obstetrics and Gynecology*, **17**, 39–46.

Westesson PL & Brooks SL (1992). Temporomandibular joint: relationship between MR evidence of effusion and the presence of pain and disk displacement. *American Journal of Roentgenology*, **159**, 559–63.

Wise TN, Cooper JN & Ahmed S (1982). The efficacy of group therapy for patients with irritable bowel syndrome. *Psychosomatics*, **23**, 465–9.

Wolfe F, Ross, Anderson J, Russell IJ & Herbert L (1995). The prevalence and characteristics of fibromyalgia in the general population. *Arthritis and Rheumatism*, **38**, 19–28.

Yatham LN, Morehouse RL, Chisholm BT, Haase DA, McDonald DD & Marrie TJ (1995). Neuroendocrine assessment of serotonin (5-HT) function in chronic fatigue syndrome. *Canadian Journal of Psychiatry*, **40**, 93–6.

Index